PRAISE FOR

MISTLETOE AND THE EMERGING FUTURE OF INTEGRATIVE ONCOLOGY

"In this pioneering book, doctors and patients will discover the incredible power of mistletoe therapy and its foundational place within integrative cancer care. As this book demonstrates, plant-based supplements that stimulate the immune system's own power—such as mistletoe—are a welcome addition to current cancer treatments and may eventually become first-line treatments (with fewer side effects)." —**Kelly A. Turner**, PhD, *New York Times* bestselling author of *Radical Hope: 10 Key Healing Factors from Exceptional Survivors of Cancer & Other Diseases*

"Mistletoe was a cornerstone of my integrative oncology practice for over 35 years. This exciting collaboration by leading integrative physicians is not only a comprehensive deep-dive into the science and practice of mistletoe therapies, it provides a context in holistic cancer care. Nutrition, spirituality, metabolic therapies, naturopathy, and other natural medicines are given voice as the new paradigm of integrative medicine." —**Neil McKinney, ND**, author, *Naturopathic Oncology: An Encyclopedic Guide for Patients and Physicians*

"This new resource is an excellent and needed addition to the world of naturopathic and integrative oncology. Using Mistletoe as a therapy is something my colleagues and I have done for many years, and like all therapies there are so many subtleties to the art of its use. This book will take the practitioner from not only a safe and entry level position using mistletoe therapies but also elevate their technical and clinical competence. All the chapters are amazing, and ones such as chapter 5, 'Test, Assess, Address...Don't Guess! Adjusting Treatment Priorities in Response to the Patient's Unique Terrain' gets to the heart of elevating patient outcomes. This is an invaluable resource!" — **Dr. Paul S. Anderson**, coauthor, *Outside the Box Cancer Therapies*; author, *Cancer: The Journey from Diagnosis to Empowerment*

"Although future cancer therapies may involve cutting-edge science such as gene therapy it may also be that ancient wisdom will be just as important. Mistletoe has been used in traditional healing therapies for centuries, if not thousands of years and may prove to be one of our greatest tools in the treatment of cancer."
—**Robb Wolf,** *New York Times* bestselling author, *The Paleo Solution and Wired to Eat,* co-host "The Healthy Rebellion Radio"

"I cannot imagine a better introduction to mistletoe than the current volume. It is fascinating, clearly organized, and well written . . . a real page-turner for anyone interested in the tortuous journey of this widely misunderstood form of complementary treatment. Visitors to Germany are often amazed to discover the respect that physicians and patients have for a botanical treatment almost unknown in America—that is, mistletoe therapy and the broader category of anthroposophic medicine. Mistletoe has been approved for cancer in Germany since the 1960s. Even the U.S. National Cancer Institute states that mistletoe extracts are among the most widely prescribed drugs for cancer patients in Europe. Yet, in the U.S. mistletoe is either unknown or carelessly maligned. This situation is now changing because of a clinical trial at the renowned Johns Hopkins University in Baltimore. This fact alone is causing greater awareness of mistletoe therapy and may help usher in a bright future for cancer patients seeking a more holistic form of treatment."
—**Ralph W. Moss, PhD**

"What a treasure this book is—for patients and practitioners alike. It's time to shed the war metaphor and acknowledge that comprehensive healing must incorporate spirit, soul, and body. These authors provide an expansive and inclusive view of how we can approach and accomplish healing the whole person. As more of us embrace and practice the approaches introduced in this book, we will truly have actual healthcare rather than disease management."
—**Jan Adrian, MSW,** founder and director of Healing Journeys

MISTLETOE

AND THE EMERGING FUTURE
OF INTEGRATIVE ONCOLOGY

MISTLETOE
and the Emerging Future
of Integrative Oncology

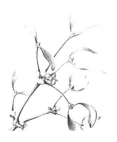

STEVEN JOHNSON, DO
NASHA WINTERS, ND, FABNO

with ADAM BLANNING, MD
MARION DEBUS, MD
PAUL FAUST, ND, FABNO
MARK HANCOCK, MD
PETER HINDERBERGER, MD

Portalbooks

Portalbooks

An imprint of SteinerBooks | Anthroposophic Press, Inc.
834 Main Street, PO Box 358, Spencertown, NY 12165
www.steinerbooks.org

DISCLAIMER

This book is intended to introduce the reader to mistletoe therapy,
anthroposophic care, naturopathic medicine, and basic principles of
integrative oncology. It is not intended as a comprehensive mistletoe
training manual, nor is it intended to diagnose, prevent, or treat cancer
or any other disease. The information presented within cannot substi-
tute for the advice of your family physician or other trained healthcare
professionals.

Mistletoe therapy, although well researched, is not an FDA-
approved therapy. It should be administered only under the advice of
your doctor and is not intended to replace current standard of care
(SOC) treatments. Patients interested in European mistletoe should
consult with a licensed practitioner who has received focused training
in both integrative medicine and mistletoe therapy. Anthroposophic,
naturopathic, and integrative therapies should be administered only
under the guidance of a practitioner trained in their appropriate use.

Several case stories are included throughout. The diagnoses, treatment strategies, and outcomes are all factual, although personal details
have been veiled to protect patient privacy.

Cover design: Mary Giddens
Design: William Michael Jensen

LIBRARY OF CONGRESS CONTROL NUMBER: 2021943206
ISBN: 978-1-938685-33-0 (hardcover)
ISBN: 978-1-938685-35-4 (paperback)
ISBN: 978-1-938685-34-7 (eBook)

CONTENTS

PART 4: WEAVING IT ALL TOGETHER: SPECIAL APPLICATIONS IN CLINICAL PRACTICE

APPENDICES

In the midst of writing this book,
the anthroposophic community said
goodbye to two shining leaders.
They are dearly missed.

Gene Gollogly (1950–2021)

Gene inspired many authors in his lifetime. This book was his last project and remains a symbol of his encouragement and dedication. That dedication to unveil the possibilities of the human spirit will live on in these pages.

Dr. Maurice Orange (1953–2021)

Dr. Orange treated patients and inspired doctors around the world. As a researcher and courageous physician, he is responsible for many of the groundbreaking applications of mistletoe therapy.

How to Use this Book

This book was structured following the syllabus for a three-day practitioner training hosted by the Physicians' Association for Anthroposophic Medicine (PAAM). The chapters highlight several of our key lectures in a condensed form. The book serves as an introductory summary of—and not a replacement for—those intensive professional trainings. While this book should not be regarded as a treatment or diagnostic manual, it is intended to better prepare practitioners to begin mistletoe therapy training. Practitioners who read this book before attending a PAAM training will glean more from their experience and have greater confidence as they begin the one-to-one mentoring phase of their training.

As we foster a community where practitioners and patients work together to cultivate health, we welcome patients to read this work as well! Patients who read this book will be empowered with a deeper awareness of the immune system's role in cancer treatment, a foundational understanding of mistletoe therapy, and a basic introduction to integrative medicine concepts.

The text is science-rich, but intentionally written with enough contextual cues that a self-educated patient should follow along well. You do not need a science background to understand the majority of the content. But it helps if you tend to take a deep interest in your own health concerns. It is always good to take notes. After reading this book, follow-up by asking questions of a clinician well trained in these extensions of modern medicine.

The book is constructed as a journey, and it is ideal to read it in its entirety. We hope that every reader, whether a patient, practitioner, or supporter of integrative oncology, has a chance to do that. We also realize that, whatever way your life has been altered by cancer, your days are full of dueling priorities. Here are a few tips that can help you journey through this book along the most efficient path.

Practitioners

Part 1: If you have specialized in oncology, immunology, and immunotherapy, and you have some basic familiarity with mistletoe, you may wish to skim chapters 1 through 3. Chapter 2 is not intended as medical textbook content or as an in-depth exploration of immunologic changes in the presence of cancer. Rather it is a basic review of immunology, appropriate for sharing with patients who want a deeper understanding of the immune system and how mistletoe components interact with the immune response. Regardless, do take some time with the second half of chapter 2, which focuses on mistletoe's constituents and specific methods of action.

Parts 2–4: If you are new to mistletoe therapy and integrative care, you will spend the lion's share of your time reading and digesting chapters 4 through 7. If you want to take a much deeper dive into anthroposophic medicine, mistletoe therapy, and integrative principles, you may wish to focus more on the robust clinical material in chapters 8 through 11.

- Chapters 4 and 5 will provide a foundational understanding of how VAE products are selected for each patient and how to monitor patients' labs with a more holistic mindset.
- Chapters 6 and 7 open the door to anthroposophic medicine (AM) and principles. If you pursue training in VAE therapy, your mentor will likely be an AM practitioner. Please take time to learn about our medical philosophy; this will help you better understand how to administer mistletoe effectively for far better outcomes.

- Chapters 8–11 include several detailed case stories, along with the science and lab-informed insights behind integrative care choices. These chapters elucidate real-world clinical decisions regarding how and when to use mistletoe therapy and other anthroposophic remedies that may be new to you, as well as common integrative modalities. Dedicate significant time to digesting these chapters, and you will find yourself far better equipped to discuss individualized patient care plans with a PAAM-assigned mentor from the course or other trained professionals.

At the end of this book, chapter 12 provides vision-casting resources and ways to become involved with the integrative and anthroposophic oncology community. It takes time to network with other like-minded physicians, but we all have better patient outcomes when we work together and share insights!

Patients and Loved Ones

Part 1: Chapters 1 and 2 provide an overview of integrative oncology and a mistletoe practitioner's perspective on immunology. The immunology content is written in an accessible style that does not require a science background. We encourage you to take time with this material to self-educate on how mistletoe therapy affects your body. You may wish to skim the Study Summaries in chapter 3, but do take time to read the Implications sections. The two case story reports toward the end of this chapter are captivating and encouraging as well.

Parts 2–3: Chapter 4 examines the importance of mistletoe host trees. Your VAE therapy practitioner will choose the right host tree for you. Take time with this chapter so you can understand this nuanced decision. Know that all practitioners have their own personalized approach to treatment choices. Chapters 5 through 9 describe your mistletoe practitioner's strategies, treatment recommendations, and care philosophy. You may wish to skim these chapters, but do take time to familiarize yourself with the general principles in each one.

Particularly, chapters 5, 8, and 9 describe how mistletoe therapy fits within your larger integrative care plan.

Part 4: Chapters 10 and 11 explore more complex mistletoe administration methods and AM principles related to specific cancer types and scenarios. This material may be a stretch for lay readers. If the theoretical content is too heavy, it's fine to skip through to the case stories at the end of these two chapters. Chapter 12 is highly practical. It provides specific actions you may take and organizations you may connect with to learn more about mistletoe and integrative care. There is a whole community caring for each other and sharing tips about mistletoe access. Please join us!

FOREWORD

Human disease is an elaborate dance between behavior, our environment, and chance. Medicine tries to tame human disease with science, but when our knowledge falls short, disease wins. This is too often the case with cancer. We spend billions of dollars each year trying to better understand it and develop tools to ease its effects.

I am a cancer doctor. I have treated patients for over twenty years and trained and worked at some of the most prestigious medical institutions in the world. I have had the opportunity to work with amazing colleagues—nurses, doctors, social workers, administrators, and many others who made a tremendous impact on cancer and other diseases and who truly helped humanity. I focus on cancer genetics and use this information to help design new ways to diagnose and treat cancer. I am fortunate to have had some great successes in conventional cancer research and treatment.

I have also had the privilege of meeting some of the most wonderful people as patients, along with their families. One can never predict how the shock of a cancer diagnosis will impact a person. I have seen the full range of human emotions from fear to courage to indifference. The human spirit is so diverse, and each individual is unique in how they confront this challenge.

It was through such a connection with one of my patients that I came to learn about mistletoe. As a faculty member at Johns Hopkins in Baltimore, I met Ivelisse Page, a young woman with Stage IV colon cancer. When cancer reaches this stage, it is a lethal condition. I was trained in and had investigated modern colon cancer treatments, but

Ivelisse declined most of the standard approaches. She was open to surgery, but wanted no chemotherapy or radiation. She did not want experimental targeted therapies. Rather Ivelisse focused on naturopathic approaches including an alkaline diet, mistletoe therapy, and most importantly, her faith.

This approach was certainly unconventional to me. It wasn't within the guidelines at Johns Hopkins or any other academic medical center in the United States. I could honestly say that no one at that time at my institution was using or had used mistletoe in their management of cancer. I would never have thought of mistletoe therapy, or taken it seriously, if I hadn't met Ivelisse. She was the spark that introduced me to a new world.

Ivelisse had a cancer that has a notoriously high death rate and rapid recurrence and progression rate. She'd seen the disease take multiple family members. Instead of fighting what seemed a losing battle, Ivelisse opted for an integrative approach that might support her quality of life during whatever remaining time she had. In partnership with Dr. Peter Hinderberger, who specializes in anthroposophic cancer care, we treated Ivelisse with mistletoe therapy. Dr. Hinderberger managed the mistletoe therapy and I, with modern tools, monitored her progress after surgery and during her anthroposophic care. I was uncomfortable at times. But with each CT scan and lab test, we continued to see no sign of cancer recurrence. None of her care providers had expected this. The science was not obvious to me. But now, more than a decade later, Ivelisse is disease-free and thriving.

I can only speculate at this point regarding the biologic basis of how mistletoe therapy affected Ivelisse's body and, more importantly, her cancer. I suspect it helped activate her immune system, so it could fight the cancer.

Because of Ivelisse's experience, and that of many other patients like her, we initiated a clinical trial at Johns Hopkins to study mistletoe's mechanism of action in patients with advanced cancer. The study is ongoing, and much more work is needed in the laboratory and at a clinical level. But I am pleased to see conventional cancer researchers seriously exploring this therapeutic option.

While I have learned a lot throughout my career, one of the most important lessons is this: *We can grow in unexpected ways when we listen to new perspectives.* Ivelisse and Dr. Hinderberger taught me that there may be other ways to care for patients with cancer, and we need to explore these options with the same passion with which we explore conventional approaches. As a physician and a professor, one who is used to being the teacher, it is important to me to keep an open mind. I strive to listen, so I may continue to learn. The best and most important lessons often come from where I least expect them.

Luis A. Diaz, MD
Head, Division of Solid Tumor Oncology
Memorial Sloan Kettering Cancer Center
New York City

INTRODUCTION

Dr. Steven Johnson, DO

I was on summer break from college, and I went to a conference for medical students and doctors at the Hague in Holland. People were there from all over the world, including some students we secretly assisted to come from Poland and Russia. Back then this was forbidden, as it was before the fall of the Berlin wall in 1989. The event took on an aura of excitement and importance.

I remember Dr. Mees, an MD at the meeting who lectured on how the human skeleton related to the mathematical intervals of the musical scales. Exploring such mysteries was intriguing to say the least. I also met Dr. Joop Van Dam, a physician who would later have an extraordinary impact on my way of practicing medicine. He helped me to appreciate the power of meditation through the book *How to Know Higher Worlds* by Rudolf Steiner.[1] (This is the same Rudolf Steiner who, along with Dr. Ita Wegman, introduced mistletoe to the medical world as a potential cancer therapy.) I also visited the facilities where mistletoe extract is manufactured. It was impressive to see the precise and methodical methods of mixing and separating the winter and summer juices of this ancient plant.

I returned to Europe many times over the following years to visit several anthroposophic and integrative hospitals. I learned about *anthroposophic medicine (AM)*, a practice that integrated conventional medicine with herbal medicine, homeopathy, and what I considered "soul-care" therapies. All were considered equally valuable and needed therapeutic treatments. At these hospitals, nurses applied herbal compresses post-operatively for surgical patients. Eurythmy (a movement therapy based on speech and tone) and music therapy were provided in the Intensive Care Units. Therapeutic massage helped center and nourish patients. Anthroposophic, homeopathic, and natural medicines were prescribed alongside state-of-the-art conventional medications, as an integral part of the treatment protocols. Can you imagine this? Even the cleaning fluids contained essential oils giving the hospital a pleasant smell of rosemary, lavender, and rose. If I close my eyes, I can still smell the aroma. Patients clearly felt cared for, and no one seemed to think this scenario was odd or out of the ordinary. I truly wanted to see hospitals and clinics like this in North America.

> *Anthroposophic Medicine:* Anthroposophically extended medicine brings deeper insights to the care of the whole human being. It is practiced by conventionally trained physicians and nurses who have undergone additional specialized training, learning to apply a broad array of effective natural medicines. This whole-person approach also incorporates art, music, movement, and massage therapies as elements of collaborative, multidisciplinary healthcare.
> —According to the Physicians' Association
> for Anthroposophic Medicine.

Though conventional practitioners and patients in the U.S. are often not aware of homeopathy, naturopathic care, and anthroposophic medicine, studies show the excellent safety and positive clinical outcomes for these modalities.[2] Even the World Health Organization has identified many aspects of integrative and holistic health as potentially crucial for the sustainable delivery of effective medicine and global public health initiatives.[3,4] The conventional medicine community is increasingly aware that it doesn't have all the answers. Conventional practitioners are seeking out more connection with holistic and integrative practitioners. This is a positive new direction.

I hope that this book, along with introducing you to one specific therapy, also makes a good case for integrative health in general, including AM, naturopathy, and other holistic sciences. All of these can extend the reach and efficacy of modern medicine. Integrative medicine is an approach that combines all the best therapeutic tools and applies them based on each patient's unique needs. There is a growing body of research noting the benefits of an integrative healthcare model, and more patients seem to be searching for an individualized and human-centered healthcare philosophy. That philosophy is central to integrative oncology.

I kept visiting European clinics over the years, and it was always profound to witness practitioners administering mistletoe therapy before radiation treatments, alongside chemotherapy, and with local and systemic hyperthermia. I was impressed by how doctors, nurses, and patients worked as a team. The patients felt empowered because they were being treated as individual human beings. They understood that mistletoe and other naturopathic medicines were modulating their immune defenses to fight the cancer, alongside the best that modern oncology had to offer. Studies have demonstrated that this treatment approach improves quality of life (QOL)[5] and decreases the side effects of conventional therapies.[6]

I eventually opened my own clinic in Louisville, Kentucky, where we administered mistletoe therapies alongside AM, naturopathy, and other integrative treatments. At one point, we almost received insurance approval, and we thought the idea of a European-style clinic would become a reality. However, as with almost all such endeavors, the powers that be would not risk becoming the first to support an integrative hospital model. Yet, for 17 years, I did get to manage various aspects of an outpatient and retreat-model clinic. I witnessed so many instances where mistletoe therapy, other natural therapies, and integrative treatments had incredible impacts on people's lives. I was fortunate to have good people around me and even a couple of open-minded conventional oncologists who were willing to work with me, even if they were skeptical at first. I also had incredible teachers and mentors who empowered me to trust these treatments, such as the late Dr. Maurice Orange, MD (1953–2021), a brilliant anthroposophic leader in Europe. I also gleaned so much from Dr. Phillip Incao, MD and Dr. Paul Scharff, MD, whose courage to heal in the face of difficult illnesses gave me the courage to think outside the box. They inspired me early on to work with mistletoe and integrative oncology.

Although mistletoe is one of the most researched integrative cancer treatments in Western Europe, it is still a lesser-known offering in North American integrative oncology. There have already been over 150 published clinical studies on mistletoe therapy,[7] but North American awareness is just beginning to grow. An ongoing trial of Helixor® Mistletoe at the Sidney Kimmel Comprehensive Cancer Center at Johns Hopkins is definitely driving the new awareness and curiosity about this therapy. Until now, mistletoe therapy has been largely a niche therapy in North America, limited to a small group of anthroposophic physicians, who were trained in Europe or directly mentored by members of the Physicians' Association for Anthroposophic Medicine (PAAM). Now, with the publication of stronger mistletoe research, and with integrative oncology emerging as a specialized field, many new medical doctors and talented naturopathic doctors are learning about this treatment. There is an expanding interest throughout the integrative oncology world.

It is important to note that mistletoe therapy, while safe and effective, has many nuances, sub-types, and potential patient responses, which necessitate professional training. Learning these nuances and sub-types of mistletoe can be the difference between an effective treatment and a sub-par or failed treatment. That is the reason for this book. The authors are a dedicated group of clinicians who originally came together to create a training course for the safe and professional administration of mistletoe therapy in integrative oncology. It is our hope that mistletoe becomes an accepted standard of care (SOC) *adjuvant* (additional, supportive therapy) for cancer treatment in the U.S.—just as it already is in Germany and Switzerland. I believe mistletoe therapy can serve as a bridge between conventional and integrative oncology. The coauthors of this book are sincere in this quest. We have written the book as a nonprofit endeavor, to further the cause and promote best-practices training for new mistletoe therapy practitioners.

As a practitioner-author group, the first training we co-led evolved into the initial outline for this book. That first U.S. Mistletoe Therapy Training took place in 2019, in Baltimore, not far from Johns Hopkins Hospital. Since then, we have trained or mentored more than 200 other licensed doctors. This success is due to the incredible synergy and unselfish effort and collaboration of our unique group.

Truth be told, back in 2018, I was not even thinking of planning a course on integrative oncology and mistletoe. I was getting ready to launch a new public health project called the Foundation for Health Creation (www.FoundationForHealthCreation.org). In that context, I was visiting the oncology wing at Klinik Arlesheim (near Basel, Switzerland) and speaking with Dr. Maurice Orange and Dr. Marion Debus. (At the time, I didn't know this would be my last opportunity to meet with Dr. Orange.) I complained to them about how mistletoe was often used improperly all over the U.S. because doctors had no access to good training, and yet patients were demanding mistletoe therapy. Of course, my colleagues put this right back on my shoulders, as all good mentors do! Dr. Debus said, "Perhaps you should go back to America and start a best-practices course."

I reluctantly agreed to do this, but only if my two mentors participated. Unfortunately, Dr. Orange's health was not good enough to travel, but Dr. Debus became an inspirational anchor and mentor for the new American course. Dr. Debus is an oncologist who practiced for many years in Germany and is now at the Klinik Arlesheim in Switzerland. She is both an inspiring teacher and a practitioner of anthroposophic medicine and oncology. The course we eventually developed is unusual in that it is co-taught by medical, osteopathic, and naturopathic doctors, who are all expert clinicians in their fields. We all wanted it to be this way because we believe the future of an individualized integrative oncology practice requires the collaboration of diverse clinicians and therapists.

When I returned home from Europe in 2018, I had a sense that I wanted to assemble such a diverse team—but I wasn't sure who the individuals were yet! I was fairly certain that one of the first people I should reach out to was Dr. Nasha Winters. She was already a well-known integrative oncology practitioner, author, and mistletoe therapy educator. Like me, she had also bridged mistletoe therapy with metabolic and functional medicine concepts.

Dr. Winters had developed a four-hour introduction to the basics of mistletoe therapy, which she provided through practitioner training sessions, sponsored by Helixor (the primary mistletoe extract brand available in the U.S.). In addition to her own case consulting, Dr. Winters had founded an integrative oncology training program for doctors and had also trained 175 practitioners specifically in mistletoe therapy in the past year. Her book, *The Metabolic Approach to Cancer Care*, was a bestseller. My colleague, Dr. Peter Hinderberger, already knew Dr. Winters. The two of them had been instrumental in setting up the mistletoe trial at Johns Hopkins. Dr. Hinderberger told me that Dr. Winters was a very strong and talented physician, well-known throughout the naturopathic community and beyond. She was clearly a fantastic resource for my multi-day course. I just needed to get brave enough to call her.

That moment came while I was in Wisconsin visiting Mark McKibben, a pharmacist responsible for distributing Helixor mistletoe products and many other adjuvant remedies for U.S. practitioners. It was a rainy autumn night and, after visiting with Mark much of that day, I had some time to myself. I was nervous that Dr. Winters would not be interested in this training, as she clearly already had a full plate! Finally, I made the call.

My worries were quickly disarmed. Dr. Winters wholeheartedly agreed to join the training, and she quickly became a wonderful colleague and inspiration for the course. As the rain poured down outside, I listened to her share some of her own story. She had fought her own battle with cancer, and so she could speak from a very special place of experience.

So, the initial team began to take shape: Dr. Hinderberger was also interested and, along with Dr. Debus, provided MD representation. I provided the osteopathic physician (DO) perspective, and Dr. Winters came from a naturopathic (ND) point of view. We had the foundation for a truly collaborative training. Dr. Paul Faust, ND also agreed to join the faculty. He was a close colleague of Dr. Hinderberger and knew Dr. Winters. He proved to be a fantastic teacher with a keen ability to present scientific concepts. The synergy between the five of us set the stage for a truly integrated course curriculum. It was amazing how our topics and teaching styles complemented each other. Everything felt like it fell into place. We completed that first three-day training in Baltimore in 2019, and we immediately began to receive requests for more.

For the 2020 course, we were blessed to add Dr. Mark Hancock, MD, a protege of Dr. Orange. Dr. Hancock was building a new clinic model for mistletoe therapy and integrative oncology. We were also fortunate to have Dr. Adam Blanning, MD join our crew, teaching the foundations of anthroposophic and holistic medicine. The synergy continued. The faculty contributed invaluable expertise and personality to the mistletoe training and, eventually, to this book. It is a blessing to have such generous and dedicated colleagues.

Dr. Winters first suggested the possibility of this book shortly after our first training in Baltimore. She'd actually been incubating the idea of a cowritten book about mistletoe therapy for a few years. She was sure it needed to be team-written, from multiple perspectives, and here we were: a diverse team of integrative oncologists. *Would we be interested in coauthoring a book about mistletoe therapy in the U.S.?*

If a book was going to be written, I personally was convinced we were the group to write it. The book needed to be written by those who were truly experts in the field and had extensive clinical experience. In 2020, with our faculty now numbering seven in total, everyone unanimously agreed to sacrifice their time and energy for this project. It was impressive to witness all the authors agreeing to donate all the profits of the book to mistletoe-related research, education, and treatment.

Nasha introduced us to an editor known for her expertise in natural health, and she agreed to organize our lectures and contributions into the book. The final piece of the puzzle was now in place, and everyone agreed to move forward with this special project.

As this is a nonprofit initiative, the fundraising task fell to me. However, there was so much enthusiasm for the idea, that the task was much less difficult than expected. This is where the lasting influence of Gene Gollogly (1950–2021) comes in. Gene was an inspiring leader in the anthroposophic world and an influential member of the publishing industry in New York. He so much wanted this book to come into being. He became an early champion of the project and helped us get it off the ground, even offering to help fund the book himself. In January 2021, with our team only a few months into writing, Gene unexpectedly died. In the following weeks, as we processed this shock, many of Gene's associates manifested, stepping in to maintain funding and enthusiasm for the project. One of those connections were the people at SteinerBooks and their expressed desire to serve as our publisher. It feels like Gene continues watching over this book, like a guardian angel. We hope it is worthy of his approval.

Our author team experienced yet another shock when, only weeks later, Dr. Orange passed away. All of us were connected to him either directly, as colleagues and proteges, or indirectly through often reading his research and recommendations. This double loss hit us hard, and yet it also fanned into flame our dedication to completing this book. Both of these men were true leaders: they helped people find their personal purpose and empowered them through mentoring and one-to-one encouragement. Ultimately, everyone has a short time here. It is on each of us to mentor others, just as we have been mentored, to pass along every good thing we have learned.

My experience of writing this book with my coauthors has been extraordinary. One after another, every setback that we've encountered has translated itself into an even greater strength. New helpers and solutions have appeared right when we needed them. Even our editor remarked on this unusual quality: *It almost seems like your book-writing journey has modeled itself after an integrative healing process.* This book was written and published in roughly one year, by seven busy and very diverse physicians all with different personalities. It is no less than a miracle. It is a testament to the collegiality that has formed between us all. Also, the enthusiasm from so many others supporting the project has carried and inspired us through the difficult times.

We coauthors have strived to lay a path toward a practice of truly integrative oncology, a care environment where MDs, NDs, DOs, and many others work together in the patient's best interest. We believe this is the future of cancer care. Patient outcomes improve when a diverse and integrative faculty of experts work together to enhance care. We have all experienced this firsthand. We hope to inspire others, both clinicians and patients, to insist on this model of care. It is the only way things will continue to change for the better. We hope readers will gain some appreciation for anthroposophic, naturopathic, and integrative medicine and will support these practices in the future.

We hope this book helps to establish best-practice standards for the use of mistletoe therapy in cancer care. We hope to inspire further research, education, and the clinical practice of integrative oncology, including mistletoe therapy. We have all seen the potential with our own patients and hope that many, many others will share the same experience. This book is for both doctors and patients. We hope it serves as a doorway to new possibilities for yourselves and your loved ones. We hope it facilitates your journey to a better state of health. Further, we hope this book sheds light on that fundamental question: "What is health?"

As you'll soon see, the mistletoe plant possesses many remarkable properties. As a therapy, it represents a rediscovery of ancient wisdom. It shows us how the science of modern medicine might expand its reach and reconnect with a more human-centered medicine.

PART 1

THE LANDSCAPE OF MISTLETOE THERAPY

"Often, times of crisis are times of discovery, periods when we cannot maintain our old ways of doing things and enter into a steep learning curve. Sometimes it takes a crisis to initiate growth."
—RACHEL NAOMI REMEN, from
Kitchen Table Wisdom: Stories that Heal

CHAPTER 1

ANCIENT PLANT, MODERN THERAPY

A Brief History of Mistletoe and Modern Oncology

*Dr. Steven Johnson, DO
and Dr. Nasha Winters, ND, FABNO*

*Special thanks to Dr. Marion Debus for advisory consultation
and historic summaries included in this chapter.*

*"There are two principal methods of treating disease. One
is combative, the other preventative."*
—HENRY LINDLAHR, MD (1862–1924),
author of *Nature Cure*

*"The good physician treats the disease; the great physician
treats the patient who has the disease."*
—SIR WILLIAM OSLER (1849–1919),
Founding Member Johns Hopkins Hospital

When patients come to us interested in mistletoe therapy, they are often entirely new to the concept. They're surprised that a plant they've known only as a holiday decoration is also a well-studied natural medicine. There's often a mix of skepticism and genuine curiosity in their questions. In the coming pages, we hope to provide helpful insights for other patients with cancer and their loved ones who have similar questions. We also hope to provide a solid introduction for clinicians who are curious about mistletoe therapy and integrative oncology.

Let's first expand our perspective through a brief exploration of humankind's relationship with mistletoe, as well as the history and evolution of cancer treatment. Then we'll find out how mistletoe fits into the modern picture of integrative oncology and other emerging holistic paradigms. After that historical tour, we'll look at the basics of how conventional oncologists, integrative medical doctors (MDs), doctors of osteopathic medicine (DOs), naturopathic doctors (NDs), and anthroposophic practitioners use mistletoe as an *adjuvant*—a therapy that complements and enhances the effects of standard of care (SOC) therapies.

Primitive parallel lives:
Mistletoe legends and the disease with no treatment

You might know mistletoe only as a curious holiday decoration—that evergreen sprig with wintery-white berries, hanging in a doorway. For some reason couples kiss under it to celebrate their love. Long before it showed up in holiday traditions, mistletoe was highly regarded in Norse and Greek mythology and in Roman epic poems. Mistletoe appeared as a wand or a key, allowing a few legendary heroes to travel safely back and forth between the land of the living and the Underworld—something not normally possible for living souls.

The ancient Druids were familiar with European mistletoe, *Viscum album*, which we use in therapeutic extracts today. In their traditions, mistletoe was considered magical because of its blooming and bearing fruit in the wintertime and for its unusual appearance: beautiful evergreen orbs growing in the winter months in an otherwise bare deciduous tree. It was highly valued when found growing in sacred oak trees. The Druids harvested mistletoe only in the winter, near solstice, and with elaborate rituals involved. For them, mistletoe was a potent promoter of fertility and longevity.[1]

In another mythic tradition, Baldur—the most beloved of the Norse gods, son of the god Odin and his wife Frigg—was killed by an arrow made of mistletoe. Baldur was later resurrected, and mistletoe was transformed into an emblem of love. This story may be the origin of today's holiday mistletoe tradition.[2]

In ancient times, such stories were a way to communicate sacred wisdom. Today, it is all too easy to dismiss them as quaint or primitive. But as we look at mistletoe's earliest uses as an herbal medicine, we begin to see some of the mistletoe benefits that contemporary researchers have now verified. Early European herbalists came to recommend mistletoe for epilepsy and as a general medicine to calm the nerves, particularly to comfort those who were incapacitated by great grief.[3] We'll see later on that many of the herbalists' observational uses have found scientific support today.

Though mistletoe had many applications in early herbal medicine, it would be centuries before it intersected with oncology. It has taken thousands of years to unlock the modern secrets of mistletoe. Our understanding of cancer has had a similar rocky evolution, fraught with mystery, fear, misunderstanding, and wonderful breakthroughs.

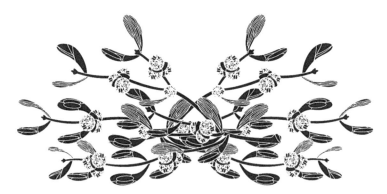

Humankind's early encounters with cancer

Some of the earliest known cancer cases are found in Egyptian mummies that show evidence of bone and breast cancer. There are also Egyptian medical texts by the physician Imhotep (2600 BCE), which likely describe cancerous conditions and refer to tumors as a disease with no treatment.[4] That was the general attitude toward cancer for millennia, though Greek and Latin physicians at least developed a theory of cancer's cause and the vernacular that we find recognizable today. From the Greeks we received the term *carcinoma*—a Greek word meaning "crab," likely referring to the crab-like shape of some tumors. They also coined *oncos*, meaning swelling, from which we get the term *oncology*. The Romans first referred to the disease as *cancer*, a Latin translation of carcinoma.[5] These early Western physicians developed the theory of "balancing humors" in the body to cure disease and regarded cancer specifically as stemming from an excess of "black bile." Believe it or not, that opinion prevailed for much of written medical history, from about 400 BCE until the 1600s CE.[6,7]

Long after the early Greek and Roman physicians, but still prehistory in terms of modern oncology, we find the story of St. Peregrine Laziosi (1260–1345), who suffered from a cancerous tumor on one of his legs when he was a young man. The lesion ulcerated and became severely infected, warranting amputation. But by the time the surgeon arrived, the infection had lessened, and the tumor had miraculously shrunk.[8] The wound soon healed, the young Peregrine kept his leg, and he lived till he was 85 with no cancer recurrence. Centuries later he was canonized and is now regarded as the Patron Saint of Cancer Patients.

The St. Peregrine story would be solely the stuff of legends, except for the fact that Western medical literature continued to accumulate similar stories. Very occasionally, a cancer patient would develop a feverish infection and, if they survived the infection, their tumor had subsequently shrunk or gone into complete remission.[9,10] The physicians didn't have the scientific capacity to describe the phenomenon at the time, but it would seem they were witnessing an early clue regarding *immunotherapy*. Only in recent years would researchers begin to consider the role of warmth and fever in immune-modulation as a potential treatment for cancer. Is it possible the heightened immune activity of St. Peregrine's infection managed to breach the barriers of the tumor's microenvironment and eliminate the cancerous cells?

We'll never know for sure. But this phenomenon would be witnessed again in the future!

No one wants to reproduce such a risky experience. But the fact that such "miracles" were documented is fascinating. While conventional oncology often regards immunotherapy as new and leading-edge, the basic principles have been noted for centuries and were even practiced with intention in the 1800s and 1900s, as we'll see shortly. The roots of immunotherapy run far deeper than the recent emergence of checkpoint inhibitors.

Regardless, those lucky cancer remissions were the exception and not the rule. For centuries, in Europe and around the world, cancer was a known and named disease. It was feared, veiled in mystery, and physicians rarely recommended any effective treatments.

Mistletoe establishes itself in European herbalism

Throughout the middle ages, herbalists continued to respect mistletoe for its ancient mystical associations. They also began to keep more detailed records about its effects based on specific preparations and dosages. European herbalists continued to use mistletoe for epilepsy and other nervous system imbalances, as well as for pain management and balancing mood. The leaves, twigs and berries were harvested and dried, then tinctures were made from the dried plant material. Topical applications were used for pain as well.[11,12]

These practitioners noticed the importance of dosage. While lower mistletoe dosages were often highly effective for nervous system disorders, higher doses could actually aggravate them.[13] In the 1700s and 1800s, herbalism, like any medical practice of that time, started to apply the new scientific method throughout its treatment observations and recommendations. There was far less of a divide between conventional and herbal medicine at that time. In many regions there wouldn't have been a divide at all. Indeed, herbs comprised the primary pharmacopeia. Though the medical community didn't yet have access to the technology needed to identify the active constituents in mistletoe, the herbalists were keen observers of its effects.

Today, we now know about mistletoe's identified medicinal constituents, including *lectins* and *viscotoxins* (see chapter 2), as well as anti-inflammatory *flavonoids* and compounds that appear to interact with *GABA receptors* (nerve cell receptors involved in self-calming).[14-20] This diverse phytoactive profile explains the historic results seen when classical herbalists provided mistletoe for pain management, epilepsy, and mood balancing effects.

Renaissance to early twentieth century: Setting the stage for contemporary cancer care and research

From the mid-1500s to the early 1600s, Western medicine underwent a transformation. Da Vinci, Galileo, and Vesalius opened doors to new knowledge about health and disease as a result of their dissections and anatomy illustrations. In the 1700s, Giovanni Battista Morgagni expanded on the practice of cadaver dissection to include "determining the likely cause of death." This new understanding of anatomy and pathology made it possible for physicians to learn much more about the structures and progression of cancer.[21] This, in turn, made it possible to consider surgery as a cancer treatment option. In the mid-1700s, London surgeon John Hunter made some of the first recommendations classifying operable and inoperable tumors. He was also known for his pathology research and some of the earliest observations about tumor metastases, though no one had the language to describe that progression yet.[22]

Around the same time, medical researchers and practitioners began to revisit and question the Four Humors theory of cancer. Upon discovering the lymphatic system in the early 1600s, Gaspare Aselli hypothesized that cancer was a lymphatic disease.[23] Others postulated that cancer might be infectious, leading to unfortunate quarantining of people who had cancer from the sixteenth through the eighteenth centuries. In the late 1700s, there was one new theory of cancer that was eventually proven accurate. Physicians throughout Europe started to notice a new kind of cancer prevalent only among chimney sweeps, particularly those who began as boy apprentices and were required to climb chimneys mostly naked—a horrifying but common practice. By the time they were young men, they developed a rare testicular cancer not seen in any other population group. Practitioners and researchers caught on: *This particular cancer was due to repeat exposure to an environmental toxin.* Somehow, the soot was causing it.[24] Though scientific validation for this assertion would not come until mouse model studies in the 1920s and '30s,[25,26] the initial conclusion still held. It even provided motivation for implementing new child labor laws, protective clothing for these workers, and other social and legal changes.[27]

From the mid 1800s through the first half of the twentieth century, the medical community laid the foundation for the modern-day practice of oncology. During that time, a wide range of treatment innovations flourished, and new laboratory technologies made significant discoveries possible. A German pathologist, Johannes Müller (1801–1858), countered the dominant theory that cancer came from degenerating lymph, and proved instead that all cancers were made up of human cells.[28] Müller's student, Rudolf Virchow (1821–1902), extended that line of inquiry even further and developed the study of cellular pathology in the 1850s.[29] Müller and Virchow opened the door to studying cancer as a cellular disease, one in which cells begin to grow out of control with a *centrifugal* (spreading outward) tendency.

Another pathologist living around the same time in England, Stephen Paget (1855–1926), introduced the "Seed and Soil" hypothesis in 1889.[30] He looked at the deceased as a pathologist, and he found that certain tumors tended to metastasize to certain organs. Particularly, he noticed that breast cancer tumors routinely metastasized to visceral organs and the bones. He believed there must be a certain "soil" where these tumors preferred to grow.

"When a plant goes to seed, its seeds are carried in all directions; but they can live and grow only if they fall on congenial soil," Paget said. "While many researchers have been studying 'the seeds,' the properties of 'the soils' may reveal valuable insights into the metastatic peculiarities of cancer cases." Paget observed that each cancer's behavior and progression depended on *the condition of the whole person* and not solely on the aberrant cells.[31] He was thinking in a holistic way.

Paget's Seed and Soil Theory got attention in its time but wound up utterly forgotten by the mid twentieth century, replaced in the 1920s by the idea that metastasis was an entirely random process, driven only by the circulatory and lymphatic systems. Almost a hundred years after Paget shared his original hypothesis, modern medicine returned to it in the 1980s. Today researchers tend to refer to Paget's "seed cells" as *progenitor cells* or *metastatic clones* and his "soil" concept is preserved in language about the *tumor microenvironment* or *tumor niche.*[32]

In the early 1900s, Paul Ehrlich (1854–1915), a microbiologist and early immunologist working in Frankfurt and Berlin, developed the theory that the immune system may be involved in controlling cancer and eliminating cancer cells in their earliest stages.[33,34] He could not prove his intuitive theory essentially because the lab technology we have today hadn't been developed yet. Like Paget's ideas, Ehrlich's concepts were forgotten until the recent explosion of research into immunotherapy.

Surveying this time period yields many more pioneering cancer researchers who developed brilliant immunological, genetic, and metabolic theories, while lacking the technology to prove, disprove, or evolve their ideas. In addition to Paget and Ehrlich, one finds the cellular metabolism researcher Otto Warburg in Germany in the early 1900s. Warburg made the impressive discovery that tumor cells could live and thrive in the absence of oxygen. They had an *anaerobic metabolism.*[35] This theory could have inspired the next century of research, but it fell out of the limelight, even though Warburg received the Nobel Prize for his work. In recent years, innovative cancer researchers have returned to Warburg's findings, rediscovering the abnormal metabolic pathways of cancer cells. There are keys here to fighting cancer by taking advantage of its unique metabolic quirks.

In the early 1900s, one also notices geneticists like Theodor Boveri in Germany and R. C. Whitman in the U.S., developing and honing a *somatic theory* of cancer cell mutation: Perhaps cancer cells became cancerous because of a critical mass of genetic mutations accumulated over time.[36,37] Unlike Paget's and Ehrlich's ideas, which were highly accurate but hard to prove, Somatic Mutation Theory (SMT) earned the trust of the research community and became the dominant cancer origin theory for decades. Only recently have we learned that this theory may have put the cart before the horse. It's true that cancer cells have many mutations, but it's possible that many of the mutations come about *after* they've turned cancerous.[38]

While cancer researchers were developing new theories of what caused cancer and how cancer progressed, practitioners and surgeons were forging new approaches for treatment. In Europe, Wilhelm Conrad Röntgen discovered X-rays in 1895.[39] A year later, Emil Grubbe began the first radiotherapy treatments in the United States for breast cancer.[40] Also in the U.S., William Stewart Halsted (1852–1922) introduced radical mastectomy for breast cancer—which became a feasible option with the advent of anesthesia.[41] Halsted was sure that the more radical the operation, the higher the cure rate. Even in his time, this was found to not be the case, but it would remain the dominant opinion until the 1980s.

In the first decades of the twentieth century, perhaps the most fascinating and high-risk cancer treatment innovation was pioneered by William B. Coley. As a cancer surgeon, Coley had seen the unpredictable efficacy of treating with surgery alone. Rather than ask only what had happened to the patients who did poorly, he began to wonder *what went right* for the patients whose cancers had shrunk or gone into remission. He went through medical files and found all the healthy cancer survivors. He discovered that, at some point in their cancer journeys, all of them had developed and fought off a major infection, usually accompanied with a high fever. After recovering from the infection, their cancers had shrunk or were in complete remission.

Coley took this information and began what would become highly controversial experimental treatments. He initially injected his first few cancer patients' tumors with live *Streptococcus* bacteria to induce fever. Most of his patients survived the therapy—as crude as it seems—and

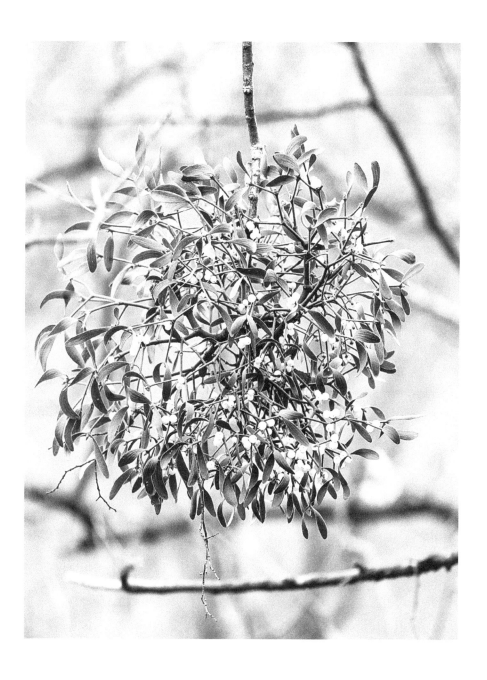

*Mistletoe is best known as a holiday decoration. Few know
that it has a one-hundred-year history of use in cancer care.*

the survivors did indeed experience tumor shrinkage or remissions.[42,43] Coley later developed a safer, heat-treated preparation from killed bacteria, going on to use this in over one thousand patients. "Coley's Toxin" can be considered one of science's earliest immunotherapies. Several contemporaries of Coley utilized thirteen different versions of these preparations. But the toxins were not well-standardized, and patient outcomes were not always tracked well. This led to Coley's toxins being abandoned by mainstream oncology.[44] Still, one hundred years later, science did return to the idea of *immunotherapy*, the concept of triggering a heightened and more efficient immune response in the battle against cancer.

Mistletoe meets cancer care:
Viscum album *at the turn of the twentieth century*

In the early 1900s, the Austrian philosopher, scholar, and social reformer Rudolf Steiner (1861–1925) collaborated with his protégé, the physician Ita Wegman, MD (1876–1943), to develop the principles of anthroposophic medicine (AM). Together, they founded one of the most well-known integrative approaches to medicine in Western Europe. They also pioneered mistletoe therapy for cancer care. AM physicians were, and are, medical doctors who complete additional training in treating the whole human being. Steiner particularly emphasized the concept of "spiritual science," the idea that both spiritual awareness and science can be (and need to be) united for medical treatment to be fully effective. Both Steiner and Wegman spoke about the importance of caring for the soul and spirit of the person as well as the physical and functional aspects of the body.[45]

Our European colleagues suggest that Steiner began mentioning mistletoe as a possible cancer therapy in his lectures as early as 1904. In 1917, Dr. Wegman first administered a *Viscum album* mistletoe extract via subcutaneous injection to several of her cancer patients in Zurich and saw positive results.[46] In 1921, she founded the first anthroposophic clinic, Klinisch-Therapeutisches Institut, in Arlesheim, Switzerland, which is still a thriving AM center today. This clinic ultimately spurred the development of many integrative hospitals in northern Europe, where conventional academic medicine, surgery, critical care, and integrative AM therapies are practiced side-by-side. Today, many physicians travel to this region from around the world to learn and train in integrative and anthroposophic medicine.

Klinik Arlesheim was founded particularly to focus on care for Dr. Wegman's patients who had cancer. Mistletoe was one of several holistic treatments she used, alongside other herbal therapies, homeopathy, anthroposophic medicines, and therapies that we might regard as soul or psychological care. These therapies include art therapy, rhythmic massage, and eurythmy (therapeutic movement).

One striking perspective in AM cancer care, then and now, was the idea that malignant cancer was the result of a decades-long process that disrupted the *rhythmic balance* in multiple body systems. This included the metabolism, nervous system, and immune system, as well as the patient's emotions and sense of spiritual purpose. The physician's role was to assist the patient in restoring a sense of rhythm and coherence within the body's regulatory systems.[47]

Most of the cancer research community was barely aware of immunotherapy and didn't yet have the language to describe the role of the immune system in preventing or inhibiting cancer growth. Yet Dr. Wegman indeed used mistletoe to encourage a heightened immune response—known today as *immune surveillance*. She and Steiner spoke of the importance of creating a "mantle of warmth" around the tumor area, and Steiner mentioned in his lectures that little result could be seen in cancer treatment unless a fever or a *warmth response* was induced.[48] Early AM physicians pioneered what they called "fever therapies" to increase whole-body systemic warmth in the patient. The warmth, whether local (focused on the tumor site) or systemic (whole body), was indicative of heightened immune activity. We'll look at the science behind these ideas in the next chapter.

Mistletoe, as a "warming therapy," came to be a core feature of AM cancer care from 1920 onward. AM physicians paired mistletoe therapy with other botanical and mineral remedies (see chapter 8) that supported immune regulation and other aspects of health needed to recover from both cancer and conventional treatment side effects. The goal was and is to create warmth, immune balance, and systemic regulation throughout the body to support optimal conditions for remission and healing. This strategy retrains a dysregulated immune system to initiate and complete its own cycles of heightened response and resolution.[49,50] This systemic and holistic approach to cancer was ahead of its time. Recently, conventional medicine and research have rediscovered these concepts, but only after exhausting a primarily disease-centric approach.

Today's terrain: Cancer care heads to war... and returns to heal its wounds

At the dawn of the twentieth century, AM's holistic care principles did not run entirely counter to the greater world of cancer research. In both the conventional and anthroposophic realm, cancer researchers were asking what went wrong in the body to allow the cancer to take root in the first place. This cause-oriented line of inquiry was inherently more constitutional, more holistic. But conventional cancer research was quickly changing, and the biggest shift wasn't due to advances in laboratory technology and methods. It's possible that the biggest shift was philosophical and cultural. It came from a world shaken by two World Wars. In the wake, "war" became a dominant cultural metaphor. Pick any challenge in modern life, and the metaphor of "waging war" or "defeating the enemy" became the modern mindset. While war metaphors had been applied to humanity's relationship to disease before (especially with the advent of germ theory), the U.S. involvement in two World Wars seemed to cement a war mindset in much of our medical research initiatives and patient care. Disease needed to be eradicated. The idea of "cultivating health" rapidly lost ground and favor. A new massive economy developed alongside our wars on cancer and other diseases.

But cancer is unique. It's not a bacterium that we can annihilate, an infection we can kill off. Cancer cells are *our own cells.*

By adopting a war mentality toward cancer, we began to seek out potential therapies (usually chemical) that could destroy all cancer cells. We couldn't see that a war on cancer might become a war on ourselves. We disregarded the power of the body, soul, and spirit to assist in our human healing.

Sometimes the war on cancer was quite literal, as chemists who were knowledgeable in chemical warfare (and sometimes the chemicals themselves) transitioned directly from the military into early chemotherapy research labs. The first chemotherapeutic drugs were inspired by the bone marrow damages caused by mustard gas.[51] Between deeply entrenched war metaphors and the chemical revolution, cancer care in the U.S. was about to turn aggressive in its techniques and results. The idea of immunotherapy was, for a time, set aside.

Cancer treatment in the late 1940s and early 50s was defined by the work of Sidney Farber, who trialed the first chemotherapeutic agents for childhood leukemia. At the time, this cancer usually translated into a six-month life expectancy upon diagnosis. Farber was the first one to develop therapeutic courage and the will to help these children. Yet many of Farber's experimental treatments, after dramatic initial remissions, ended in fatal recurrences months later.[52,53] While chemotherapy treatments for childhood leukemia would eventually become highly effective and both life-saving and life-extending, these initial experimental treatments did not meet expectations. Despite the mixed results of early chemotherapy, most of cancer research homed in on these new synthetic solutions as oncology's shining hope.

There were occasional novel insights. From the late 1940s until the late '60s, Frank Macfarlane Burnet (1899–1985) introduced more nuanced immunological theories of cancer. His Immunosurveillance Theory pointed out how cancer might be able to hide from the immune system.[54,55] This initiated a search for *tumor-associated antigens* (TAA), the ID keys that a healthy immune system could use to identify cancerous cells and destroy them.[56]

Then, in the 1980s, the work of Mina Bissell appeared, identifying the tumor "microenvironment"—the vessels, tissues, and extracellular matrix around the tumor—and how that space might hold clues for unmasking the cancer. If the cancer could be unmasked, perhaps the immune system could find and eliminate it. But it would be another thirty years before Bissell's work was revisited and examined for possible treatment alternatives.[57-60]

Apart from a small handful of independent thinkers, cancer treatment in the U.S. became defined by the triad that materialized in the World War era: surgery, chemotherapy, and radiation. In 1971, then-President Nixon formalized the dominant mindset by signing the National Cancer Act—publicly referred to as the War on Cancer. This would provide national funding for decades of research, though the focus remained on "fighting" cancer instead of searching for varied root causes.

Mistletoe research blossoms alongside shifts in conventional care

Founded as an *Institut* (Klinisch-Therapeutisches Institut), Dr. Wegman's Arlesheim clinic was intended as a research hospital. In 1924, Dr. Eberhard Schickler was commissioned with tracking twenty-two case studies. These cancer patients were provided what we would now consider high doses of mistletoe. Ten to twenty milligrams were injected subcutaneously near the tumor or, in some cases, as *intratumoral injections* (into the tumor). These high doses induced moderate fever. Treatments and the associated fever reaction were provided rhythmically over years-long treatment courses, with breaks in between. These cyclic fevers helped to invigorate and reeducate the immune system.[61,62]

Dr. Schickler tracked three treatment groups:

- Late-Stage Cancers: For those with inoperable conditions, mistletoe provided palliative (pain-reducing) effects and significant improvement of the "general condition." They experienced improved energy, weight stabilization, improvement of sleep and appetite, and sometimes the ability to work again.

- Adjuvant Treatment: When mistletoe was used as an adjuvant (a supportive therapy alongside conventional treatment), patients felt less fatigue and fewer side effects from radiotherapy.

Schickler noticed mistletoe's usefulness in helping conventional therapies work better, while maintaining the patient's quality of life (QOL) during treatment.

- Prophylactic Treatment: Mistletoe was also provided to patients who had a family history of cancer or constitutionally showed symptoms typical for carcinomas, for example: accelerated aging, fatigue, and constipation that were not responsive to other AM therapies. These patients became stronger and less anxious, and they came back on their own requesting follow-up injections.[63]

Schickler's preliminary case study notes were eventually joined by the research of Alexandre Leroi, who also improved mistletoe extract processing, and Georg Salzer, who oversaw and published the first randomized, controlled mistletoe trials.[64] In the 1940s and '50s lab research identified some of the most active phytochemicals in mistletoe extract, and multiple animal model studies noted the extract's ability to shrink tumor size and alter immune activity—effects that have been similarly observed in recent research.[65] The pioneering work of Schickler, Leroi, and Salzer laid the foundation for the abundance of mistletoe lab research and clinical studies since then.

Today, mistletoe is one of the most well-researched and clinically tested integrative cancer therapies in the Western world. In addition to the effects noted in human clinical findings, lab testing has identified multiple compounds in the extract, primarily the *viscotoxins* and *lectins*, which are, in varying ways, both directly cytotoxic to cancer cells, as well as immune stimulating.[66] The combination of active compounds in mistletoe extract appears to result in a general *immune surveillance* effect. Mistletoe therapy assists in breaching the tumor's microenvironment and damaging the cancer cells (see chapter 2). Simultaneously, it supports the white blood cells' ability to identify the tumor as a threat and take that information throughout the body, to educate the rest of the immune system. This leads to more efficient destruction of the cancer cells.[67]

Shifts in US research return our attention to immunotherapy

By the late 1990s, mistletoe therapy had acquired significant aware-ness and a research base in Europe. Meanwhile, across the Atlantic, cancer research in the U.S. had begun to come full circle, returning to questions about how a healthy immune system interacted with and eliminated cancer cells. While treatment options remained limited from the 1960s through the turn of the 21st century, we have seen recent shifts regarding cancer-cause theories. Mina Bissell's work on the tumor microenvironment would take a couple decades to gain trac-tion. But the Two-Hit Theory of cancer appeared in the 1970s and was mainstream by the '80s and '90s. We began to view cancer as caused by a genetic susceptibility (Hit One) aggravated by an environmental risk factor (Hit Two).[68] This theory held some truth for some cancers but did little to alter dominant treatment strategies.

Meanwhile, the patients themselves began to lead the way in seek-ing out alternative cancer care options, often while still carrying out the recommended conventional treatment protocols. Conventional medi-cine and research communities began to pay attention when certain "alternative approaches" began to regularly yield positive outcomes. In 1992, the National Institutes of Health (NIH) formally established the Office of Alternative Medicine (OAM) to evaluate such practices—not only in oncology, but also in all fields of healthcare. In 1998, the OAM expanded its umbrella to become the National Center for Complemen-tary and Alternative Medicine (NCCAM). In a more recent metamor-phosis in 2014, it became the National Center for Complementary and Integrative Medicine (NCCIM). Its funding for research exploring the science and efficacy of such approaches continues to grow today.[69]

More than one-third of Americans use some form of alternative or integrative medicine in general.[70] That figure holds steady for patients who have cancer,[71] though some research suggests those numbers are much higher—possibly closer to 80 percent.[72] It's very likely that alter-native medicine usage is underreported due to perceived backlash from the SOC establishment. Whatever the true number, the interest in complementary options is common enough that conventional oncology had to take notice. A formalized definition of *integrative oncology* was published in the fall of 2017 in Oxford Academic's *JNCI Monographs*:

> Integrative oncology is a patient-centered, evidence-informed field of cancer care that utilizes mind and body practices, natural products, and/or lifestyle modifications from different traditions alongside conventional cancer treatments. Integrative oncology aims to optimize health, quality of life, and clinical outcomes across the cancer care continuum, and to empower people to prevent cancer and become active participants before, during, and beyond cancer treatment.[73]

This is the definition approved and used by The Society for Integrative Oncology (SIO), which was founded in 2003.[74] In part because of SIO initiatives and research, integrative offerings are quickly becoming commonplace in major cancer treatment centers. There is still a lot of work to be done, but we have come far in bridging the gap, particularly in the past twenty years!

The primarily patient-led shift has inspired researchers to ask more holistic questions. What if cancer is more systemic in nature? In the early 2000s, Dr. Thomas Seyfried of Boston College theorized that cancer was a metabolic disease, one whose course could be changed by altering the patient's metabolism, usually through dietary choices and fasting.[75] Today, cancer research is widening its lens and thinking more creatively, more systemically and holistically. The living questions are, "What if cancer is both metabolic and immunologic? What if there are multiple intertwined causes?"

Recent years have ushered in resurrected or newly emerging ideas ranging from *deutenomics* (which introduces quantum mechanics into cancer theory),[76] to TOFT (Tissue Organization Field Theory),[77] to Dr. Seyfried's expansions on his Metabolic Theory of Cancer.[78] All of these are interested in the patient's *terrain* as the focal point. They focus particularly on the mitochondria, the energy-production centers in human cells, and how mitochondrial function differs greatly in tumor cells, compared to healthy cells. These new theories explore mitochondrial health and wellbeing as both cancer's cause and its potential remedy. For the sake of this book, we will not go into the details of each of these theories, but we do want you to be on the lookout for what the future of integrative oncology holds. Overall, this deeper questioning and sense of cancer as a systemic disease has fostered greater openness among conventional oncologists to consider the value of *systemic adjuvant therapies* like mistletoe. Contemporary researchers and practitioners alike now refer to Steven Paget's Seed and Soil hypothesis and discuss therapies that build up the body systemically, in addition to treatments that attack the cancer.

The current shift has also led to the blossoming of immunotherapy and functional medicine. In that environment of curiosity and receptivity, conventional oncologists in the U.S. are now interested in the mistletoe immunotherapy that is more commonly used in German and Swiss cancer care. After over one hundred years of research and safe use in Europe, the U.S. is beginning to research mistletoe. This therapy is finally the focus of the first clinical trial of its kind at the Sidney Kimmel Comprehensive Cancer Center at Johns Hopkins, now underway as of the publication of this book.[79] Meanwhile there are also hyperfocused efforts to research new cancer immunotherapy drugs across the nation.[80,81]

As the saying goes, what was old is new again. It's true that many new immunotherapy drugs, from checkpoint inhibitors to modified oncolytic viruses, often wind up mimicking the activity of herbal and nutritional therapies. But the latter have been around far longer and have fewer side effects. In the case of mistletoe, we have an herbal immunotherapy with over one hundred years of clinical use. Even if the earliest practitioners did not have the immunotherapy vernacular, their approach was certainly immunotherapeutic in nature. They used mistletoe to provoke a "warming" response in the body—to awaken the immune system. Mistletoe therapy improves autonomic self-regulation, therefore providing other metabolic and functional support as well. In the U.S., we are finally beginning to see some recognition of the science that supports this unique systemic therapy.

Currently, there are several smaller integrative oncology clinics across the country that follow integrative, functional, or anthroposophic models of care. The larger medical insurers have not, for the most part, been willing to support integrative oncology, and so they remain very modest initiatives. But Dr. Winters and her colleagues have recently founded the Metabolic Terrain Institute of Health (see chapter 12). This institute is unique; it brings together metabolic and integrative approaches to healthcare with many similarities to those European anthroposophic hospitals that integrate mistletoe and conventional care. The institute is also developing a robust algorithmic and multivariant database to collect patient data and outcomes from clinics that emphasize metabolic and integrative cancer care.[82] We envision this project as a sustainable model that will go far to ensure credibility, cooperation, and better evidence-based practices in the emerging field of integrative oncology. We look forward to this exciting development.

Mistletoe today: Basics of administration and use

To clarify, when we refer to mistletoe for cancer care, we mean European mistletoe, clinically referred to as *Viscum album* extract (VAE). In this book, we use the terms *mistletoe therapy* and *VAE therapy* interchangeably. There are numerous species of mistletoe worldwide, but *Viscum album* is best known for conveying supportive or even life-prolonging benefits in cancer care and for other chronic health conditions. As of publication of this book, over 150 studies have been conducted on anthroposophic mistletoe preparations,[83] and many patients who have cancer in Germany choose to include it as an adjuvant in their treatment plan.[84] Continental Europe is home to the largest concentration of cancer care centers that offer mistletoe therapy—used on its own or alongside conventional treatments, depending on the oncological situation. It is a rapidly growing therapeutic option in Asia and South America as well.

VAE is recognized as a homeopathic remedy in the U.S. It is listed in the homeopathic pharmacopeia as a remedy taken orally for headache—another well-studied mistletoe benefit.[85,86] This is why, when we purchase VAE, it arrives in sterile ampules labeled as "sips." Administering mistletoe therapy for immune support during cancer care is respected as a legitimate Off-Label Drug Use (OLDU), supported by extensive European research and SOC guidelines. Indeed, even recent articles published by the U.S. National Cancer Institute recognize and respect VAE therapy.[87] Of course, practitioners must inquire within their own jurisdiction, as guidelines may vary from state to state.

Practitioners who are trained in VAE therapy for cancer care teach their patients how to open the ampules and administer the extract through *subcutaneous injections* (injected just below the surface of the skin), usually in the skin of the abdomen. After in-office training, most patients opt to complete their injection series at home. At certified infusion centers, VAE may also be administered intravenously (IV) for intensified systemic effects. There are other methods for administering VAE (see chapter 10), but subcutaneous injection and IV are the most common. Method and dosage are personalized to each patient based on the individual's state of health; the type of cancer, its stage, and how aggressive it is; and the patient's greater hopes for their treatment outcome.

The goal with all VAE therapy is to *enhance warmth* in the patient, which coincides with immune activity, autonomic regulation, and other holistic QOL benefits we'll discuss in chapters 6 and 7. With subcutaneous injections, the enhanced warmth is tangible. The injections begin at a low dosage and increase incrementally until there is a small local reaction, a reddening or darkening at the injection site, about the size of a silver dollar, and often mild to moderate itching (see appendix A). This reaction is good! It means the VAE has awakened the immune response. With IV mistletoe, we often attempt to trigger a moderate fever of no more than 100.2 degrees Fahrenheit (37.9° Celsius). More experienced providers, usually in a hospital setting, may prompt much higher fevers. This too, is a desired clinical response, though it is not always achieved. The fever typically lasts a few hours or, rarely, up to 24 hours. It is this "warming response" that indicates heightened immune activity, awakening immune cells to their larger task. We'll look more at how VAE interacts with the immune system in the next chapter, and we'll explore more of the nuances of when and how to use subcutaneous and IV administration throughout the rest of this book, especially within the case stories shared in Parts 3 and 4.

A note on orally consumed mistletoe

There is not substantial research on orally consumed forms of mistletoe. It is possible the immune-stimulating lectins are broken down in the GI tract, limiting their immune effects. There are some promising case stories that involve providing oral mistletoe (specifically as *anthroposophic sips* produced by Helixor®) for children with brain cancers and a single case report on astrocytoma in an adult.[88-90] In such delicate situations, oral administration of anthroposophic mistletoe products might be a safe, gentle adjuvant that still conveys some benefit. But over one hundred years of successful clinical administration indicates that subcutaneous injection, IV, and similar injected applications are the most efficacious for adults.

Mistletoe as a gateway to true holistic care

We often say in our VAE trainings, "Mistletoe is not a protocol plant." There isn't a dosage chart based on height and weight and cancer type. Rather there are starting dose recommendations, followed by a process in which the practitioner and patient together determine the patient's optimal dosage based on the physical response to the injections. So VAE inherently requires individualized administration.[91] As such, for many conventional and integrative physicians, mistletoe therapy is a first encounter with truly patient-led, response-guided care. It requires active cooperation and communication between the clinician and the patient.

Personalizing mistletoe therapy begins even before the first dose. Practitioners are trained in how to pick the best mistletoe extract for the patient based on qualities of the mistletoe *host trees* (see chapter 4) and specific manufacturer nuances. European mistletoe, *Viscum album*, is cultivated on numerous types of host trees. VAE manufacturers harvest mistletoe from more than a dozen different host tree species. They pay close attention to the time of year when they harvest and give special care to branded processing techniques. Each extract has a different lectin composition and viscotoxin concentration. Chapter 4 will describe these differences in depth, but for now it's good to be aware that host trees affect VAE composition, and this is a significant factor in personalizing the therapy for each patient.

The holistic nature of mistletoe therapy is also reflected in the plant's multitude of phytonutrients. While a handful of isolates have communicated some benefits in preliminary studies,[92] it's clear that mistletoe therapy is more effective when the whole extract is used.[93] The diverse compounds work in synergy on multiple body systems. They activate immune cells, selectively damage tumor cells, and enhance mood. Collectively they are responsible for mistletoe's best-known benefit: supporting patient QOL during conventional treatments.

Just as mistletoe works better when used as a whole extract, VAE can provide enhanced effects when paired with other natural remedies and conventional treatment options. It contains within it an orchestra of compounds that work very well in synergy with other therapies. Though it is employed as a stand-alone therapy in some parts of the world, it is a strong and adaptable adjuvant. Just as VAE therapy introduces practitioners to personalized response-guided care, it also provides an introduction to more involved *systemic thinking* when choosing additional adjuvants.

VAE shows up in diverse contexts, whether it is one natural therapy among many in complex, whole-person care or as the sole integrative adjuvant in a conventional care plan. Mistletoe can be used safely as an adjuvant therapy along with almost all other conventional and integrative treatments. Its power is in its ability to enhance the effects of other treatments and mitigate side effects during more aggressive conventional treatments.[94] That includes tempering leukopenia, thrombocytopenia, anemia, nausea, pain, fatigue, and hepatotoxicity.[95] In addition to mitigating side effects, VAE therapy also conveys QOL effects that are harder to quantify, including an increased sense of purpose and greater spiritual clarity. We'll explore possible roots of these effects in chapter 7.

The world of anthroposophic cancer care in Europe and the U.S.

As you explore the rest of this book, keep in mind that European cancer care differs from SOC in the U.S.—especially when one looks at cancer treatment centers in Germany, where AM is more established. In AM cancer care, VAE therapy is routinely provided alone or alongside conventional treatments, but care does not stop there. In fact, soul- and spirit-care are given equal regard. In AM, the therapies that affect the *function of the physical body* include: VAE therapy, chemotherapy, radiation, personalized medicine, and immunotherapies, as well as other AM homeopathy, herbs, and nutritional changes. All these work in tandem with therapies that *cultivate soul and spirit*, such as: art therapy, music therapy, journaling (biography work), rhythmic movement (eurythmy), trauma resolution, and purpose exploration. We'll explore these concepts more in the second half of this book. The importance of soul- and spirit-care will be evident in our case stories throughout.

AM cancer care does exist in the U.S. There are about 300 AM-trained physicians in the U.S., many of whom studied in Europe and are trained in VAE therapy. These doctors often incorporate integrative and conventional medicine into their practices. Some are listed in the PAAM Provider Directory at www.AnthroposophicMedicine.org. Additionally, there is a growing number of practitioners who provide VAE therapy who are not anthroposophic doctors—though they have often trained with AM physicians on the specifics of administering VAE.

The AM community has welcomed partnerships with other practitioner communities to participate in VAE training and exchange knowledge with each other on treatment strategies. We regularly connect with practitioners with backgrounds in conventional oncology as well as Ayurveda, traditional Chinese medicine, functional medicine, homeopathy, and naturopathy. What we all have in common is a desire to cultivate health—not solely fight disease. Even if a patient can't find an AM physician in their region, they should be able to find a naturopath or integrative physician who is trained in mistletoe administration and other aspects of integrative oncology. Clinicians who want to learn more about VAE therapy may reach out for training and mentoring through PAAM. Fortunately, the number of doctors interested in VAE therapy is growing, and the training has become more accessible and comprehensive.

Meanwhile, cancer research has expanded its scope from Somatic Mutation Theory (in which cancer is a linear progression and your genes are your destiny) to include highly layered metabolic and immunologic questions. In the Metabolic Theory, the commonality shared by all cancer cells is not defective DNA, but rather a warped *anaerobic metabolism*. Cancer cells make their energy without oxygen.[96] That cellular defect is both their strength and a weakness that we can target with strategic dietary and immune-supporting therapies. From a metabolic standpoint, cancer is a dynamic process with many points of influence. It's not your destiny at all. Early cancers come and go often, and established cancers can go dormant. Changing your inner terrain and manipulating the tumor microenvironment can starve and stunt or even regress a cancer. As the research expands, we're seeing more openness to holism and systems thinking in medical practice.

Studies around the world are making new paradigm-shifting discoveries every year: lifestyle choices affect metabolism and metabolic shift can affect cancer growth,[97,98] meditation can alter immune markers,[99] our response to stress can alter our epigenetics,[100,101] and even disturbed circadian rhythms can affect cancer risk.[102,103] The new Blue Zone studies, looking at regions with high densities of people living to one hundred years or more, have identified nine essential determinants of health. They're all lifestyle factors related to nutrition, daily rhythms, and connection to the natural world.[104] That's just the tip of the iceberg. Breakthrough findings regarding the power of integrative care and lifestyle choices are spurring U.S. cancer centers to look to their European colleagues for recommendations. What's happening right now is another massive and beautiful shift, from a care model that's focused on fighting disease to one that addresses the disease while cultivating health. It's the difference between *pathogenesis* and *salutogenesis*—instead of asking only, "What is the cause of the disease?" we also ask, "What is required to *create health*?" Mistletoe is a powerful addition to the collection of therapies within that health-creation paradigm.

Learn more about Anthroposophic Medicine, find Anthroposophic Practitioners, and learn about upcoming mistletoe trainings for U.S. practitioners at: www.AnthroposophicMedicine.org.

CHAPTER 2

THE IMMUNOLOGY AND SCIENCE OF MISTLETOE

Dr. Paul Faust, ND, FABNO

"The best and most efficient pharmacy is within your own system."
– ROBERT C. PEALE, UK Prime Minister, mid-1800s

Plant extracts are inherently unique. Unlike synthetic drugs, which typically provide a single hoped-for targeted effect, botanical extracts naturally contain an array of compounds with multiple synergetic effects. Mistletoe therapy provides a range of constituents that simultaneously heighten immune system activity, increase the quantity of some immune cells, and directly inhibit tumor cells. In this chapter, while we explore the specifics of each effect, keep in mind that it's the synergy of all those effects together that result in substantial benefits for the patient.

This chapter is not intended as an in-depth textbook exploration of immune escape, cellular mutations, or cancer's manipulation of the immune system. All such clinical and investigative concepts are relevant to mistletoe therapy, and we do discuss them at PAAM-sponsored practitioner trainings (see "Resources"). For the purpose of this book, we will review the basics of immunology: the immune cell categories and their varied tasks. Then we'll look at mistletoe, its many active constituents, and how those constituents influence the immune response and the tumor itself.

Immunology basics: An overview

You might remember the primary immune cell categories from high school or college. The human immune system, its cells and other components, are divided into two primary groups: *Innate* and *Adaptive*. *Innate immunity* refers to the immune system components, barriers, and cells that have always been present in you. *Adaptive immunity* involves cells that are able to learn about, identify, and address all the new pathogens you encounter from birth onward. Let's review these two classes of cells, so we can better understand how mistletoe interacts with them.

Innate immune system

Natural and non-specific, I think of innate immunity as a multipurpose pocketknife. It has many tools to complete a wide array of jobs, but it probably will not work as well for a more specialized task. The innate immune system is broken down into four parts:

Physical barriers: Skin and mucous membranes. Our most basic first line of defense against external pathogens.

Immune cells: Specifically neutrophils, lymphocytes, dendritic cells, and macrophages. These diverse cells can engulf (through phagocytosis) or otherwise kill pathogens and cancer cells. This category includes natural killer (NK) cells—so called because they can kill a pathogen or cancer cell on their own, without activation from another cell or antibody.

Complement: A vital part of the immune response consisting of circulating blood proteins. These proteins can attach to, degrade, and attract additional immune response toward pathogens. These proteins are produced by the liver; this is the reason that patients with late-stage liver disease can become prone to infection.[1]

Alert and Communication System: Information shared between immune cells, particularly through messenger chemicals called cytokines. There are several types of cytokines with varied roles including mediating local inflammation, addressing viral infection, and stimulating NK cells and macrophages. A variety of immune cells can produce cytokines, including macrophages and mast cells, as well as B-cells and T-cells from the adaptive immune system.

When considering the innate immune system's role in cancer treatment, we're especially interested in NK cells. These cells are able to recognize stressed and unhealthy cells even in the absence of antibodies. This is important because tumor cells, in an active cancer process, are often able to hide from the immune system. Since cancer cells originate from our own cells, they are often overlooked by the immune system, which is surveilling the body for foreign pathogens. But NK cells can potentially work around that and still recognize the tumor cell as a problem. The activated NK cell releases cytokines, including *tumor necrosis factor-alpha* (TNF-α). Activated NK cells also increase the activity of macrophages, dendritic cells, and neutrophils. They prompt T-cell activity and antibody-producing B-cells. They are a powerful ally, and later we'll learn how mistletoe therapy affects them.[2]

Adaptive immune system

Also called the *specific* or *acquired immune response*, adaptive immunity is composed of T- and B-lymphocytes. Though highly specified in their purpose, these cells (about 2 trillion in the human body) make up 20 to 40 percent of the white blood cell mass, equivalent to the mass of the brain! There are a lot of these cells circulating in the body.

> *B Cells:* Involved in *humoral immunity*. B cells create antibodies in response to newly recognized pathogens. Antibodies are pathogen-specific; they recognize and latch onto unique proteins on the surface of a specific pathogen. This identification process can help the immune system recognize and eliminate the problem faster if ever exposed to it again in the future.
>
> *T Cells:* Involved in *cell-mediated immunity*. T cells are further differentiated into CD4+ cells and cytotoxic CD8+ cells. CD4+ cells are also referred to as *helper T cells*. They "help" by activating the

CD8+ cells, which are also called *killer T cells*. Those killer T cells do the actual work of eliminating pathogens (especially viruses and cancer cells), but first a helper T cell activates them. CD8+ killer T cells are of particular interest in cancer immunotherapy, because of their ability to kill tumor cells.[3]

Difference Between Innate & Adaptive Immunity

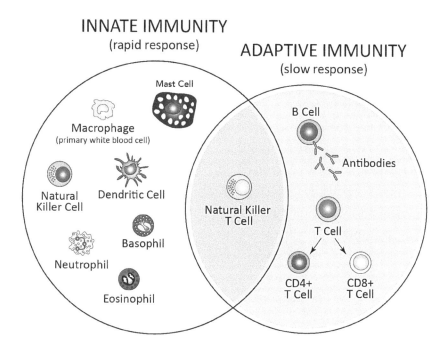

INNATE IMMUNITY
(rapid response)

ADAPTIVE IMMUNITY
(slow response)

Mast Cell

Macrophage
(primary white blood cell)

B Cell

Antibodies

Natural Killer Cell

Dendritic Cell

Natural Killer T Cell

T Cell

Basophil

Neutrophil

Eosinophil

CD4+ T Cell

CD8+ T Cell

A healthy immune cascade

As you can see, the entire immune system is divided into two major classes, and those classes contain multiple cell types and components. We think of all these cells having individual, specified roles, but there's a lot of overlap, redundancy, and cooperation between all parts of the immune system. Some immune cells can directly kill a pathogen by inserting cytotoxic chemicals into it. Others are able to engulf parts of a pathogen, or the entire pathogen. They can destroy the problem and "educate" the rest of the immune system about it. Yet other immune cells excel at recruiting help from the rest of the immune system. Ultimately, it's the concerted effort of all these immune system constituents that results in a successful response.

Let's consider how this works in a single pathogen encounter. For instance, when your body is exposed to a bacterial infection that it hasn't seen before, components of the innate immune system are frequently the first to find it. Circulating blood complement attaches to the bacterium. These proteins both create a "flag" of sorts and begin to degrade the surface of the pathogen. Innate immune system cells now notice the problem and proceed to destroy it. In that elimination process, macrophages and dendritic cells can present parts of the dead bacteria to the adaptive immune cells. They hold up the pathogen parts, essentially on display, so other immune cells can learn about the problem. See the image (bottom of page 33) for the detailed steps in this MHC Class II process. In this way, the *innate cells* begin sharing information with the *adaptive cells*. The adaptive cells are the ones who then record a memory of this bacterial threat. They generate and circulate antibodies for future use. In short, the *innate immune cells* begin the process of threat elimination, then the *adaptive cells* complete that process and create a record of the pathogen encounter.

Weeks, months, or years later, if this bacterium shows up again, you can actually get reinfected. "Immunity" doesn't mean you don't get infected. You do technically become infected, but your immune system memory (in the form of circulating antibodies) ensures that both innate and adaptive immune cells can attack the problem immediately. That makes for such an efficient immune response, you never even notice the infection. Your immune cells eliminated the problem before any symptoms could occur.

In the case of a viral infection, the process is similar, but with an important deviation. With viral infection, the pathogen is often *already inside* a cell—that's how viruses replicate; they need a cellular host. They're not going to be floating around outside the cells waiting to be found. This is an immune threat that's already inside the human cell.

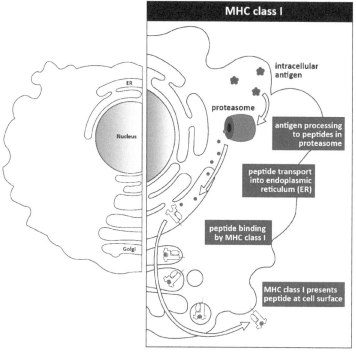

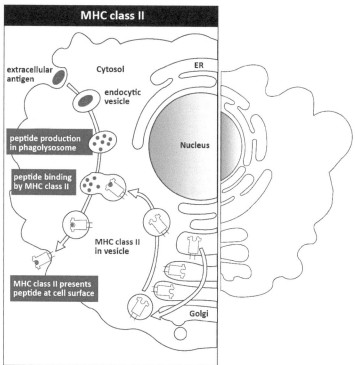

That's called an *intracellular pathogen*. It's possible for any human cell, not just immune cells, to recognize that it has a viral problem and then present parts of that virus on its own exterior surface. (See top of page 33 for the MHC Class I process.) In this scenario, there is a specific adaptive immune cell that needs to arrive on the scene to educate itself about this viral threat: *a cytotoxic T cell*, or CD8+ killer T cell.[4]

These details about virus recognition and elimination are important because *the process by which the immune system eliminates a virus is very similar to the process by which it recognizes and eliminates cancerous cells.*[5] Just as a virus can hide inside an otherwise normal human cell, so an *oncogene* can hide inside and alter a human cell. The immune system uses a similar pathway to handle both of these threats, and both scenarios lean heavily on CD8+ killer T cells. That CD8+ presence will become more significant as we look at how mistletoe interacts with the immune system.[6]

Where is the immune system?

It's common to assume that all these complex responses and interactions are all happening within the circulatory system. But that's not actually the case. Only about two percent of your lymphocytes are in circulation with your blood. The rest, the vast majority, are dispersed throughout your body tissues and in your lymphatic system.[7] That makes sense, since most pathogenic threats are going to enter the body through mucosal membranes or through an insult to the skin—external pathogens don't just suddenly appear in the blood. So immune cells are present throughout body tissues. They're just below the surface of your skin, they're patrolling organs, and they're especially concentrated in the mucosal membranes of the respiratory tract and the gastrointestinal tract.

It's important to note this nuance, as it becomes quite relevant when we consider how to best administer mistletoe therapy. We'll get to that shortly. Let's first look at the active constituents in mistletoe extract and how they interact with the complexities and layers of the human immune system.

Mistletoe's activities:
Modulating immune response and damaging the tumor itself

Mistletoe has been used as medicine for one hundred years. For quite some time, practitioners and patients have been experiencing and observing the clinical effects. But it's really in the past decade that there's been an explosion in *Viscum album* research and investigation into how it works at a cellular and molecular level. As with any scientific inquiry, we're quickly learning what we don't know! This is an evolving knowledge base, and we hope that this chapter simply brings you up to speed on the most recent discoveries about mistletoe's best-known active constituents and their effects.

Mistletoe's primary constituents

There are several significant phytochemicals in mistletoe extract, but there are two groups that appear to be doing most of the heavy lifting when we use VAE therapy. These are the *lectins* and the *viscotoxins*. The lectin proteins and polypeptide viscotoxins collectively convey both destructive effects on tumor cells and modulatory effects on the immune system. Let's define and learn a little more about these unique compounds and a few of mistletoe's other active constituents.

Mistletoe Lectins: The word *lectin* comes from the same Latin root as the words *select* and *elect;* it means "to choose." A lectin is, indeed, a complex protein whose molecular structure "chooses" to bind to specific carbohydrate groups on the surface of certain cells. The three primary lectins in VAE are commonly referred to as Mistletoe Lectins I, II, and III. Those three lectins have a demonstrated *apoptotic* (destructive) effect on cancer cells, with Lectin III having the strongest effect and Lectin I being milder.[8–11]

Mistletoe not only provides these three primary lectins; it is also one of the first plants ever identified to contain two classes of lectin. The three closely related lectins are joined by a fourth unique lectin, known as *chitin-binding agglutinin*. This additional lectin is less researched, but structurally similar to a lectin in stinging nettle.

In animal studies, the lectin in stinging nettle is known as a *super-antigen*, which is a substance that can provoke a dramatically heightened T-cell response.[12-14] The animal studies show that even small exposure to this lectin can activate up to 20 percent of their T cells. This may explain why it takes such small doses of VAE to elicit such striking immune system effects in patients. While Mistletoe Lectins I through III potentially convey apoptotic effects directly at cancer cells, this additional lectin appears to interact more with the immune cells, heightening their activities.[15-17]

Mistletoe viscotoxins: Viscotoxins are regarded as plant *defensins*, compounds that plants produce to protect themselves against parasites, bacteria, and fungal infections. Human immune cells produce some similar defensin compounds, too.

Viscotoxins are especially fascinating because they preferentially bind to more depolarized or negatively charged cell membranes.[18] This is where things get quite interesting. The external surface of a healthy cell membrane is usually positively charged relative to the surface inside of the cell. The external membranes of fast-dividing problem cells (such as cancer cells) are usually more negatively charged than healthy cells.[19] That means that viscotoxins have a preference for binding to and harming the membranes of cancer cells. Once attached to the cell membrane, the viscotoxin creates a pore (hole) in the membrane. This opening allows a flood of calcium into the cell. The cell loses its structural integrity and cellular lysis (breakdown) begins. Once the pore is wide enough, the viscotoxin itself can also enter the cell space and begin binding with and destroying other cellular components.[20-24]

The most important point to take away from this introduction concerning mistletoe lectins and viscotoxins is their *selectivity*. The lectins choose (elect) to bind to specific carbohydrate structures, particularly those associated with tumor cells. Meanwhile, viscotoxins have a preference for binding with fast-dividing negatively charged cell surfaces, which are common among cancer cells.[25,26]

Other Mistletoe Constituents: Table 2.1 provides a list of known VAE constituents and their studied effects. The highlights include

Structural Types	Substance Class	Effects on Tumor Cells	Effects on Immune Cells
Glycoproteins	Mistletoe Lectins I, II, and III (RIP II)	Cytotoxicity through inhibition of ribosomal protein synthesis and induction of apoptosis (intrinsic pathway).	Macrophage activation, release of TNF-α, IL-1, IL-2, IL-6, eosinophilia
	VisalbCBL = cbML	Weak cytotoxicity	Adjuvant increase in immune response
Polypeptides	Viscotoxins	Cytotoxicity through cell membrane leakage	Macrophage activation, increased phagocytosis activity of granulocytes
Oligo- and polysaccharides	Arabinogalactans, galacturonans	Indirect, immune-mediated tumor inhibition	Stimulation of T helper cells, increased NK cell activity
Flavonoids	Quercetin derivatives	Induction of apoptosis	Anti-inflammatory, antioxidant, and antinociceptive (pain relieving) effects
Phenylpropane glycosides	Syringin	NA	Antioxidant, stress protection, and immunoprotection (adaptogenic effects)
Triterpenes	Oleanolic, ursolic, betulinic acid	Induction of apoptosis and cell differentiation, anti-angiogenesis	Anti-inflammatory and antioxidant effects, immunoprotection

Table 2.1: Mistletoe extract (VAE) constituents and studied effects[36]
(*Source:* Helixor Heilmittel, *used with permission*)

several oligosaccharides and polysaccharides that appear to stimulate helper T cells and heighten NK cell activity. They also help to stabilize the mistletoe lectins.[27–29] Mistletoe extract contains flavonoids like quercetin, which is known to help induce healthy *apoptosis* (normal cell death).[30,31] Mistletoe also contains a high concentration of *thiols*, including *glutathione*—which is regarded as the body's "master antioxidant" and has an important regulatory role in lymphocyte function,[32] as well as detoxification processes in the liver. Finally, mistletoe contains several triterpenes, which have been studied for their antiproliferative effects (preventing cancer from spreading) and their ability to help induce normal apoptosis.[33]

What is most striking about mistletoe extract is the complementary and synergetic nature of the entire list of actives. The power of VAE therapy doesn't rest in a single active constituent. It's the whole plant, all its actives, that work together to produce multiple apoptotic and immunomodulatory effects. There have been some cell line studies that have seen beneficial effects conveyed by a single constituent isolated from mistletoe. However, in practice, the whole plant extract seems to be the most effective.[34,35]

Variation in mistletoe extract content

Lectin content is typically more concentrated in the center of the plant, in the stems and sinker root. Lectin levels also tend to be higher in plant material that's harvested in the winter. Conversely, viscotoxins are more concentrated in the peripheral parts of the plant, not in the sinker root, and the viscotoxin levels are higher in plants harvested at midsummer.[37,38]

Harvest season matters. Plant parts matter. Whether harvest takes place during winter or summer and whether a manufacturer harvests the leaves, flowers, buds, stem, or sinker root—all these factors affect the lectin and viscotoxin content. All anthroposophic VAE manufacturers use the whole plant, combining both winter- and summer-harvested mistletoe, to acquire the broadest range of actives. When crafting their extracts, each manufacturer uses its own unique process to acquire specific active ratios. That's why pine mistletoe from two different manufacturers will differ in lectin concentration. This is actually quite useful for most mistletoe practitioners as it provides a more varied tool set when addressing diverse cancer types and patient scenarios. Chapter 4 discusses these manufacturer and host-tree differences in greater detail.

Mistletoe's activities as an adjuvant cancer therapy

Now that we know some basics about the immune system, and we're aware of mistletoe's known active compounds, let's look at how VAE interacts with the immune system in the context of cancer care. In general, VAE alters multiple immune system activities, resulting in a net effect that is considered *immunomodulatory*. It neither overstimulates nor suppresses the immune system. It helps the immune system work more efficiently.

Direct anti-cancer effects

As noted, when we looked at the mistletoe lectins and viscotoxins, VAE therapy provides some adjuvant (additional and supportive) effects that are directly harmful to the tumor itself. It can help:

Induce Apoptosis: This is achieved through *direct* cytotoxic effects (lectins and viscotoxins can directly break down tumor cell membranes[39]) and *indirectly* by supporting the immune cells that are able to kill cancer cells (i.e., NK and CD8+ cells).[40–42]

Limit Metastasis: We're still learning about the method of action, but VAE appears to reduce the cancer's ability to expand its own blood supply (anti-angiogenic effect)[43] by lowering *VEGF* (Vascular Endothelial Growth Factor, involved in blood vessel formation).[44] VAE also appears to inhibit proliferation and inhibit protein synthesis by the tumor cells.[45] All of these effects hamper the cancer's ability to spread.

Repair and Stabilize DNA: When healthy cells are stressed or damaged, whether through the disease process or due to conventional treatment side effects, VAE appears to help stabilize and even repair DNA. In a *European Journal of Cancer* article, researchers postulated that "the increase of DNA repair could be due to a stimulation of repair enzymes by lymphokines or cytokines secreted by activated leukocytes or an alteration in the susceptibility to exogenic agents resulting in less damage."[46,47]

These direct anti-cancer effects are accompanied by effects on multiple immune cells. VAE therapy both damages the tumor and empowers the immune system to join in with that process of identifying and eliminating tumor cells.

Innate and adaptive immune system effects

As a patient, the first tangible effect of VAE therapy is the *cytokine release*. This manifests as reddening or darkening at the injection site, which may be accompanied by some warmth and itching. This is good; it's a sign that the mistletoe therapy is working. It's activating the immune cells, prompting them to release cytokine messengers to communicate with each other.[48] That cytokine release is just the beginning. Mistletoe's full cascade of effects on the *innate immune system* includes:

- An increase in all white blood cells, including lymphocytes, neutrophils, and monocytes[49-51]
- Improved anti-tumoral efficacy of macrophages and monocytes[52]
- Activated dendritic cells[53,54]
- Increased NK cell formation in the bone marrow and increased NK cell activity and cytotoxicity[55]

Regarding that last benefit, remember that NK cells are the ones that can work around the "masking" behavior of tumor cells. They directly identify and destroy problem cells without needing to be induced by a specific antigen. Increasing the number and activity of NK cells is highly beneficial during cancer treatment. We know from animal studies that low numbers of NK cells are associated with tumor development and progression.[56,57] Human lab studies have seen a similar connection: peripheral blood NK cell activity is significantly reduced in patients with cancer, compared to control subjects who do not have cancer.[58]

Along with these effects on innate immune system cells, VAE has simultaneous effects on the *adaptive immune response*. Mistletoe therapy appears to:

- Increase activity of CD4+ cells (helper T cells)[59]
- Increase cytotoxicity of CD8+ cells (killer T cells)[60]

VAE stimulates both helper T cells and killer T cells. While cytotoxic killer T cells are recognized for their ability to directly damage cancer cells, the helper T cells are also important. Remember, a killer T cell cannot do its work unless it is activated by a helper T cell. Because of this, the CD4+ helper T cells are sometimes referred to as the "brains" of the adaptive immune response.

As VAE therapy progresses, depending on the patient's specific treatment plan and goals, mistletoe dosage may be increased to the point of prompting temporary fever (see chapter 10). As we discussed in chapter 1, and we'll continue to touch on throughout this book, fever is an indication of a healthy, active immune response. Fever is not a disease or something we should constantly suppress. In fact, spontaneous remission and regression of cancer due to fever has been documented in hundreds of publications.[61]

Anti-inflammatory effects

Within integrative oncology and anthroposophic medicine, mistletoe is perhaps best-known for prompting that initial acute cytokine release and for its use as a fever therapy. Cytokine release and fever are regarded as *pro-inflammatory* effects. So, what's this about *anti-inflammatory* effects? Realize that inflammation is not a one-step, binary process. Ideally it is a multi-step cycle within a healthy immune response, involving a constantly changing list of cells and mediators. Cytokine release is only one of several steps within an initial acute inflammatory response. So is achieving a fever. These *acute inflammatory states* can be healthy when they're part of a flowing process, when they're transient. These are actually highly desired effects in a situation where immune response (including a healthy inflammation cycle) has become compromised.

That said, yes, VAE has also been found to convey selective *COX-2 inhibition*—a well-researched and defined *anti-inflammatory* benefit. When considering multiple effects that seem both pro-inflammatory and anti-inflammatory, it's useful to understand the difference between *acute* and *chronic* inflammation:

> *Acute inflammation* is a transient state that can involve cytokine release and fever. These states actually promote heightened immune function. We see a cycle of heightened immune activity, followed by full resolution and reduced activity.

> *Chronic inflammation* occurs when the body gets stuck at a certain point in the inflammatory process. This type of inflammation

is degenerating and does not promote overall health. Upregulated COX-2 is often a sign of chronic degenerating inflammation.

COX-2 is often highly induced and upregulated in cases of poor cancer prognosis. We need more research to elucidate how VAE helps tamp down COX-2, and we're still learning about the connections between chronic inflammation and cancer. For now, it's one of mistletoe's many fascinating side-benefits: COX-2 inhibition without the side effects of common pharmaceutical inhibitors.[62] This is especially relevant for colon cancer where we do know that upregulated COX-2 is a hallmark of that cancer's progression.[63]

Overall immunomodulation

The net effect of all these activities is immunomodulatory in nature. Looking at table 1 (page 37) we notice the stimulation of B cells and T cells, cytokines and granulocytes, and NK cells and macrophages. We see VAE helping to unmask tumor cells that are hiding from the immune system. We see immune stabilization—neither overstimulating nor suppressing the response. Simultaneously, some of the mistletoe compounds are directly cytotoxic to tumor cells. Others provide DNA stabilization and neuroendocrine effects. The entire array translates into VAE's best known net benefit: *increased quality of life (QOL)*. Whatever the primary treatment course, providing VAE therapy as an adjuvant can provide better treatment outcomes[64,65] and mitigate common conventional treatment side effects.[66–68]

Administration considerations: Applying a better understanding of the immune system and VAE composition

We've taken a brisk journey through the immune system, the mistletoe extract constituents, and how those constituents interact with tumor cells and immune cells. This understanding equips us to address some more nuanced questions that often come up regarding VAE therapy.

Subcutaneous vs. IV administration

As practitioners, we often hear from patients and other practitioners who want to know if they should even bother with subcutaneous (SC) VAE injections. Isn't it always more effective to administer natural therapies via IV? That's not necessarily the case with mistletoe. Remember, 98 percent of your T cells are in your body tissues—not in the blood—and SC injections target the immune cells that are embedded in that space just below the surface of the skin.

The answer to the question is that both administration routes (SC and IV) are highly valuable, but in different ways. SC injections should not be viewed as a "lesser therapy." In addition to targeting immune cells in the tissue space, SC injections are useful for priming the body for a more systemic IV administration. This is especially beneficial for patients who are in a seriously weakened state. SC injections are also portable; they can be done at home, which makes it easier to complete treatment if the patient lives far from the mistletoe practitioner's clinic. IV administration can deliver higher concentrations of VAE, which is desirable in certain clinical situations. Some patients experience more hoped-for results through SC injections, some through IV therapy. More often I see the best success with patients who utilize both administration methods. Reaction to SC VAE injections can also be enhanced directly by administering IV mistletoe on the same day, which can be experienced as deeply strengthening for the patient.

Allergy concerns

Latex, banana, avocado, kiwi, and chestnuts have lectin structures similar to those found in mistletoe extract. Cross-reactive allergy is a concern, even though it is quite rare. The Anamnestic Form from Helixor® (see appendix C) screens for allergy concerns. Additionally, a skin prick and intradermal test are recommended prior to starting any patient on VAE therapy. If allergy potential is mild, I know of practitioners who will give patients the option to move forward with IV mistletoe, but preload the IV with *Quercus Cinis*, an anthroposophic remedy that inhibits the allergic response.

Choosing mistletoe extracts based on lectin content

After ruling out allergy and deciding on administration routes, the next priority is choosing the right extract based on lectin concentration and host tree species. This book devotes a whole chapter to that matter (see chapter 4). We'll look at VAE brands available in the U.S., the specific host tree extracts, and how they all differ in composition. Those differences do matter. Mistletoe practitioners are trained to select the right extract for the right patient based on tumor type and based on the patient's entire constitution, their treatment goals, and their greatest obstacles at this point in their cancer journey.

Before we head into that exploration, chapter 3 will share recent clinical studies investigating VAE therapy. Using what we've learned in this chapter, we can better understand the research methods and studied outcomes, along with the implications for us as we use mistletoe in cancer care today. Let's take a look at how all the active constituents in mistletoe manifest as measurable outcomes in cancer research, tangible benefits in the lives of patients, and successful strategies at integrative oncology centers around the world.

CHAPTER 3

The State of Current Mistletoe Research

Dr. Paul Faust, ND, FABNO and Dr. Marion Debus, MD

*Special thanks to Dr. Nasha Winters
for additional contributions to this chapter*

"The words question *and* quest *are cognates. Only through inquiry can we discover truth."* —Carl Sagan

"By disregarding intuition in favor of science, or science in favor of instincts, we limit ourselves." —Bernie Siegel, MD

Mistletoe therapy is supported by a foundation of over one hundred years of research and safe clinical use, from initial studies looking at observed effects only, through current research elucidating complex immunological methods of action. This chapter shares only a handful of the most recent and compelling studies. We'll look at seven clinical studies, one case report series, and one qualitative study. It was challenging to limit our selection, but these are some of the most recent (2004–2020) leading-edge and informative studies in the growing pool of VAE research today. With each, we'll share a brief summary of the study and its findings, as well as our own observations about clinical implications.

This is by no means a full systematic review of all the existing research. Please see the Resources and Endnotes sections at the end of this book to find many more studies. A comprehensive compilation of mistletoe research can be found at www.Mistletoe-Therapy.org. The authors of this book will also regularly update a list of VAE therapy case stories and links to published studies at www.TheMistletoeBook.com.

1. A. Longhi, et al. "Long-term follow-up of a randomized study of oral etoposide versus viscum album fermentatum pini as maintenance therapy in osteosarcoma patients in complete surgical remission after second relapse" (Sarcoma, Apr. 2020)

Background and Overview: Osteosarcoma (bone cancer) remains an especially challenging cancer when relapse occurs. Surgical treatment is often regarded as the primary standard of care (SOC) treatment. There are no standard post-surgery maintenance therapies recommended. Chemotherapy does not appear to convey any benefit that would outweigh its risks. Typically, the five-year post-relapse, disease-free survival (PRDFS) for this cancer is around 20 percent after a second recurrence.[1-4] There has been one randomized study evaluating metronomic chemotherapy (oral cyclophosphamide + methotrexate) as a maintenance strategy following surgical remission of osteosarcoma. But that study found that chemotherapy conveyed no benefit as far as disease-free survival or overall survival.[5]

With these concerns in mind, researchers in Italy set out in 2007 to test oral etoposide and VAE therapy as two possible maintenance therapies for osteosarcoma patients who are in surgical complete remission after a second relapse. There is not yet a broad scientific base for etoposide in this situation, but it is used as an adjuvant to help prevent further recurrences. We know that oral etoposide (50 mg/m2/daily), as a 14-day monotherapy, has demonstrated a 15 percent response rate (RR) in relapsed pediatric patients with metastatic disease.[6]

This randomized study was small and should be considered a pilot study. However, its results were striking, and the long-term follow-up is highly valuable. Ten patients received daily etoposide for three-week stretches every 28 days for six months. Nine other patients received subcutaneous VAE therapy three times per week for a year. Researchers checked all patients' white blood cell counts at baseline (beginning of study) and at three, six, nine, and twelve months.

Results and Conclusions: In 2019, 12 years after the study began, researchers found a median PRDFS of 106 months (more than eight years) among the patients who had been provided VAE therapy. The ten-year PRDFS was 55.6 percent in the VAE arm and zero in the etoposide arm. Thus, in this long-term evaluation, more than half of the patients in the subcutaneous mistletoe group had not relapsed, while 100 percent of the patients receiving chemotherapy relapsed. The ten-year overall survival forecast was 64 percent for VAE therapy and 33 percent for etoposide. Just as striking were the effects on white blood cells. At six months, the mistletoe group experienced an increase in T-cell categories (CD3, CD4, and NK cells), while the etoposide group experienced a decrease in those categories.

The study authors concluded that since chemotherapeutic maintenance therapies have so far proven ineffective when this cancer recurs, "an inexpensive maintenance treatment like *Viscum* should be...further evaluated in post-relapsed osteosarcoma." They ended with a call for a larger randomized controlled trial.

Implications: The five-year overall survival for patients with relapsed osteosarcoma is around 20 percent,[7] and that has remained unchanged for the past three decades.[8] The use of immune stimulating therapy for osteosarcoma was first pioneered by Coley who injected a mixture of streptococcal bacteria into unresectable bone sarcomas in 1891, achieving an immunological reaction and tumor regression.[9] Mistletoe acts similarly (minus the potential risks) to stimulate the immune system. This study also found that the T-cell and NK (natural killer) cell lymphocyte populations increased with mistletoe but decreased with chemotherapy.

This study compared mistletoe and etoposide as individual, separate treatments. It is fascinating to note that a previous preclinical study has shown that mistletoe has a synergistic action in osteosarcoma when *combined with* etoposide.[10] Regardless, subcutaneous mistletoe alone was highly effective for this aggressive cancer and was safely administered for a year without serious side effects.

2. M. Mabed, et al. *"Phase II study of viscum fraxini-2 in patients with advanced hepatocellular carcinoma"* (British Journal of Cancer *90 no. 1, Jan. 2004:65–9)*

Background and overview: Liver cancer, or hepatocellular carcinoma (HCC), is the sixth most common cancer (diagnosed in approximately half a million people per year)[11] and the second leading cause of cancer mortality worldwide.[12] With a five-year survival of 18 percent, liver cancer is the second most lethal tumor, after pancreatic cancer. Surgery is often the most effective treatment option, but HCC is frequently inoperable by the time it is diagnosed.

Since mistletoe extracts are immunologically active, the Hematology and Medical Oncology Unit at Mansoura University in Egypt sought to determine whether mistletoe therapy might be a viable alternative treatment option in advanced HCC. This was a small study (23 participants) of patients with advanced liver cancer who had not previously received systemic therapies. In all cases, their HCC was considered inoperable, and they were not candidates for transcatheter arterial chemoembolization (TACE) or percutaneous ethanol injection (PEI). All participants received a fixed dose of *Viscum album* extract from the ash (fraxini) host tree, administered subcutaneously once weekly.

Results and conclusions: While the study was small, three patients (13.1 percent) did experience a complete response (CR, defined as the complete disappearance of all known lesions on radiological imaging for at least four weeks). When evaluating all participants in this study who experienced either CR or partial response (PR), the total response rate came to 21.74 percent. This comes close to the response rate of the above mentioned atezolizumab plus bevacizumab which is 27.3 percent.[13] The median overall survival time was 29 months for the CR group.

Implications: Palliative treatment for HCC provides a modest survival benefit (two to three months) and today typically comprises tyrosine kinase inhibitors—sorafenib (or lenvatinib) and others.[14] Immune therapies (checkpoint modification, vaccines, and cell-based therapies), either alone, or in combination with loco-regional thera-pies, are showing some promise in modifying the occurrence of meta-static disease and regressions.[15–17] Two extension trials (Keynote-240 and CheckMate 459) failed to show statistically significant survival benefit.[18,19] Recently though, combination therapy with atezolizumab plus bevacizumab was FDA-approved for patients with unresectable or metastatic HCC, who had no prior therapy. This Phase III trial showed significantly longer overall and progression-free survival, as well as better patient-reported outcomes than sorafenib. This combi-nation is now a benchmark for first line treatment of advanced HCC.[20] That said, we do need to research additional adjuvants for this highly aggressive cancer.

Mistletoe is not a "protocol therapy." Ideally it is always provided at a highly personalized dosage and administration frequency, based on the individual patient's response. This foundational requirement for ideal VAE administration makes it inherently challenging to study in typical clinical study models—which depend on dosages that are iden-tical for all study participants.

This study is a perfect example of this research challenge. The study was designed with a fixed dosage of mistletoe at a fixed interval of only once weekly. In actual clinical practice, the dosage of mistle-toe is routinely escalated over time to maintain responsiveness and the interval of dosing is optimized based on patient tolerance and response. In this study, there were no measures of patient tolerance such as localized skin reaction (a hallmark of patient response used to guide clinical application), fever, or immune system response (such as lymphocyte subpopulations).

All those challenges noted, the less-than-ideal administration of mistletoe still elicited a significant positive response. It is likely that the impressive results in this study could have been even better if the design included a method of dose escalation and optimal timing similar to what is actually used in clinical practice. The study did present a chance to observe the effects of VAE as a sole therapy in a very challenging cancer. Once again, the power of a simple, inexpensive, and well-tolerated therapy (even for those with advanced liver disease) was clearly demonstrated with subcutaneous mistletoe. Overall, *Viscum album fraxini* extract showed more than double the response rate (21.74 percent, versus less than 10 percent) compared to the usual response to chemotherapy (which was standard at the time of the study).[21-24] The response rate was similar to that achieved with expensive modern immunotherapies, which can cause serious side effects. A more recent case report series, with a similar patient population, also observed this activity of AbnobaViscum® Fraxini in advanced HCC.[25]

3. B. K. Piao BK, et al. *"Impact of complementary mistletoe extract treatment on quality of life in breast, ovarian, and non-small cell lung cancer patients: A prospective randomized controlled clinical trial"* (Anticancer Research 24 no. 1, Jan.–Feb. 2004:303–9)

Background and overview: In Europe, *Viscum album* extract is often used as an adjuvant to chemotherapy, in part to improve quality of life (QOL) and to mitigate conventional treatment side effects. *Lentinan* is a shiitake mushroom preparation containing the immunomodulatory active ingredient β-1,3 beta-glucan. It is similarly used as a cancer treatment adjuvant in China, and has been the subject of numerous human clinical studies.[26-33] A 2019 review of 9,474 lentinan-associated cancer treatment cases concluded that the "overall clinical data show solid effect of lentinan on improving the QOL and on promoting the efficacy of chemotherapy and radiation therapy during cancer treatment."[34] Mistletoe therapy and lentinan are applied in similar ways and are known to convey some similar benefits.

This multi-center, randomized, open, prospective, clinical trial examined the QOL and tolerability of polychemotherapy in combination with mistletoe therapy. It compared the effects of standardized mistletoe extract (sME) Helixor® A to the effects of lentinan as an adjuvant to recommended chemotherapeutic treatment for 233 breast, ovarian, and non-small cell lung cancer patients at three major cancer care centers in Beijing, Shenyang, and Tianjin. Both adjuvants were administered via injection. The lentinan group received daily 4 mg intramuscular injections. sME was administered via subcutaneous injections three times per week, administered in escalating dosages from 1 mg to a maximum of 200 mg, depending on patient response.

The study authors acknowledged that complete "blinding" was not possible for this comparative study, since most practitioners and many patients would be aware of the typical local inflammatory reaction associated with subcutaneous sME. The lentinan group also could not be considered a true control group, since lentinan conveys its own beneficial effects.[35]

Results and conclusions: Of the original 233 patients, 224 met the requirements for final analysis. Improvement of QOL was significantly better under adjuvant mistletoe therapy compared to control therapy with adjuvant lentinan (p < 0.05). There were also significantly fewer chemotherapy-related side effects under add-on mistletoe therapy. The Karnofsky index, which measures a patient's general condition (and therefore ability to tolerate chemotherapy), improved in 50.4 percent of patients in the mistletoe group and in 32.4 percent in the control group, which was statistically significant (p = 0.002).

As a result of mistletoe therapy, fatigue, insomnia, loss of appetite, nausea, and pain in particular improved. A total of 52 adverse events (AEs) occurred in the mistletoe therapy group and 90 in the lentinan group. Respectively, 28 and 77 were chemotherapy-related. In 5 and 10 cases, respectively, the AEs were considered severe. Most mistletoe therapy-specific AEs were overreactions at the injection site, which were self-limiting and did not need therapeutic intervention. Subcutaneous mistletoe was found to be generally safe and well-tolerated.[36]

Conclusion: In this study, patients with breast, ovarian, and non-small cell lung carcinoma showed a significant improvement in QOL and a reduction in chemotherapy-related side effects when treated with chemotherapy plus mistletoe therapy, when compared to chemotherapy plus lentinan.

Implications: This study is valuable for both its administration methods and its sheer number of participants. Many mistletoe studies do not utilize personalized escalating dosages. It's common to see a fixed-dose protocol, which generally does not work as optimally and skews the study results. It's refreshing to see that these researchers intentionally provided an escalating dosage schedule, basing the VAE dosage on patient response. This provides VAE therapy results and data that better reflect those seen in clinical practice. The larger data set is also appreciated. Mistletoe therapy is still growing its research base, and many clinical studies are admittedly small, often under 100 participants. This study's multicenter aspect and larger population (over 200 patients in the final analysis) have provided us with stronger statistics.

The primary challenge with this study, as noted by the authors themselves, is the issue with the "control group." This is more of a comparative study than a true controlled study. The substance used as a control in any study should be indistinguishable to both the participant and investigators, and it should also have a negligible effect on the study outcomes. In this study, the control has itself been shown to improve QOL and efficacy of chemotherapy, so the mistletoe extract had to overcome this positive effect in order to establish a statistical benefit. However, even with this stacked deck, the mistletoe extract was shown to significantly improve QOL and reduce AEs when compared to lentinan. Several other studies appear to observe similar results, including the study summarized next and a recent study by the Society for Cancer Research at the Hiscia Institute in Arlesheim, Switzerland.[37]

4. V. F. Semiglazov, et al. "Quality of life is improved in breast cancer patients by standardised mistletoe extract PS76A2 during chemotherapy and follow-up: A randomised, placebo-controlled, double-blind, multicentre clinical trial" (Anticancer Research 26, no. 2B, Mar.–Apr. 2006:1519–29)

Background and overview: As we have seen in the previous study, which looked at multiple cancer types, mistletoe therapy appears to enhance QOL and mitigate side effects during chemotherapy. This multi-center study further explored these benefits, focusing on the effects of mistletoe extract in breast cancer patients during chemotherapy and during a chemotherapy-free follow-up period. 331 patients from six cancer centers completed four to six cycles of chemotherapy (CMF: cyclophosphamide, methotrexate, fluorouracil) and began the follow-up period. Participants were women ages 18 to 55 with operable breast cancer (Stages II and III), who underwent surgery one to four weeks before starting adjuvant chemotherapy.

Because much attention has been given to the lectin component of mistletoe, the study authors selected a VAE product standardized to mistletoe lectin.[38–40] Participants were divided equally into two groups, one group receiving a placebo and the other receiving 0.5 mg of a VAE providing 30 ng mistletoe lectin/ml. Both the VAE and the placebo were administered subcutaneously, twice weekly for 16 to 24 weeks, depending on the patient's chemotherapy course. Mistletoe treatment or placebo were continued during a two-month chemotherapy-free follow-up phase.

QOL was assessed in terms of physical, emotional, and functional wellbeing. Researchers used the FACT-G Scale (Functional Assessment of Cancer Therapy-General) as a primary assessment tool.[41–43] The GLQ-8 (Global Quality of Life Scale) and Spitzer's uniscale served as secondary evaluating tools.[44–48]

Results and Conclusions: Physical, emotional, and functional wellbeing improved by 9.5 percent in the mistletoe-treated group compared to an 11.1 percent decline with the placebo. Most of the GLQ-8 factors were better in the mistletoe group as well, particularly related to tiredness, anxiety, and depression. Nausea and vomiting, common chemotherapy side effects, were also improved in the mistletoe group. VAE therapy was found to be tolerable and safe. The only reactions noted were those associated with a normal, mild reaction at the mistletoe injection site. The only adverse events that were observed were those associated with CMF chemotherapy.

Implications: When looking at the supportive effect of VAE therapy and the decline in wellbeing in the placebo group, the difference between the two groups is over 20 percent. This is a significant course-altering difference. The side effects of CMF chemotherapy can be harsh enough that patients discontinue their treatment plan. Improving general wellbeing by 20 percent can be the difference between staying the course or discontinuing conventional treatment.

We've witnessed this indirect benefit frequently in clinical practice. When wellbeing is bolstered and side effects are held at bay, patients are able to persist with more aggressive conventional treatment. Hopefully in the future we will see even larger studies that analyze this effect on treatment completion.

5. A. Rose, et al. "Mistletoe plant extract in patients with nonmuscle invasive bladder cancer: Results of a phase Ib/IIa single group dose escalation study" (Journal of Urology 194 no. 4, Oct. 2015:939–43)

Background and overview: Most bladder cancer cases (75 to 85 percent) can be classified as nonmuscle invasive bladder cancer (NIBC), meaning limited to the mucosa inside the bladder and not invaded into surrounding muscle tissue.[49] Standard treatment focuses on surgery (transurethral bladder resection or TURB). Recurrence after TURB ranges from 50 to 70 percent depending on tumor stage and grading. Historically, intravesical chemotherapy (for intermediate and high-risk cases) or immunotherapy with Bacillus Calmette-Guerin (BCG, for high-risk) has been found to significantly reduce this risk of recurrence.[50,51] These therapies can have unwanted side effects (for example, generalized mycobacterial infection after BCG or severe symptoms of cystitis), which has motivated exploration of other adjuvant therapies that could possibly reduce recurrence.[52,53]

Mistletoe extract can be administered as an intravesical therapy (also referred to as bladder instillation). Intravesical therapies are administered directly into the bladder through a catheter. The therapeutic agent is held in the bladder for a planned duration of time, usually up to two hours, then released through urinating. This administration route can provide direct cytotoxic effects at the tumor site.

The focus of the study was to determine the upper-limit dosage (due to side effects or toxicity) of mistletoe that could be used in this manner. While this was a dose tolerance and safety study, some efficacy evaluation data were also provided "to be interpreted in a strictly exploratory sense." A standard 3 + 3 design was used to determine the upper-limit dose. In this design, three patients at a time were given a starting dosage (in this study, 45 mg for the first group) for six weeks, then if no toxicity was seen, another group of three patients were provided the next higher dose. This was repeated until the final group received the maximum dosage studied of 675 mg.

Before the study, all 36 participants had their bladder tumors removed, except for one small marker tumor that could be checked as a reference for treatment efficacy. Starting two weeks after the resection, patients were treated with weekly instillations of mistletoe extract for six weeks. Twelve weeks after the start of instillation therapy, the patients underwent transurethral resection of the marker tumor or a biopsy of the former marker tumor location, so they were tumor-free when entering the follow-up period, which lasted until week 48. During the follow up, cystoscopy was done every 12 weeks to monitor for recurrence.

Results and conclusions: The dosages ranged from 45 to 675 mg with no observed toxicity. Furthermore, it was concluded that a dose limiting toxicity "could not be expected at higher doses." Bladder instillation of VAE was determined to be safe and well-tolerated, even though the 3+3 study design meant that the dosages were provided in a fashion that was nothing like the individualized approach used in normal clinical practice.

After 12 weeks, the marker tumor had disappeared in 55.6 percent of the patients and, at a one-year follow-up, the recurrence rate for all the patients was 26.3 percent. According to European Association of Urology (EAU) guidelines, the forecasted one-year recurrence rate for these patients would have been 24 to 38 percent.[54,55] It seems even this very limited administration of mistletoe may have helped patients reach the low end of their typical recurrence range.

Implications: Bladder instillation of VAE is considered a novel administration method in the U.S. (see chapter 10). This tolerable dose study helps to establish the credibility and safety of this alternate administration route. This study highlights the versatility of mistletoe, since we now have reviewed studies that show a dramatic impact on cancer using subcutaneous, IV, and now bladder instillation. Keep in mind that, in clinical practice, these various routes of administration are often combined to achieve maximal benefit for the patient.

Despite the fact that VAE was not administered in a typical clinical fashion, participants still experienced some benefit from the therapy. This is a remarkable result given the wide range of dosages. The study did not report response-dosage correlation since that was not the intent. A confirmatory Phase III trial is currently underway.

6. W. Tröger, et al. *"Viscum album (L.) extract therapy in patients with locally advanced or metastatic pancreatic cancer: A randomised clinical trial on overall survival"* (European Journal of Cancer 49, no. 18, Dec. 2013:3788–97)

Background and overview: Patients with late-stage pancreatic cancer have few treatment options. Possible chemotherapies typically include FOLFIRINOX, gemcitabine and nab-paclitaxel, which show some benefit in terms of disease control, but side effects can be severe, and treatment is not possible or effective in many of the patients.[56,57] The research community has been exploring therapeutic alternatives that may be gentler, but still provide some level of efficacy. As far as VAE's effects in pancreatic cancer, at the time of this 2013 study, one animal study and one human study had already seen some benefits, but these studies focused on intratumoral injection. Little was known about the effects of subcutaneous VAE in pancreatic cancer care.[58,59]

This study looked at the effects of subcutaneous VAE (Iscador® Quercus) in locally advanced (Stage III) or metastatic (Stage IV) pancreatic cancer, compared to a control group that was provided "best supportive care." Study participants had at least a one-month life expectancy but were determined ineligible for any chemotherapeutic options. While randomized and controlled, the study was open label (not blinded). Per FDA guidelines, blinding is not necessary in "studies with overall survival as a primary end point."

The mistletoe was administered three times per week in a fixed escalation schedule up to a maximum of 10 mg per injection. If patient reaction to the VAE therapy exceeded clinically expected parameters (for injection site reaction or body temperature), the dosage for that patient "was to be reduced to the last well-tolerated dosage."

Results and conclusions: 220 patients were analyzed at the interim (mid-study) evaluation. The median overall survival (OS) in the mistletoe group was 4.8 months compared to 2.7 months in the control group (hazard ratio [HR] = 0.49; $p < 0.0001$)—with control group OS found to be consistent with life expectancy for similar pancreatic cancer cases in the literature. In two following subgroup analyses, in which the patients were divided according to a prognosis index, the median survival time in the group with "good prognosis" was 6.6 months for the patients with mistletoe therapy and 3.2 months for the control group (HR = 0.43; $p < 0.0001$). In the group of patients with "poor prognosis" the corresponding survival times were 3.4 and 2.0 months respectively (HR = 0.55; $p < 0.0031$). Additionally, 15 percent of the mistletoe treated group were able to finish the 12-month study with a regular follow-up visit, while none of the placebo group were well enough to do this.

The interim results were so dramatic that the independent reviewing organization stopped recruitment into the study early due to the proven effectiveness of the mistletoe. *They also decided to provide mistletoe to all the remaining patients in the study, since it was deemed "medically unethical" to not provide mistletoe to everyone.*

Most of the parameters for QOL were also significantly different between the two groups. For example, a QOL questionnaire designed for patients with cancer (the EORTC QLQ-C30) showed a significant and clinically relevant advantage in the mistletoe therapy group in 13 of its 15 dimensions. The significant improvement was also reflected in the reduced number and severity of cancer-related symptoms during treatment. In particular, cancer-related pain was significantly lower, which was accompanied by a significant reduction in analgesics. In addition, nausea and vomiting as well as loss of energy and appetite were significantly less severe. Despite all expectations, the investigators even observed a slight weight gain in patients of the mistletoe therapy group.[60]

Implications: This study found that, even with one of the most aggressive forms of cancer, VAE therapy can improve OS. The positive effects on tumor-related symptoms, notably pain and weight loss, were striking. It is good to see that the personalized escalating-dosage method typically used in clinical practice was indeed applied in this study, though the study design did limit the maximum dosage to 10 mg per injection. In actual clinical practice, the dosage would likely be increased over time to maintain patient response. Regardless, the findings in this study are striking and the larger participant base affords us some stronger statistics.

This study validates VAE therapy as an extremely valuable therapy, with minimal side effects, for one of the most difficult cancers. A study designed in a similar way to investigate these results is currently underway in Sweden.[61]

7. F. Schad, et al. Overall survival of stage IV non-small cell lung cancer patients treated with Viscum album L. in addition to chemotherapy, a real-world observational multicenter analysis (PLoS One, Aug. 2018)

Background and overview: Accounting for 25.9 percent of all cancer-related deaths in 2017, lung and bronchial cancer ranks first position, followed by breast, colon and rectum, prostate, and pancreatic cancer. Over one half of primary non-small cell lung cancer (NSCLC) patients are already diagnosed with Stage IV lung cancer. Median overall survival (OS) for these patients ranges between 7.0 and 12.2 months.[62]

The authors of this study noted that "stage IV NSCLC is one of the most devastating diagnoses of lung cancer, [and so] worldwide great effort is done in the search for new treatment solutions—i.e., reflected by the vast clinical research on CTX-combinations in the past and accelerated approval of new immuno-oncological treatment in the U.S. and Europe in recent years."[63,64] Despite reported efficacy, the tolerability of current modern oncological treatment with respect to side effects, QOL, and palliative care, remains an important issue.[65] The medical community continues to look for a treatment regimen that is both effective and safe.

Mistletoe extracts are applied in integrative oncology alongside conventional SOC to improve QOL. The potential beneficial effects on cancer patient survival are accumulating.[66] This observational study aimed to evaluate the effect of adjuvant mistletoe therapy on the survival of Stage IV NSCLC patients who also received SOC treatment.

This non-randomized, multi-center, observational study analyzed 158 patients with histologically confirmed Stage IV NSCLC. The data were obtained from the clinical register of the Network Oncology (NO) database. To determine the influence of mistletoe therapy on survival time, data from two patient groups were included. One group of 108 patients received only chemotherapy, and the other group of 50 patients received a combination of chemotherapy and mistletoe therapy. Only patients who were still alive for at least 28 days after diagnosis were analyzed. The average age was about 64 years; there were no statistically significant differences between the two groups.

First-line chemotherapy consisted of platinum compounds (73.4 percent), often in combination with gemcitabine, pemetrexed, vinorelbine or etoposide. Patients receiving additional mistletoe therapy (with AbnobaViscum, Helixor, or Iscador) typically received subcutaneous administration, sometimes in combination with IV infusions (off-label).[67]

Results and conclusion: Median overall survival was 17 months in the group with additional mistletoe therapy compared to 8 months in the group receiving chemotherapy alone. The difference was statistically significant (p = 0.007). The one-year survival rate was 35.5 percent in the chemotherapy group compared to 60.2 percent in the group with additional mistletoe therapy, and the three-year survival rate was 14.2 percent compared to 25.7 percent.

The results of this real-world data study suggest that patients with Stage IV NSCLC who received combined chemotherapy and mistletoe therapy have a significantly longer survival than patients who received chemotherapy alone. The authors suggest that these real-world observational findings should be complemented by prospective randomized studies.

Implications: The merit of this study is the fact that it examines findings from everyday clinical practice. It's not a randomized trial, which would be affected by inclusion and exclusion criteria. This was not a selected population, rather it looked at the overall effects of adjuvant mistletoe therapy as applied by clinicians.

The statistics were calculated in a conservative manner, and the authors were astonished to find a survival benefit this significant. Palliative chemotherapy for metastasized lung cancer, on average, improves survival by two months. That is a modest benefit. When speaking with an individual patient, it is powerful to be able to offer a simple therapy in this palliative situation that could significantly enhance the chance of one-year and three-year survival.

8. M. Orange, et al., "Durable regression of primary cutaneous b-cell lymphoma following fever-inducing mistletoe treatment: Two case reports" (Phytomedicine 20, Issues 3-4, Feb. 2013: 324–27)

Background and overview: Primary cutaneous lymphomas account for 5 percent of non-Hodgkin's lymphoma. Among the subtypes, primary cutaneous B-cell lymphomas (PCBCL) are even less common, accounting for up to 25 percent of primary cutaneous lymphomas.[68–70] Some of the subtypes occur alongside an autoimmune tendency (i.e., rheumatoid arthritis).[71–75] These lymphomas respond best to immunological treatments such as intratumoral injections of interferon-α.[76] Intratumoral therapies, in which a therapeutic agent is injected into the tumor itself, are occasionally seen to convey an *abscopal effect*—when treatment of a primary tumor results in reduction or full remission of other lesions.[77]

Mistletoe therapy is typically administered via subcutaneous (SC) injections, but it has also been studied and administered as an intratumoral (IT) therapy (see chapter 10). Higher doses, through IT, SC, and intravenous (IV) therapy, have been shown to induce therapeutic fever in *mistletoe-naïve patients* (those who have not received VAE therapy before). These fever-inducing dosages have been associated with tumor reduction and remission.

In 2008, two patients with primary cutaneous lymphoma sought integrative treatment at Park Attwood Clinic (PAC) in England. Both patients had, of their own volition, decided to forego or delay conventional treatment options, wishing to try mistletoe therapy first.

CASE 1

A 51-year-old female, in good health otherwise, presented with two lesions on the lower part of her left leg. One lesion had developed smaller satellite lesions. This was confirmed as grade 1 follicular B-cell lymphoma. The patient was generally healthy with no allergies or history of infections. She did not smoke or drink and wasn't taking any medications. A bone marrow biopsy was normal, but she did have one swollen inguinal lymph node. SOC recommendations were: systemic immunochemotherapy followed by radiation. The patient came to PAC wishing to delay the SOC plan and "keep it in reserve," while trying VAE therapies first.

Treatment and Outcomes: The patient and her practitioner team developed a plan combining IV, IT, and SC mistletoe over the course of one year, and then continued IV and SC mistletoe for another eight months (*AbnobaViscum Fraxini*). She also received multiple treatments of whole-body hyperthermia (WBHT, medical hyperthermia; see chapter 9). No other cancer treatments were administered during this time.

IT injections were administered from the margins of the lesions, to avoid the very thin skin over the tumors. The patient experienced four febrile (fever) responses during the initial fever induction phase. The lesions swelled (as expected) initially, then began to regress. Regression accelerated with WBHT, and after four months the lesions were significantly reduced. Remission was assessed by three independent clinicians and confirmed by scans in May 2009. IT therapy was stopped at this time, and the patient continued with the eight months of IV and SC therapy along with WBHT. Complete remission had been maintained as of reviews in both June and December 2011.

All therapies were generally well tolerated. IV and IT therapies caused some transient fatigue, and swelling from the IT injections caused discomfort, but not enough to warrant analgesics. The patient referred to the fever therapies as intense and "the only thing I could do during that time." She also stated that, "During one of the high fevers an old traumatic experience became disentangled, and I have felt freed up since; I now feel better than before my cancer, physically and emotionally."

CASE 2

A 52-year-old male was diagnosed with stage 2A primary cutaneous marginal zone B-cell lymphoma (PCMZL). An initial lesion on the inside of his left elbow (left antecubital fossa) was excised and found to show evidence of nodal marginal zone lymphoma. Shortly thereafter, another lesion formed on his chest, near his right shoulder. The patient was otherwise asymptomatic with no signs of systemic disease on a CT scan. However, he did have a history of other conditions including: two basal cell carcinomas (excised), actinic keratoses (precancerous condition) on his back, rosacea, and keratitis, as well as facial cutaneous scleroderma (autoimmune condition). He reported no allergies or recent infections and was not taking any medications. He did use nicotine and drank moderately. SOC recommended either R-CVP chemotherapy followed by radiation or six months of pulsed chlorambucil. The patient had declined both options.

Treatment: The patient and his practitioner team decided on combined IV, IT, and SC mistletoe therapy *(AbnobaViscum Fraxini)*. The patient understood that mistletoe could possibly aggravate his autoimmune condition. The combination therapy schedule lasted a little over eight months, and no signs of autoimmune reactivation or hypersensitivity were observed. During the induction phase, the patient experienced six febrile responses. The lymphoma lesion showed expected swelling after IT injections. The lesion initially increased in size (referred to as *pseudo progression*, see appendix B) and then, when the IT dose reached 100 mg, the tumor began to regress. Complete remission was reached at 8.5 months and confirmed by three independent clinicians. IT injections were discontinued in April 2009, while IV and SC mistletoe continued until November 2010.

The patient described the first three months of fever therapies and inflammatory responses as challenging and fatiguing. But after six months, he was stronger and regularly reported "improved vitality and wellbeing." When commenting on his treatment choice, he said, "The treatment itself, whilst challenging, confirmed my feeling that it was the bedrock, the main stay [sic] of being healed."

Implications *(Contributed by Dr. Nasha Winters)*: Both patients were still in remission three years later when these case reports were published. This response seems quite consistent with every person with lymphoma whom I have supported. Most patients and practitioners are under the impression that solid tumor types are the only cancers that best respond to mistletoe therapy. However, in my personal clinical experience, along with that of many of my colleagues, lymphomas seem to respond beautifully to this powerful remedy.

VAE is normally used alongside conventional treatment. I have also seen it offer some rather extraordinary outcomes with lymphoma, both as a treatment *after* SOC has failed the patient, and *before* SOC is initiated. When I first used VAE therapy in a lymphoma case, patients wanted to prepare and support their body for chemotherapy by using subcutaneous mistletoe for two months prior to SOC treatment. Instead, toward the end of their VAE course, the enlarged lymph nodes and other symptoms had resolved and were no longer visible on scans. All the Terrain-based Core Lab Tests (see chapter 5) had normalized, including LDH (which can be elevated in more aggressive lymphomas).[78] None of us had expected that. This experience, and case stories like those above, have led me to use VAE therapy as a "first resort" in patients rather than a last. Each patient reports improved QOL in addition to symptom resolution and reduction in tumor burden. It is highly unusual for mistletoe therapy to be used as a stand-alone therapy, but we do see some preliminary successes like these with B-cell lymphoma cases. Much more research is clearly needed.

9. G. S. Kienle, et al. "Intravenous mistletoe treatment in integrative cancer care: A qualitative study exploring the procedures, concepts, and observations of expert doctors" (Evidence-based Complementary Alternative Medicine, 2016, ePub, Apr. 2016)

Background and Overview: Mistletoe therapy is innately difficult to research because it is the most effective when administered in a highly individualized fashion. As mentioned earlier, quantitative clinical research models frequently depend on fixed dosages and treatment timelines for all study participants—the opposite of individualized dosing. In contrast, this particular research initiative was a qualitative study, meaning the researchers interviewed doctors who provide mistletoe therapy, to learn more about the actual use and possible effects of VAE therapy in clinical practice. The research team hoped to discover commonalities in administration choices and possible treatment effects that are harder to draw out of randomized, controlled trials.

Originally the team sought to explore more broadly "the concepts, goals, procedures, and observations associated with individualized cancer care" as well as specific uses of mistletoe therapy in practice. Initial inquiries yielded the finding that "physicians often stress the importance and potential of intravenous application of [VAE], which differs from normal subcutaneous...treatment." That discovery led to the development of this focused inquiry regarding intravenous (IV) administration of mistletoe extracts.

Interview subjects came from a pool of doctors highly experienced in the use of IV mistletoe therapy for cancer. They were selected through purposive sampling to ensure a broad range of specializations and countries. Intensive interviews (up to five hours) were conducted with 35 physicians between 2009 and 2012. Interviews began with a warm-up question, then commenced with the subjects first providing un-influenced case stories, then completing a consistent checklist interview. The interviews were transcribed and charted to find thematic repetitions. Two members of the research team conducted data analysis using MAXQDA (qualitative data analysis software).

Findings: The research team found a consensus on the reasons for applying IV mistletoe. Reasons focused on the IV therapy's ability to:

- address diminished responsiveness to subcutaneous mistletoe injections;
- stimulate the immune system with induction of a fever reaction;
- support patients who have a high risk of recurrent disease;
- improve tolerability of chemotherapy and enhance overall QOL;
- stabilize the patient during advanced or progressive disease;
- address specific tumor situations that have responded poorly to other treatments.

As far as the effects of IV mistletoe, physicians were careful about pinpointing specific causal relationships. This is, indeed, hard to do within a truly integrative setting: *Did the patient's improvement occur because of mistletoe or some other therapy, or the synergy of multiple therapies?* Still, several observed benefits were noted repeatedly throughout the interviews, namely: overall improved QOL and patient vitality demonstrated through improved day-to-day activities (i.e., walking farther or with less assistance); increased strength, energy, and focus; improved appetite and sleep; and often improved toleration of chemotherapy. Interestingly, IV mistletoe was not regarded as a pain-reducing therapy unless pain was associated with bone metastases, in which case it did seem to help. Physicians also did not regard IV mistletoe as a specific therapy for tumor reduction or remission. However, they consistently shared examples of IV mistletoe helping with "long-term disease stabilization." It appeared to help people live longer with greater QOL, while managing an aggressive disease.

Implications: Mistletoe therapy is best utilized as a therapeutic system that synergizes with all other aspects of integrative care. It needs to be individually applied, personalizing dosage and dosage rhythm, as well as administration route. In this way, physicians tailor VAE therapy to the specific medical condition and complaints of the patient; to his or her emotional, mental, spiritual, and social needs; and to his or her respective goals. Experienced doctors recognize that IV mistletoe should not be used in a formulaic or highly standardized manner (i.e., "green chemo"), but must be incorporated within a holistic approach to healing.

This on-the-ground patient-centric understanding is crucial for any new mistletoe practitioner. Such nuances are impossible to learn from reading quantitative study findings only. New practitioners become skillful in mistletoe therapy through long-term mentoring. As stated by the authors, "The main strength of this study is the richness of information, arising directly from everyday clinical practice and from doctors who took care of their patients, often over years or even decades." Such narrative knowledge is invaluable when learning how to effectively administer such a nuanced therapy.

Still, both quantitative and qualitative research findings are needed. Both approaches help grow mistletoe's research base and our own understanding of its effects. Indeed, the study authors ended with a call for more *quantitative* clinical studies focused on some of the specific topics that emerged from their interviews. This includes exploring whether and how VAE might mitigate: cancer-related fatigue, weakness, and cachexia; pain from bone metastases; and chemotherapy side effects. As future researchers continue to explore these lines of inquiry, through both quantitative and qualitative means, new findings will empower practitioners to administer mistletoe with even greater insight and skill.

PART 2:

MISTLETOE IN CLINICAL PRACTICE

"If we treat people as they are, we make them worse. If we treat people as they ought to be, we help them become what they are capable of becoming."
—JOHANN WOLFGANG VON GOETHE

CHAPTER 4

UNDERSTANDING HOST TREES

Best Practices in Choosing Mistletoe Therapies

Dr. Peter Hinderberger, MD

Special thanks to Dr. Steven Johnson of Collaborative Medical Arts (Chatham, NY) for summary material included in this chapter

"Do not get so taken up by the cancerous condition that you forget the most essential part of your treatment— the general condition."—DR. ELI JONES (1850–1933)

Mistletoe is an eye-catching presence in a winter forest. Deciduous trees, like oak or birch, have no leaves in wintertime, so mistletoe plants appear as vibrant green orbs hanging among the bare branches. Each of those mistletoe plants has a single *sinker root* tapped into and drawing nourishment from its host tree. European mistletoe is technically a parasite, but it doesn't destroy its host. Rather, *Viscum album* has a relatively benign impact on its host. In contrast, the impact of the host tree on the mistletoe plant is significant.

Through multiple lab studies, we now know that mistletoe takes on some qualities of its host. Whether it grows in pine or fir or a variety of deciduous trees, the specific host tree species influences the phytochemical composition of the mistletoe plant.[1,2] That, in turn, affects the composition of each mistletoe extract. The gesture of the host tree is conveyed into the specific *Viscum album* extract (VAE). In this chapter, we'll learn how host trees influence VAE composition and how to choose the right extract for the right patient and for specific cancers. Through this exploration we'll begin to better understand why mistletoe is most effective when administered with a whole person anthroposophic approach.

Why host trees matter

Researchers have identified just over 80 confirmed species of mistletoe,[3] but only *Viscum album*, European mistletoe, is used in VAE therapy. *Viscum album* can grow in more than 450 known host tree and shrub species,[4] and we've learned that the individual host species does affect the composition of each mistletoe plant. Fourteen host tree varieties (two coniferous, twelve deciduous) are harvested for the VAE products that are available to U.S. practitioners. Rudolf Steiner suggested that the benefits of VAE therapy could be significantly increased by mindfully choosing the right host tree and the appropriate homeopathic metal to administer alongside it (see chapter 8). It is crucial to match the right host tree to the individual patient, their constitution, past and present spiritual patterns, and hopes and goals. The right host tree will mesh harmoniously with the person's immune system and their life forces (or *etheric body*, see chapters 6 and 7).[5,6]

The host tree species directly influences the phytochemical content and ratios in the final VAE extract. Other factors result in additional extract variations between manufacturers. The bioactive substances in the leaves and berries will vary from winter to summer, and processing methods also affect the composition of the final extract. Phytochemical actives vary depending on what time of year the plant is harvested, where the host trees are grown, the climate and soil of that region, and the proprietary processing methods of each manufacturer including mixing, temperature, and fermentation technique.

Because manufacturers have unique processing techniques, not only do lectin concentrations (see chapter 2) vary between host tree origins, but also between brands for the same host tree. For instance, for one manufacturer (Helixor®), their pine VAE has one of the *highest* lectin contents. But pine VAE in any other brand tends to provide one of the *lowest* lectin levels.[7] Let's look at the four major VAE manufacturers, the host tree options they provide, and their associated phytochemical constituents. Then we'll observe the individual host trees themselves and begin to understand how mistletoe practitioners match each patient to their best host tree.

The mistletoe extract manufacturers

Helixor mistletoe is the most easily acquired VAE brand in the U.S. Helixor-type mistletoe is available through Uriel Pharmacy and is provided in three different host trees, with a variety of potencies: Apple (*mali*), fir (*abietis*), and pine (*pini*). Helixor's pine VAE (Helixor P) is the one that has that remarkably high lectin content (1900 ng/mL; see table 04.01). Helixor also provides a VAE with one of the lowest lectin contents—their abietis mistletoe extract (Helixor A). Lectin content is a strong consideration in many clinical situations. But more is not always better. Lectins drive a strong, positive inflammatory response, awakening the immune system. This is desirable for many people who have cancer. But there are situations where "less is more." With highly weakened patients, those who are completely new to VAE therapy, and for certain cancers, Helixor A (low-lectin abietis) is the best option. When practitioners are first mentored in VAE therapy, they often begin with Helixor A. It is a gentle but highly effective low-lectin VAE, regarded as a safe starting point for almost any cancer.

Like Helixor, Iscador® offers VAE from three different host trees in the U.S.: Apple (*mali*), oak (*quercus*), and pine (*pini*). (A preparation from the elm tree, Iscador U, is available in Europe as well.) With Iscador, their pine mistletoe extract has the lowest lectin content (table 04.01) in their trio. Then, instead of providing fir (*abietis*), they offer an oak (*quercus*) mistletoe extract that has an exceptionally high lectin content. All three of these extracts are available in two different potencies. Iscador's apple and oak mistletoe extracts are also available in forms enriched with homeopathic metals (see chapter 8), which can enhance VAE therapy's effects. Between Helixor and Iscador, we have access to four of the most commonly prescribed mistletoe host trees (pine, fir, apple, and oak).

Mistletoe Type	A Chain Mistletoe Lectin ng/ml	A-B Chain Mistletoe Lectin ng/ml
AbnobaViscum abietis 20 mg		730
AbnobaViscum fraxini 20 mg	15,300	13,000
AbnobaViscum mali 20 mg	7,100	4,200
AbnobaViscum pini 20 mg	200	70
Helixor abietis 10 mg	30	Undetectable
Helixor abietis 50 mg	300	100
Helixor mali 50 mg	800	600
Helixor pini 50 mg(11)	1,900	900
Iscador mali 20 mg	500	300
Iscador pini 20 mg	3	Undetectable
Iscador quercus	*U.S. data unavailable*	
Iscucin abietis, H Strength	2,000	1,600
Iscucin mali, H Strength	8,100	8,000
Iscucin pini, H Strength	1,000	800

Key: Host Tree Species, Common Names

Abietis = Fir	Mali = Apple	Quercus = Oak
Fraxini = Ash	Pini = Pine	

Table 4.1: Lectin contents of common mistletoe products, by brand and host tree (compiled by Dr. Mark Hancock, MD, per K. Mulsow data, 2017)

Two other companies harvest mistletoe from a broader range of host trees. AbnobaViscum® provides extracts in four potencies from nine host trees: Almond (amygdali), apple (mali), ash (fraxini), birch (betulae), fir (abietis), hawthorn (crataegus), maple (aceris), oak (quercus), and pine (pini). AbnobaViscum is unique in that no other VAE manufacturer provides extracts from almond, ash, birch, or maple. Meanwhile, Iscucin® provides VAE in two potencies from eight host trees: Apple (mali), fir (abietis), hawthorn (crataegus), linden (tiliae), oak (quercus), pine (pini), poplar (populi), and willow (salicis). Linden, poplar, and willow are the unique options in this list. Though the unique host trees in the AbnobaViscum and Iscucin lists can give us more options for fine-tuning host tree selection for each patient, these two companies occasionally run into supply shortages in the U.S. I am careful about relying on their products as a sole mistletoe therapy and tend to use them as a complement to a Helixor extract as the primary VAE.

More is not always better:
Phytochemical concentrations and host tree selection

Table 4.1 shows lectin levels for several extracts. Looking at the range of lectin concentrations across all four brands, it's useful to note that AbnobaViscum fraxini provides the highest and Iscador pini is the lowest. Far too often, patients say, "Whatever provides the highest lectin concentration, put me on that!" Keep in mind that lectins and viscotoxins are not the be-all components of VAE therapy. Patients respond to the full complement of constituents in an extract, and high lectin content does not always equal optimal response. Mistletoe extracts contain other less-studied but bioactive compounds including ferulic acid, caffeic acid, and various flavonoids. High lectin and viscotoxin levels are beneficial for certain cancers, but not all. For instance, in cell line studies, apple (*mali*) VAE, with its moderate lectin content, produced slightly better results in fresh post-op breast cancer cells, when compared to lectin-rich oak (*quercus*).[8] In another cell line study, bladder cancer cells responded more optimally to hawthorn (*crataegus*) and linden (*tiliae*), compared to oak (*quercus*) or fir (*abietis*).[9] We do have a growing clinical and lab knowledge base to draw from when matching host tree to cancer type, but in many cases the specific methods of action are not yet known.

All that said, we do tend to look to higher-lectin preparations in situations where we wish to achieve an intensified warming response and when the cancer is especially aggressive. Lower-lectin extracts are more often used alongside chemotherapy or radiation, or when the patient is highly sensitive or weak. It is also common to alternate rhythmically between host tree types and brands, as we'll see in several of the case stories throughout this book.

Foundations of constitutional prescribing

For practitioners and patients familiar with homeopathic, Ayurvedic, or Chinese medicine, studying the qualities of the mistletoe host trees can provide an opportunity to further personalize treatment on a constitutional level. Chapters 6 and 7 will dive much deeper into constitutional factors when evaluating the individual patient. For now, we want to provide a gentle overview of what it means when an AM physician matches the gesture of the tree to the patient's constitution.

The first factor we look at when considering host tree options is the choice between *coniferous trees* (those with evergreen needles) versus *deciduous trees* (those with leaves that shed in autumn). If you think of the sheltering nature of a stand of pine or fir trees in a storm, the way one can often remain warm and dry underneath their dense and sturdy boughs, then you have a sense of the *general gesture* of coniferous host trees. This sheltering quality seems evident in the situations in which pine (*pini*) and fir (*abietis*) VAE wind up being especially effective. We use these extracts when patients are in the midst of aggressive conventional treatments or feeling weak afterward. Pini and abietis are indicated where there is reduced vitality, cachexia, or excessive sensitivity to lectin-rich VAE. These lower-lectin mistletoe extracts are appropriate for brain tumors and for immune system cancers like lymphoma and leukemia. Of course, that's all with the exception of

Helixor P, which, although it is a pine mistletoe, actually has a higher lectin content. We wind up using Helixor P more like a high-lectin deciduous mistletoe variety.

Deciduous mistletoe extracts are used more often to induce strong warmth response and fever. They are frequently used for metabolic and reproductive cancers, especially where the tumors are quite aggressive. We do sometimes look to deciduous host trees when caring for glioma and glioblastoma (brain tumor) patients if there is no edema (swelling). Some gliomas respond better to a higher lectin mistletoe extract if the patient can tolerate it. That depends on where the tumor is in relation to brain structures and whether the patient is on a steroid to reduce brain swelling and inflammation. We'll look at glioma strategies more closely in chapter 10.

As we begin to venture into *constitutional host tree matching*, one of the easiest places to start is with Helixor's constitutional overview (table 04.02). Helixor intentionally provides three host tree extracts that line up with the three *somatotypes* (or metabolic types). This is another factor we consider when selecting VAE by host tree. Not only do we look at tumor type tables (see appendix E); we also look at the person, for we are actually treating and assisting the person, not the cancer! The somatotypes are fairly accessible and often well-known even among conventional practitioners. In table 4.2, we see the somatotypes noted alongside the AM constitutional types. In this comparison, the *ectomorphic* person is typically slim, with a fast metabolism and possibly nervous disposition; the *endomorphic* person is more stocky, possibly overweight, and tends toward a slower metabolism; and the *mesomorph* is someone in between the two, often described as being athletic and having an intermediate metabolism. These three individuals align with particular mistletoe host trees. Those trees possess qualities similar to these human constitutions. You might think of the towering fir tree alongside the slim ectomorph, the round fruit of the apple tree associated with the endomorphic person, and the densely packed pine tree in relation to a sturdy, muscular mesomorph.

Product	Helixor A (Abietis, fir)	Helixor M (Mali, apple)	Helixor P (Pini, pine)
Constitutional Type	Nerve-Sense – Slim, lower energy, introverted tendency	Metabolic – Stocky or overweight, ruddy, extroverted tendency	Balanced – Athletic, intermediate build and energy levels
Somatotype	Ectomorphic	Endomorphic	Mesomorphic
Lectin Content	Lowest	Mid-range	Highest

Table 4.2: Constitutional aspects of Helixor products, by host tree (compiled by Dr. Steven Johnson, MD. Anthroposophic constitutional types according to Ernst Kretschmer)

As you can see, it is possible to select host trees based on documented *scientific, biochemical data*. We know that the host tree, its soil, and product-processing influence the composition and the quantity of bioactive substances in the mistletoe extract. We can also look at host tree selection empirically, based on a century of documented clinical experiences from hundreds of practitioners. There is a wealth of case stories and retrospective studies noting which host tree worked best for different cancers.[12]

We can also select extracts based on the *signature of the host tree*, matching it to the patient's constitutional characteristics or the signature of the cancer. For example, let's consider quercus VAE, from the oak tree. The Latin name for oak is *Quercus robur*. Robur means strong and robust. Historically, the main square of a town in Europe was always adorned by an oak tree. Town elders would sit under the oak, leaning their backs against the trunk and feeling its strength and inspiration flowing through to help them decide the fate of their community. Judgments were made under the oak tree. The oak grows slowly and steadily. It is mighty and powerful, withstanding many storms.

The cancer patient who fits this signature is known for his or her strength. They may appear "battle-weary," goal-oriented, strong-willed, or forceful. One cancer that particularly fits this signature is prostate cancer (mostly slow-growing and with a certain relationship to the metabolic-reproductive system). Quercus VAE can also be used in cancers of the digestive tract. Imagine how much the digestive tract has to withstand—and it is lined only with a single layer of cells, the epithelium of the mucosa!

When selecting the right host tree, I always keep in mind three decision-making influences: Intellect, Imagination, and Inspiration.

Intellect: Scientific studies and clinical findings
Imagination: Drawing from anecdotal reports and one-to-one mentoring
Inspiration: The intuitive art of healing and caring for the individual

It takes all three of these influences to choose the right VAE host tree for the situation in front of me right now. With these foundational anthroposophic basics in mind, let's look at the VAE host trees one-by-one.

The trees: A closer look at individual host-tree qualities[13]

As we look more closely at the gestures and qualities of the host trees and match them to tumor types, as well as the ideal patient constitution, our path can become quite nuanced. Expect to reread this section in the future. If you are a practitioner, expect to read other resources that go into much greater depth on this topic.[14] Refer often to the Host Trees and Cancer Types table (appendix E). For now, with each host tree, commit a few key qualities to memory. It takes time and repetition before this becomes second nature. That's why, in the anthroposophic world, new mistletoe practitioners are paired one-to-one with an experienced mentor.

Frequently prescribed coniferous host trees

Fir (abietis)

Available through Helixor, Iscucin, and AbnobaViscum. Abietis mistletoe extract, with its lower lectin content, tends to be considered gentle, sheltering, and structuring (think of needles instead of leaves, and cones instead of flowers). It is a reliable choice if patients are presently completing chemotherapy or radiation treatment. Abietis is often used for patients with tumors of the brain, head, neck, stomach, esophagus, and lung. Typically, they are tumors located above the diaphragm, though abietis is also useful for prostate cancer and tolerated well by patients with lymphoma. It is also helpful in other cancers when there are bone metastases.

It's fascinating that AbnobaViscum's abietis mistletoe is recommended in eight of the twelve cancer types on the manufacturer's own host tree matching table. Across all the manufacturers, abietis is often considered the most versatile and gentlest VAE therapy. If a patient's condition is highly complex or weakened, as in an advanced palliative situation, abietis is often a safe and beneficial starting point.

The Abietis Person: This patient is often considered stubborn and reclusive, with a strong sense of responsibility. They often claim that they feel cold. They may express this as feeling cold in their core, in their stomach region or lungs, or they may express that they feel cold more systemically, like they cannot keep their blood warm.

Pine (pini)

Available through all four VAE manufacturers. Pini mistletoe is typically lower lectin, with the exception of Helixor P. *The following recommendations are skewed toward the lower-lectin brands.* Pini mistletoe is most commonly associated with tumors of the sense organs—with neurological cancers and tumors of the brain and skin. The affected parts of the body are organs that deal primarily with sense impressions (nervous system oriented), as opposed to organs that metabolize outside substances (such as the GI tract).

Pini mistletoe is a well-studied and widely applied standard treatment for lymphoma patients and has been especially beneficial in situations where there is a compromised immune system and recurrent infections.[15] It is also often used with certain breast cancer types and with tumors of the skin, the retroperitoneal region (kidneys, urinary tract), penis, testis, and cervix.

The Pini Person: This patient tends to suffer from guilt complexes, self-loathing, and even self-harm. They never feel adequate. They are usually lean, modest, and withdrawn, with a lot of intense thoughts and passions that they keep to themselves. Pini people see faults in others, too, but they keep these thoughts to themselves. Physically, they often have respiratory challenges and allergies. For these individuals, pini VAE has the capacity to calm and soothe, like taking a pine bath when you have been feeling exhausted or stressed.

Frequently prescribed deciduous host trees

Apple (mali)

Available through all four VAE manufacturers. Mali mistletoe extract is most commonly associated with female reproductive cancers (breast, ovarian, uterine), though it is also useful for tumors of the abdominal region, and lymphatic cancer. Mali is actually one of the most common host tree variants that we use, and its selection is more often influenced by constitutional type.

The Mali Person: These patients tend to be a little overweight, perhaps pear-shaped, but look healthy and strive to exercise or maintain an athletic lifestyle. They tend to be more phlegmatic (stolidly calm) and shorter in stature. They frequently feel under-appreciated, unattractive, or unloved. Mali patients are often female but can also include men who have a strong sense of guilt or shame. They are often perfectionistic, sometimes compulsively so.

Ash (fraxini)

A little harder to obtain in the U.S., fraxini mistletoe is available through AbnobaViscum, depending on their supply. If you connect with AbnobaViscum, you'll learn the value of this mistletoe variety because of its high lectin content. Fraxini mistletoe is especially valuable for IV therapy and for fever induction (see chapter 10). It's used with very aggressive cancers with a strong tendency toward metastasis. Specifically, we use it with sarcoma, fast-growing pediatric cancers, and breast cancer that appears after a serious trauma.

If you look at the ash tree, it is quite massive and takes up a lot of water, so much so that other trees often can't survive near it. When other trees struggle, the ash thrives. It is a massive presence, and yet it lets a lot of light through because its leaves are thin and serrated. Ash is extremely vital and, in AM practice, we believe it can impart some of this vitality (sun forces) to patients, especially in times when it seems that all is lost.

The Fraxini Person: The fraxini patient is incredibly capable and is often perceived as someone who "does it all." They are multi-tasking parents, often mothers who struggle to find and embrace their destiny. Hormone imbalances are also common. Fraxini is especially helpful for them when they have experienced excess trauma beyond the cancer diagnosis itself or when they are completely spent from surgery, chemotherapy, or radiation.

Hawthorn (crataegus)

Like fraxini, crataegus can be harder to obtain. But it is available through AbnobaViscum and Iscucin. Crataegus is high in lectins—one of the most warming—and can induce fever. Yet it is also well-tolerated by people who are in a weakened state. This mistletoe is used in complex and aggressive cancers, in situations where the patient may be too weak to tolerate fraxini. It is not so much a tumor-specific mistletoe; rather, we tend to select crataegus based on the patient's constitution and general state.

The Crataegus Person: This patient is someone who expresses that their heart or purpose has not been sufficiently nourished. There is a sense that their feminine side may be neglected. Physically, they may be bluish or show other signs of poor circulation. Often, they are in a space where they have no capacity for feeling. We use crataegus when this person has experienced a trauma or deep disappointment, are swept into a massive life transition, or are in severe shock from the cancer diagnosis. Until this trauma or shock is addressed, other therapies (conventional or integrative) will struggle to have an impact.

Oak (quercus)

Available through AbnobaViscum and Iscador. Quercus is used when there are dense, hard tumors—often of the pancreas, rectum, gall bladder, or prostate, or in hepatocellular tumors or squamous cell carcinoma of the lung. I tend to think of it as useful for tumors in any organ where an external substance is taken in, metabolized, and eliminated. That includes any tumors of the digestive tract and the kidneys and respiratory system. This is in contrast with pini mistletoe, which is associated more with organs involved in sensory impressions.

As a tree, quercus has sturdy, earthbound, and nourishing qualities (it serves as a living space for a huge variety of small animals and produces calorie-rich acorns). As mentioned earlier, it is associated with wisdom and strength, as the gathering place for community elders. This tree has a leadership quality to it and can be useful for people who are themselves strong leaders or for those who long to embrace a stronger sense of leadership.

The Quercus Person: Quercus is most often used with male patients who have cancer, but it can be used for women too, especially if they have a strong, stoic, more stereotypically male constitution. Regardless of gender, they are typically compact, strong, and athletic. Quercus people work hard for others all their lives and never complain about it. They are dedicated to a fault and never permit weakness. No one knows that they are struggling. Though they care for others' wellbeing, they are poor at paying attention to their own feelings and self-care and may have trouble experiencing joy.

Secondary host tree descriptions

The following host tree sources are available through AbnobaViscum, Iscador, or Iscucin, and supply sometimes varies. However, they can be immensely helpful adjuvants (additional supportive therapies), used alongside a primary Helixor VAE. For practitioners, it is best to learn more about each of these varieties by connecting with your mentoring practitioner. The following is only a brief introduction to these diverse options.

Almond *(amygdali)*: Associated with patients who are unwilling to address past injustice and who may overachieve to compensate for hurt or bitterness. Used for neck and skin tumors, as well as lymphoma (available through AbnobaViscum).

Birch (betulae): Works beautifully for patients who have lost their enthusiasm and buoyancy; allows light to shine into a depressive state. Often used for kidney and bladder cancer as well as melanoma (available through AbnobaViscum).

Linden (tiliae): Associated with maternal types who are social and generous. Tiliae is frequently effective when other mistletoes fail to warm the patient. Often used for soft tumors such as endometrial cancer, adenocarcinoma of the lung, and some breast tumors (available through Iscucin).

Maple (aceris): Not referred to often but can be used to help people come back to, or newly discover, their destiny; restores a capacity for action (sense of personal agency). Used especially for liver, pancreas, prostate, and breast cancers (available through AbnobaViscum).

Poplar (populi): Often recommended for people who seem fearful, superstitious, or excessively religious. Frequently used for aggressive bladder and prostate cancers (available through Iscucin).

Willow (salicis): Used for patients who lack life (etheric) forces and have a generally negative attitude; helps restore hope. Frequently used for leukemia, myelodysplasia, bladder cancer, ovarian cancer, and testicular cancer. May also be used when there are precancerous conditions or in cancer prevention strategies (available through Iscucin).

Basics of rhythmic administration and alternating host trees

As we've described in previous chapters (and appendix A), mistletoe therapy ought to elicit a mild inflammatory reaction at the subcutaneous (SC) injection site or a measurable systemic warming response with IV administration. These are signs that the VAE is successfully awakening and intensifying immune activity.

The degree of reaction will vary from patient to patient, depending on how VAE interacts with their immune system and constitution, and depending on the dosing strategy and treatment goals. With some cancers, it may be appropriate to provoke a significant fever response right at the start, but this strategy should be pursued only if the patient seems strong enough (see chapter 10). Fever requires energy and exertion from the patient. Sometimes the patient is too weak for that effort.

If the patient is quite weakened, it can be helpful to prime the immune system with a low-lectin VAE administered subcutaneously, with a "low and slow" approach to increasing dosage. I typically start patients with a Helixor mistletoe extract, as that is the best-tolerated brand for most people and is usually the most readily available too. Once the patient begins to respond to SC injections, and their body grows accustomed to the treatment rhythm, I might try adding IV treatment using VAE from the same or an alternate host tree.

It can be highly beneficial to alternate host trees along with alternating administration methods. We often see a rigidity in people who have cancer, sometimes from long-time personal patterns, sometimes influenced by the transition into a reality dominated by high-stress medical appointments and treatment schedules. Rhythmically alternating host trees can help to loosen this rigidity and nurture some inner flexibility. It is especially effective to alternate a coniferous with a deciduous host tree variety. Using two host trees can introduce a broader range of host tree qualities and beneficial phytochemicals, too.[16,17] Sometimes this translates as using one host tree variety for the SC injections and another for IV administration. Or it could involve SC injections, using one host tree extract at home and then coming into the clinic once a week for an injection of another host tree extract. Frequently the host tree extract used at home is a lower-lectin mistletoe, while the injection administered in clinic has a higher lectin content. This allows for an occasional punctuated rhythmic response and permits the practitioner to monitor the reaction to the higher-lectin extract. Whichever host trees are selected for the patient, whatever the administration route, there is definitely a rhythmic nature to VAE therapy—warming the immune response, letting the response resolve, and then encouraging the heightened immune activity again.

Dosing considerations common to all four manufacturers

With all the VAE manufacturers, there are some across-the-board similarities. All dosing guidelines start low and increase in strength as tolerated, until the patient experiences a local reaction or slight temperature increase or both. All the manufacturers recommend some variation of dosing in a cycle from low to high, again and again, with breaks in between (see appendix A). They all respect that the dosage should be modified based on the severity, stage, and symptoms of the disease process, and on the level of patient compliance.

The importance of that last factor cannot be overstated. If I set up a dosage calendar for a patient, and it's too complex for them to implement, the SC injections will happen sporadically at best. I'm always sensitive to the issues of overwhelm and poor short-term memory during cancer treatment. Sometimes I drastically simplify a SC injection calendar to accommodate the fact that a patient may be able to remember only two injections per week. I find that, in the U.S., patients often seek out integrative care after they are already well into their cancer journey. This can result in greater compliance challenges—not because they do not want to do the therapy, but because they genuinely can't keep track of it all.

Remember to spend time with the trees

Both patients and practitioners can get overwhelmed by all the facts and nuances surrounding host tree selection and rhythmic administration. Perhaps the most important thing we all can do is to spend time with some of these trees. Several of them likely grow in your region. Take time in nature, sit with coniferous or deciduous trees, and admire and learn their gestures, their innate qualities. This is the heart of anthroposophic medicine: to experience who the patient is and to experience the spirit of the medicinal substance, whether mineral or botanical. Listen to what that substance is telling you.

Ultimately, life is a miracle. Nature is a miracle. Miracles cannot be analyzed. We need to develop other sources of knowledge that are dormant in us, rather than solely finding ourselves sucked into endless internet searches or overwhelmed by lectin content tables. Powerful answers come to us when we combine both *conventional scientific knowledge* with *spiritual scientific knowledge*. Rudolf Steiner called this *spiritual science*.[18] Effective whole-person care flows from that unified awareness.

CASE STORY ONE: PAUL

When the Patient's Mistletoe Reaction Plateaus				
Physician: Dr. Peter Hinderberger	**Patient:** Paul	**First seen:** June 2015	**Age:** 53	**Sex:** Male
Cancer Type & Stage:	Non-small cell, right lung cancer with local lymph node involvement. T2bN1 at start of conventional treatment in January 2015.			
Risk Factors:	No obvious risk factors (non-smoker, non-smoking home and non-smoking family of origin). However, patient is an office worker at a feed mill (possible chronic grain dust exposure).			

When Paul came to me, he had already journeyed through the initial lung cancer diagnosis and conventional treatment. He came to me seeking guidance on preventing recurrence—which is common with non-small cell lung cancer (NSCLC). Paul shared the story of his diagnosis and treatment. He had been experiencing shortness of breath, a cough, and wheezing for about three months when he went to his primary care physician. A chest X-ray showed a mass in his right lung. There was evidence of lymph node involvement. T2bN1 lung cancer meant that treatment would be rather aggressive. Conventional treatment included a right *pneumonectomy* (removal of the right lung), followed by 16 weeks of chemotherapy.

Paul had been through a lot, but he had tolerated chemotherapy remarkably well. He had lost 18 pounds during treatment but had gained it back by the time he and his wife met with me. He was in exceptionally good health and spirits, given what he'd been through. But he and his wife were, of course, understandably anxious about recurrence.

Perhaps the biggest reason for concern was his lack of known risk factors. How could they prevent recurrence of a condition that didn't appear to have a typical cause? Paul had never smoked. No one in his house smoked, and no one in his childhood home had been a smoker. His family history was full of people in great health. I couldn't find indications of severe toxin exposure, either.

Paul ate mostly organic foods and avoided processed foods and white sugar. He drank plenty of water, avoided coffee, took a multivitamin, and took daily walks. He did have occasional alcoholic drinks, but no red flag habits. He wasn't taking any prescription medications for any other health conditions. As far as his labs, Paul's CBC w/diff and CMP (see chapter 5) were all healthy, and his follow-up CT scan showed no cancer activity. Apart from the expected "diminished breath sounds" on the right side, his physical exam was normal.

The only clear risk factor I could find was his job. Paul worked in the office of a feed mill. I had some concerns that he might be dealing with ongoing grain dust exposure. It didn't seem a major risk factor, but maybe for some reason, for Paul's body it was.[19]

If he couldn't change his job, we had to focus on supporting his body in the face of that possible risk factor. Paul had a good diet, but I shared tips for fine-tuning his nutrition and fully avoiding foods that can become quick energy for cancer cells. I'm more interested in compliance than complexity when it comes to anti-cancer diets. My dietary philosophy is to address acidity, inflammation, and sugar.

In short, I encouraged Paul to avoid all processed carbs, white sugar, fruit juices, tropical fruit, and dried fruit—all of which are exceptionally concentrated sources of sugar. He needed to avoid wheat too, though very occasional dark, sourdough, rye bread would be okay, as long as it was true fermented rye, not a pigmented white flour. As with all my patients, I asked Paul to continue avoiding caffeine and avoid alcohol (both acidify the body) and start each day with a dose of apple cider vinegar or the juice from a fresh lime or lemon to alkalize the body. Finally, I explained that he should increase his intake of organic vegetables and eat a small serving of a fermented food (kombucha, kimchi, kefir, sauerkraut, etc.) every day. Paul and his wife heard all these recommendations and seemed happy to take on the dietary adjustments. There wouldn't be any major issues with dietary compliance since they already ate so well.

Then we discussed adjuvant therapies. I recommended a gentle VAE Abietis Series 1 (Helixor), one vial every other day till Paul experienced the hoped-for local response. His condition was stable, and I recommend only SC mistletoe (not IV) when a cancer is stable. I chose abietis initially because of Paul's constitution (more nervous-sensitive type), his gender, and because of the location of the tumor (lungs). He responded to 5 mg of VAE and gradually built up to 20 mg, which became his maintenance dose, three times per week. I also recommended artemisinin SOD along with Beta 1,3 Glucan for general immune support.

Paul followed this preventive strategy for two years. In the spring of 2017, he noticed his injection site reactions had significantly decreased. A two-year follow-up CT scan in 2017 showed a subcutaneous 10 mm soft tissue nodule on the right anterior chest wall and a few sub-centimeter hypodensities in his liver. Neither were conclusively cancerous and, for the moment, Paul did not want to go through a biopsy of the chest wall mass.

He preferred pursuing our treatment course first, then re-scanning. There was nothing in the CT report that indicated anything had traveled from the lungs to the lymph nodes and, from there, jumped to the chest wall. So, I felt comfortable with this patient preference as well.

With this situation, changing host trees seemed one of the most effective strategies. Paul was no longer reacting to the 20 mg abietis. If he'd stayed on abietis, I would have at least increased his dosage to 50 mg. But I believed switching host trees might be even more effective. I switched him to Iscador Quercus because it is recommended predominantly for men, and it is also appropriate for respiratory tract cancers. It has a higher lectin content, so I knew it would have a strong chance of reinvigorating his immune system's response to the SC VAE injections.

We switched Paul to 20 mg SC Iscador Quercus, three times per week. (Iscador Quercus is a fermented product, so it is more concentrated; the 20 mg of Iscador Quercus is equivalent to 50 mg of the Helixor A.) This change—both in host tree and equivalent dosage—allowed Paul to experience an adequate reaction once again. He followed this adjusted regimen, and within six months, his CT scan normalized and showed no evidence of the mass previously seen on the right chest wall. The hypodensities in the liver were unchanged; they are most likely hemangiomas (benign vascular tumors).

Paul has continued with this adjusted course and remains in good health. He continues self-administering 20 mg Iscador Quercus, three times per week. He is breathing well, sleeping well, walking daily, and still working. He is now six years out from his original diagnosis, and he was excited to email me his most recent CT scan in November 2020: *still clear*. We may never know precisely what made him vulnerable to this particular cancer. But his therapeutic plan and lifestyle are helping him maintain his good health, and we've been able to respond successfully to setbacks along the way.

CASE STORY TWO: MARY

Matching Host Tree to a Patient's Newly Found Sense of Self				
Physician: Dr. Peter Hinderberger	**Patient**: Mary	**First seen**: April 2011, second diagnosis in 2018	**Age:** 60	**Sex:** Female
Cancer Type & Stage:	2010: right ovarian cancer, 1 positive lymph node. 2018: 1.3 cm mass found in left breast. MRI guided biopsy showed a well-differentiated ductal adenocarcinoma (ER+, PR+, HER2-negative).			
Risk Factors:	Significant personal stress; past diagnosis of Lyme disease (not currently symptomatic).			

Mary was diagnosed with ovarian cancer in 2010, and I first saw her in 2011 after she had gone through a total hysterectomy and chemotherapy. When we met, she was recently divorced and lived with two of her three children. The oldest child lived independently. Mary worked for a publisher, but her passion was her own creative writing—though she clearly didn't have time for exploring that. She cared much more for others than for herself. Her life revolved around her children. That's common for many parents, but for Mary it seemed more pronounced. She'd not had her husband's support for years, and now they were divorced. This was an incredible source of stress on top of the cancer diagnosis.

Having completed conventional care, she was exploring how to prevent recurrence. She did seem on the verge of transformation and creating a healthier life for herself. Mary was 5'9" and weighed 186 pounds at her new client appointment. In her past, she'd also been diagnosed with Lyme disease, but was symptom-free at the time. Her physical exam and labs were otherwise within normal ranges. We discussed therapeutic options and lifestyle changes.

Mary was open to mistletoe. I shared that VAE from the mali (apple) tree would be highly appropriate for her. VAE mali is frequently recommended for women, particularly those who are incredibly nurturing, yet sometimes turn bitter toward others who have perhaps taken advantage of them.[20] This is an understandably common constitutional imbalance among any people in care-providing roles. Mali is also indicated for cancers of the reproductive organs, and for people who have a "pomaceous" body type, with fat distribution tending lower, at and below the waist line.

We discussed that extra weight. Mary was 60 at the time, and I shared how extra fat tissue can be a challenge in terms of female reproductive cancers. Later in life, after the ovaries become dormant (or if they are removed), fatty tissue continues to produce hormones, and so do the adrenal glands. She was aware that this fatty tissue was a hormone-balance risk factor. It is good to lose the weight, but of course, any weight loss program needs to be pursued at a balanced pace.

Mary understood all this and wanted to start on mistletoe too. She worked up to 20 mg of *Viscum Mali* injected subcutaneously, three times weekly for the first two years, then twice weekly for the next three years. During that five-year period, Mary also transformed her life. Her children grew up and moved out, and Mary moved into a condo, creating a space that suited her well. She began working on her own writing. She lost 40 pounds and attended support programs through a community-based nonprofit that offered free services to people affected by cancer. Mary was successfully maintaining a cancer-free life, and we shifted her mistletoe schedule to reflect that: four times per year, she completed a single series of *Viscum Mali* Series 2.

Then in 2018, when Mary was 67, a mammogram and ultrasound showed a 1.3 cm mass in her left breast. An MRI-guided biopsy showed a well-differentiated ductal adenocarcinoma (ER+, PR+, HER2-negative). She had cancer again, which isn't unusual after surviving ovarian cancer. But this time Mary seemed different. She presented as a woman who was far more confident and self-assured. She had just published her first novel and seemed lighter than before, even though this new diagnosis was in her reality. She was open to adjusting her mistletoe therapy and looking at other complementary therapies too, particularly focused on hormone balance. She decided against lumpectomy, radiation, and hormone-deprivation therapy (aromatase inhibitor). She wanted to try "other options" first.

We returned to the discussion of hormone balance after menopause. In terms of whole health and cancer risk, there are multiple forms of estrogen and progesterone, and some of these forms are beneficial, some are not. Estrone, for instance, is a form of estrogen associated with higher cancer risk.[21] As we get older, we tend to produce more of the hormone intermediates—the bad forms. When an ER+, PR+ breast cancer appears years after ovarian cancer, it's common to use an aromatase inhibitor to block the bad hormone forms that would fuel the cancer. But an aromatase inhibitor cuts off *all hormone production* at the very top, even the good forms. It is possible to support healthy *hormone metabolism* instead—to help the body clear out the bad hormones and allow the useful forms to remain. This can be done with certain supplements, particularly calcium D-glucorate, a nutrient found in some citrus fruits and broccoli, and DIM, an extract from cruciferous vegetables that helps break down excess hormones.[22] With Mary, I also recommended myomin, which works similarly. Instead of blocking hormone production, this approach would activate her healthy hormone metabolism.

Mary was very interested in this. She had developed a significant supplement protocol of her own as well. She was taking melatonin, vitamin D, liposomal vitamin C, and turmeric. I saw no problem or potential toxicity with any of these, so she continued with them. I also recommended low-dose naltrexone (LDN, see chapter 9) and metformin (though her transformed diet and weight loss will likely make the latter unnecessary for her at some point). Mary had been eating a modified vegan diet: avoiding all animal products, except fish. As long as she continued to eat fish (a source of Omega-3, needed for hormonal balance), I was fine with that, too.

Then we looked at her mistletoe therapy. There was room for a couple potentially powerful changes, in terms of both host tree and dosage. Mary's life and her entire presence had shifted significantly. Constitutionally, she was happier in her own skin, more confident. It seemed *Viscum Mali* no longer suited her. She was no longer trapped in that caregiving cycle of putting others first to the point of harming her own health.

In contrast, *Viscum Pini* has been described as suitable for the person who "suffers from self-reproach, guilty feelings, and discouragement...[but when] transformed they accept their own weaknesses and can forgive themselves for their own shortcomings..."[23] Mary looked more like the "transformed pine personality" than the typical apple personality. I also wanted to increase the lectin content of her VAE therapy, given her new cancer diagnosis. Helixor's pini mistletoe (Helixor P) has a higher lectin content than their mali mistletoe. It is also generally recommended for breast cancer in postmenopausal women.

Mary switched from her seasonal 20 mg *Viscum Mali* series to *Viscum Pini* 50 mg, administered via SC injections three times per week. Because of the cancer recurrence, and particularly because it appeared as breast cancer, I recommended that she remain on a similar VAE regimen for the rest of her life. With so many other aggressive cancers (i.e., colon, pancreatic), if a patient is cancer-free at five years, they are truly "in the clear." But breast cancer is unique. It's one of the few cancers that can go dormant and then recur ten or twenty years later. It has its own agenda regarding time. I shared this with Mary, and she seemed ready to commit to making mistletoe a regular part of her ongoing wellness care.

In April 2018, Mary began both the adjusted mistletoe therapy and the new hormone-balancing supplements, in addition to continuing all the positive self-care she now had in her life. Three months later, ultrasound showed a stable situation, based on measurements where a clip had been placed in February 2018. Six months later, the tumor measured 0.9 cm (a 0.4 cm decrease). In July 2020, the area around the clip was negative. As of early 2021, Mary is stronger than ever and still cancer-free. She continues her nutritional and self-care strategies, along with SC *Viscum Pini* two times per week. Just as importantly, she is a transformed person. She lives a life that is a truer expression of her "I."

CHAPTER 5

TEST, ASSESS, ADDRESS . . . DON'T GUESS!

Adjusting Treatment Priorities in Response to the Patient's Unique Terrain

Dr. Nasha Winters, ND, FABNO

"One day, patients will say: I'm not an average patient. I am who I am. You need to understand who I am before you prescribe whatever treatment you plan to prescribe."

—EDWARD ABRAHAMS, President of
Personalized Medicine Coalition

"More information is always better than less. When people know the reason things are happening, even if it's bad news, they can adjust their expectations and react accordingly. Keeping people in the dark serves only to stir negative emotions."   —SIMON SINEK

Mistletoe is not a "protocol" treatment. As previous chapters have explained, there is no height and weight chart for administering mistletoe. Rather, VAE therapy begins with close observation of patient response: both visible and sensory reaction at the injection site. But even before that, as a mistletoe practitioner, I run dozens of lab tests on my patients and go through hours of patient intake inquiry. That initial data, along with real-time response and follow-up lab tests, guide the treatment progression, including mistletoe administration. I constantly monitor my patient's metrics and adjust all treatments responsively.

In the integrative and anthroposophic worlds, we often say, "We don't treat cancer; we support the person." In this chapter, we'll look at a holistic and *terrain-based* approach to monitoring the patient's baseline starting point and their response to therapies. We'll define several aspects of the body's inner terrain, the lab tests that effectively reveal that terrain, and the levels and ranges that define true health. (It's not worthwhile to strive for the "normal ranges" of a generally unhealthy population group!) Along the way, we'll look at how lab findings influence our choices about mistletoe therapy and other integrative care, as well as how those therapies can, over time, nudge patient labs in a positive direction.

Terrain-based care: The patient as an ecosystem

When discussing my Terrain-Based Core Lab Tests™, it's helpful to first explore my underlying medical philosophy, how I regard the body as a complex ecosystem with multiple subsystems. In Western medicine, we have cardiologists, neurologists, endocrinologists, pulmonologists, gastroenterologists, urologists... and the organ-specific list goes on and on. But the body doesn't understand these silos. The body's organs are all intricately intertwined and interdependent. Learning some basics about terrain-based thinking will make it easier to follow along when we begin looking at individual blood tests and discover their ramifications for multiple body systems.

In over 25 years of caring for myself and my patients, I have learned to evaluate health through ten terrain-focused elements. This is a way of looking at health in terms of multiple whole-body layers, which affect and involve all the organs. This is a paradigm shift away from evaluating health and disease as issues affecting a single organ only.

There are certainly more than ten systemic pathways in the human body, but these are simply the most common and critical entry points that I've experienced in my practice. These Ten Terrain Components are inspired by the book I co-authored with Jess Higgins Kelley, *The*

Metabolic Approach to Cancer Care, which defines each of these concepts in robust detail and describes their associated therapies at length.[1] For our purposes here, this is only a brief summary. We'll refer to these terrain components again in chapter 9, when we look at several integrative therapies commonly used alongside mistletoe.

1. *Epigenetics:* The genetic blueprint that you were born with. Genetic predisposition is not destiny! Gene expression can be influenced by diet, lifestyle, trauma and stress processing, medications, nutrient deficiencies, and more. The more you know about your blueprint and its vulnerabilities and strengths, the more you can rearrange your inner home and create a terrain that's more resilient to health challenges.

2. *Metabolic function and blood sugar balance:* The key to keeping your motor humming along without damaging organs, weakening immune function, promoting cancer growth factors, or rendering conventional treatments less effective. Optimizing the metabolism of your healthy cells simultaneously slows the metabolism of cancer cells![2]

3. *Toxic Burden:* The cumulative effects of living on a toxic planet. It is not a matter of *if* you have a toxic load; it is a matter of *how much*. In integrative oncology, it's a priority to remove and avoid as many toxic assaults as possible, so the body can spend more of its energy on healing.

4. *Microbiome and digestive function:* The basis of many ancient medical models like Ayurveda and traditional Chinese medicine. Indeed, we can't absorb and utilize many healing nutrients without an optimal balance of microorganisms in the gut, along with a properly functioning gut lining.

5. *Immune Function:* Long-ignored in conventional cancer care but emerging as a new focus of immunotherapy research. Chemotherapy, radiation, and surgery do a fine job at removing the tumor. However, an intact immune system is the greatest defense against progression and recurrence.[3-7]

6. *Inflammation:* The driving force of progression in most of our modern diseases, including metabolic syndrome and cancer. Inflammation is stimulated by sugar, stress, and other common contemporary lifestyle factors. Chronic inflammation is a complex response to an overwhelmed terrain.

7. *Circulation and angiogenesis:* Refers to patterns of flow or stagnation of the blood. Includes factors such as heart rate, clotting tendencies, dehydration, exercise habits, inflammation, and stress. Circulation also looks at the altered liver function that occurs during an active cancering process, and how that impacts blood viscosity, oxygenation, and blood vessel growth.

8. *Hormone balance:* One of today's greatest challenges now that we live in a swimming pool of xenoestrogens and estrogen-mimicking substances pervasive in food, water, body care products, industrial chemicals, and plastic products, as well as hormone medications like steroids, birth control pills, and hormone replacement therapy. It takes work, but it is not impossible to restore balance and function for hormone receptor sites.

9. *Stress and biorhythms:* Refers to natural cycles of activity and rest, deep sleep, daytime light exposure, appropriate darkness at night, and our experience of seasons and moon cycles. Only in the past century have humans fully disrupted our innate circadian rhythm through electric light, blue light, night shift work, overwork, medications, and a loss of connection to natural rhythms. Recent studies now show circadian disruption to be implicated in several conditions, including cancer.[8-10]

10. *Mental and emotional health:* Possibly the most under-emphasized but widely influential terrain element. Our thoughts impact our response to any situation. We are what we think. The field of psychoneuroimmunology shows direct links between our psychosocial wellbeing and our ability to ward off infection and disease.[11,12]

These Ten Terrain Components are my personal take on a terrain-based treatment philosophy. However, terrain-based thinking is not an original idea. We mentioned in chapter 1 that there were several medical thought leaders in the 1800s who viewed the body and disease processes in terms of terrain or "soil." Rudolf Virchow (1821–1902) said, "Germs seek their natural habitat—diseased tissue—rather than being the cause of dead tissue."[13] This was another reference to the body's overall terrain. Many other brilliant practitioners and researchers have kept that flame of insight alive, leading up to and including Mina Bissell's past work in the 1980s and her more recent research describing the tumor microenvironment.[14,15] *Soil, terrain,* and *microenvironment* are all words for the same concept.

So how do we monitor that terrain? And what do we do when we discover some new disturbance in it? Let's first define and explore six Core Lab Tests. Then we'll return to five of the Terrain Components that are especially relevant during mistletoe therapy. We'll connect the tests to the terrain and look at possible treatment adjustments and considerations in response to test results.

The following is not a comprehensive list of all the lab tests I use in my practice. Every cancer patient has profoundly diverse underlying conditions, which call for highly personalized testing, inquiry, and observation. For now, we'll look closely at the Core Lab Tests that I use with all my patients, regardless of condition. If you wish to take a deeper dive into nuanced cancer-related lab tests, interpretation of those tests, and what we consider truly healthy ranges, please review appendix F and the resources section.

Core labs: Tests that reveal the terrain

When patients begin their integrative care journey with me, some are surprised at how deeply I monitor their inner terrain through initial and ongoing lab tests and epigenetic testing. Some don't want that much testing—they're worried about what they might discover! For those who are hesitant, I emphasize this reality: *The more we test, the clearer the picture we obtain of your current challenges. The more we know, the more we can effectively personalize a path back toward health.* Testing empowers you. It's crucial to recognize that every test result—even discovering that you have a genetic or epigenetic challenge—can provide you only more empowering information. Becoming aware of an issue gives you options and shows you what your body needs to live at its best. Test results are not static or set in stone. Our health, even epigenetic expression, is dynamic and in a constant state of flow. The more you know, the more you can influence the direction of that flow.

You'll find you're probably already familiar with these Core Lab Tests, but we'll look at them with a more scrutinizing systems-thinking eye. With all six of the following test categories, it's crucial that you get baseline readings—*run these tests at the outset, before you begin any integrative therapy.* Rerun them monthly (or every two weeks in complex situations) for the duration of treatment and, as your terrain improves after treatment, continue running them quarterly for another two years. Then monitor them yearly thereafter.

1. CBC *with differential*

This is the blood test that everyone gets at an annual physical: The Complete Blood Count (CBC). Like it sounds, it lists and tallies the components of the blood. This includes the quantity of different cells (both blood cells and specific immune cells), number of platelets, and hemoglobin level. Integrative oncologists run this test too, but we home in on ratios and numbers that aren't so commonly discussed. If you want to learn even more about the ratios and all the health implications you can glean from a simple CBC, visit the Oncology Nutrition Institute (www.OncologyNutritionInstitute. com, see "Resources"). Their website offers a 90-minute web-based class solely on interpreting the CBC. For our purposes now, with our focus on mistletoe therapy, let's examine something called the Neutrophil-to-Lymphocyte Ratio (NLR) and then take a close look at eosinophil numbers.

The neutrophil-to-lymphocyte ratio (NLR)

Considering how well-researched NLR is in relation to cancer and all-cause mortality, it's amazing it isn't a standard listed ratio on the CBC. Thankfully, the math is easy. Simply look for the *absolute neutrophil count* (not the percentages) and divide it by the *absolute lymphocyte count* (again, not percentages). The resulting number should be close to 2, preferably a ratio of 2:1 to 1:1. That means an average of two neutrophils to one lymphocyte, or as low as one neutrophil to one lymphocyte. That's a slim range. It's a narrow therapeutic ratio, and if you're outside either end of it, you might have a problem developing.

This is one of the most prognostic immune tests we have for everyone, not just patients who have cancer. There are over two hundred studies looking at how NLR relates to modern diseases.[16–19] If you have too many neutrophils and too few lymphocytes, this is associated with higher all-cause mortality, meaning the risk of death from *any condition* goes up.[20] If the ratio flips, and you have fewer neutrophils and too many lymphocytes, blood cancers (leukemia, lymphoma, myelodysplastic syndromes) begin to manifest.[21] Cancer survivors who have a poor NLR have a higher recurrence and progression rate, while survivors who have an optimal NLR tend to experience robust maintenance of remission.[22–24] This simple ratio, which you can pull straight from your most recent CBC, is that significant.

NLR can be affected by cancer treatment, so it's important to monitor it frequently—twice a month or even weekly in highly complex situations. Patients are often treated for a primary cancer and, if treatment is especially aggressive, it can stress the immune system to the point of reversing their NLR. They have more lymphocytes than neutrophils. This leaves them vulnerable to blood dyscrasias, myelodysplastic conditions, idiopathic thrombocytopenia (ITP), lymphomas, and leukemias.[25] Any of those conditions can stem from that imbalanced NLR. We often see high incidents of secondary cancers, especially in women with breast cancer who may have had their cancer overtreated.[26,27] A reversed NLR is likely at play in these situations.

We can anticipate this issue. We can see who's vulnerable to imbalanced NLR by watching those numbers more closely. There are immunomodulatory remedies that can help the body bring the NLR back into balance. Not surprisingly, mistletoe is one of them. VAE therapy has a direct impact on NLR, balancing out both ends of the spectrum. It has a modulatory effect on immune cell generation, increasing or decreasing neutrophil or leukocyte numbers until that appropriate balance is reached.[28]

Eosinophils

Watching the eosinophil count is an effective way to determine if a patient is responding to mistletoe. Of course, to do that, you must run the CBC *prior* to starting mistletoe, to get a baseline reading. There's a narrow therapeutic window for this cell count. Ideally, eosinophil count should be at 2 or fewer.

Elevated baseline eosinophils – If eosinophils are elevated before starting mistletoe therapy, it's a clue that some TH-2 immune process is occurring, something allergy-related. The patient is eating or breathing something that's causing an allergic response. This is why we ask allergy-related questions on the Anamnestic Form (see appendix C). If there is an identified allergy, it's not necessarily a contraindication for mistletoe therapy. But it does mean I'll order an IL-8 cytokine test before the patient starts VAE therapy.[29] If eosinophils are elevated, but IL-8 is normal, I'm not concerned about VAE therapy. However, I do monitor patient response very closely and use greater caution with doses and timing. If both eosinophils and IL-8 are high, we wait on VAE therapy and do some detective work to determine what's causing the IL-8 spike. Ideally, we remove that obstacle (possibly an allergen the patient is exposed to constantly). Then we'll proceed with caution and a "low and slow" VAE schedule. Elevated IL-8 is associated with compromised response to conventional treatment, so determining and addressing its cause is a high priority.[30]

Elevated eosinophils after starting **VAE** – If eosinophils spike slightly after starting mistletoe therapy (if the number blips from 2, up

to 3 or 4) that's fine. That's expected and within a safe zone. If eosinophils weren't high to begin with, then we know that this is simply the
mistletoe creating a desired effect.[31] But if the number spikes to 5 or
more, we need to stop the VAE therapy and conduct some more detective work. We'll look at IL-8 levels, to determine whether this cytokine
spike was triggered by mistletoe. Or we look for other possible underlying medical conditions that might involve IL-8. Even so, this won't be
a complete contraindication for VAE therapy. But it does mean letting
the body come back into balance as far as IL-8 and eosinophils, then
returning to VAE with a very gentle titrating approach. As always, the
patient's body and lab metrics should guide the rate of increase and
maintenance dosage.

It's rare to see mistletoe cause an overzealous spike in eosinophils
or IL-8. But it can happen, and you can catch it with simple, affordable
tests. Catching it is paramount for patients to have good outcomes. In
20 years, I've had only two patients who couldn't go back on mistletoe
therapy after persistent eosinophil and IL-8 spikes. With them we provided *Helleborus niger* instead (see chapter 8). This is a powerful alternative to have in your toolbox, particularly for patients with hyper-
allergic patterns. In some cases, changing the mistletoe host tree, dose,
or brand can also alleviate a specific eosinophilic reaction.

Platelets and the M.D. Anderson Prognostic Scoring System: Mistletoe therapy and autoimmunity

When reviewing the baseline CBC, platelet count is another important marker to consider before any immunotherapy, including VAE.
Similar to the NLR noted above, we may also need to consider PLR
(*platelet*-to-lymphocyte ratio). When we see elevated platelets and
lower lymphocytes, outcomes and prognoses are poor.[32] Elevated
platelets alone are prognostic for many cancer types and indicate
thick and sticky blood patterns. The latter leads to higher incidence of thrombosis, which is one of the common causes of fatal-
ity secondary to a cancer diagnosis.[33] The M.D. Anderson (MDA)
Prognostic Scoring System (see appendix D) notes that "elevated

platelet count" is a possible contraindication for immunotherapy or is at least associated with poorer immunotherapy outcomes. In short, patients with elevated platelets (more than 400, according to standard of care [SOC] and over 250 by my terrain assessment) and three or more positive findings on the MDA score, should be cautious and thoughtful in implementing any immune therapies including mistletoe.[34]

2. Comprehensive metabolic panel (CMP)

The CMP provides a total picture of how the whole terrain is lining up in this moment, how the body is metabolizing fuel and eliminating waste products. This test provides measurements of blood sugar, electrolyte balance (sodium, potassium, chloride), calcium levels, acid-base balance, and organ function (liver, kidneys). Specifically, it shows levels of liver enzymes and waste products that are normally produced or removed by the liver and kidneys. This gives us a clear picture of how efficiently your body is able to clean up the typical waste products of metabolism. It also hints at whether you're staying hydrated well enough.

Over time, when taking a terrain-centric approach and incorporating VAE as part of the treatment, we would expect improvement in these testing parameters. Namely, we see improvement in organ function if the tumor burden is resolving in those areas, improved metabolic function if VAE is impacting the blood sugar and insulin response process, and more balanced inflammation cycles, as shown by improvement in various markers throughout the CMP and a trio of tests that we call the Trifecta Labs.

The "Trifecta Labs"

I can't take credit for naming this trio of labs; a few of my patients coined the phrase "Trifecta Labs" several years ago. I've continued insisting that every patient monitor these three metrics at least monthly, and the Trifecta moniker has stuck! The tests are not obscure. They're well-known measurements: Quantitative CRP, LDH, and ESR. But the way I evaluate them may be new to you.

3. Quantitative CRP

C-Reactive Protein is a well-known inflammatory marker, and it's a common add-on test when running the CMP. It picks up on chronic systemic inflammation. CRP, much like NLR, is considered prognostic regarding how a patient will respond to conventional cancer treatment. If CRP is elevated, the patient is more likely to experience multiple drug resistance,[35,36] more likely to have intensified side effects of the treatment[37] (which means they may have to stop or alter treatment timing), and they'll have a poor prognosis for survival.[38] CRP is that important. Knowing a patient's CRP level, and addressing underlying inflammation head-on through diet and lifestyle, can change the outcome of SOC treatment. It's surprising that CRP is not a standard required test prior to starting conventional treatment.[39]

4. LDH

Lactate dehydrogenase (LDH) is another add-on test that is commonly regarded as a marker of tissue damage. LDH has even more value for evaluating tumor microenvironment and whether the overall body terrain is hospitable to cancer. For leukemia and lymphoma, LDH is its own tumor marker.[40] But even for all the other solid tumors, LDH is a marker of *cellular turnover;* it can roughly tell us the rate of cell division. The higher your LDH, the more rapid your rate of cell turnover.[41,42]

LDH also tells us whether the cancer cells have shifted toward something called the *Warburg Effect.* In a healthy cell, normal metabolism—the process of using oxygen to burn glucose for energy—produces a small amount of LDH as a byproduct. But cancer cells have a method for producing energy even if they're short on oxygen. This *anaerobic metabolism* is inefficient and produces far more LDH as a byproduct (image 05.01). All that excess lactate contributes to more acidification in the tumor's microenvironment and drives out oxygen even more. This begins a vicious cycle of anaerobic metabolism.[43,44] That's the Warburg Effect, and that's why we're able to look at this one blood test and see a clue about the body's entire terrain.

Lactate Dehydrogenase (LDH)

NORMAL CELL

Glucose

Glycolysis

LDH

Pyruvate ⇌ Lactate

O_2 → Mitochondria (Krebs cycle)

→ CO_2

Oxidative phosphorylation-high ATP: glucose ratio, low LDH activity in both directions results in high energy production.

CANCER CELL

Glucose

Glycolysis

LDH

Pyruvate ⇌ Lactate

O_2 → Mitochondria (Krebs cycle)

→ CO_2

Metabolically impaired glycolysis (Warburg effect) - low ATP: glucose ratio, high LDH activity in one direction. Results in biomass incorporation and cell proliferation.

Lactate

Biomass Incorporation

Cell Proliferation

Elevated LDH can indicate that the body's terrain has become cancer friendly. It tells us about the overall metabolism. Is the metabolism primarily oxygen-rich (aerobic) and therefore hostile to cancer? Or is it mostly anaerobic and therefore friendly to cancer growth, metastasis, or recurrence? Elevated LDH can also indicate that there may be damage to the heart, lungs, kidneys, or liver. If an LDH test is elevated, I immediately order the *LDH Isoenzymes* test. This can tell us precisely which organ or tissue is damaged. Sometimes, even if LDH is normal, I will check on the isoenzymes, just to elucidate other mystery symptoms in the body. LDH Isoenzymes can show which bodily tissues are aggravated or irritated. Now, if the LDH level is abnormally low, especially if the other two Trifecta Labs are elevated, this is also a reason to test the isoenzymes. Sometimes, in a state of metabolic wasting, the LDH levels may not be able to track at normal or elevated levels, but the isoenzymes still offer clues.

5. ESR

Erythrocyte Sedimentation Rate (ESR) is also commonly added onto the CBC when a practitioner is looking for signs of inflammation. ESR refers to how quickly the erythrocytes fall out of solution, how quickly they settle out of the blood. This indicates how freely flowing or how "sticky" the blood is. Sticky blood is one of many indicators of systemic inflammation. If sedimentation takes a long time, if that number is elevated above 10, it means there is a thick, sticky blood matrix. This can indicate a toxic, sludgy, less fluid blood flow. Elevated ESR can also hint at an autoimmune process. That's because autoimmune reactions make the blood agglutinate.

As you can see, each of these Trifecta Labs is powerful on its own. There are hundreds of studies looking at each of these metrics on their own in relation to cancer. But taken together, the three tests give me an even more complete picture of the patient's inflammatory status and level of oxidative damage.

CRP by itself can tell us a lot. LDH can tell us a lot. Sedimentation rate can tell us a lot. But if all three are high, I know with certainty that *cancer is in the driver's seat.* We need to take focused and directed action immediately. If all three are within my functional ranges, then I feel confident that *the patient is in the driver's seat.* In my experience, the Trifecta Labs have consistently been more prognostic than scan results and tumor markers. I am *far more* concerned about patients who have clear scans and normal cancer markers, but all three of their Trifecta Labs are elevated. I am *far less* concerned about the patient whose scans still show tumors present, and their tumor markers are still elevated, but their Trifecta Labs are perfect. In that moment, their body is actually managing the cancer. The patient is in the driver's seat; the cancer is not.

VAE can definitely impact the dance and expression of the Trifecta Labs. If these labs are not stabilizing and trending downward, we may want to take a closer look at how the patient is responding to VAE therapy (and any other therapies). I'll ask deeper questions about their cytokine reactions and quality of life (QOL) symptoms. Despite all our best efforts, stubborn, elevated Trifecta Labs might just indicate that our goals of restoring cellular communication and overcoming the massive oxidative stress are simply out of reach. If those lab findings also coincide with loss of QOL and ability to function normally, it may be time to discuss palliative and end of life care (see chapter 11). This does not mean we have given up! It simply means we need to be realistic and continue supporting the wishes of the patient, while we determine if there are other options available to us. I find, in these moments, that more oxidative and cytotoxic therapies actually hasten death. Too often, that's all that is offered. In contrast, those who take a much-needed break from aggressive SOC or integrative care can sometimes right the ship, allowing us to reevaluate and move forward in treatment again.

Sometimes a patient will tell me that their conventional practitioner said that CRP, LDH, and ESR are normally elevated during treatment. That may be common, but it isn't healthy. My patients who proactively work on these inflammatory markers through diet, lifestyle changes, and other natural therapies are able to maintain healthy Trifecta Labs even during conventional treatment. They're able to do that because they're keeping their terrain as healthy as possible. As a result, they wind up responding better to treatment, too.

I've seen patients celebrate that they're done with chemotherapy and radiation, and their scans look good. But their Trifecta Labs are clearly off. Too often there is a recurrence or progression of cancer within months of these findings. This effect is an increasing subject of study. We know that if a cancer survivor has a high CRP, the cancer is more likely to have a fatal recurrence.[46] Conversely, I have many patients who still have a tumor present, but they're *managing it well*. The relationship between systemic inflammation, anaerobic metabolism, and cancer is that tightly interwoven.

All that said, I must clarify that every lab result needs to be regarded within the greater context of the patient's lifestyle and general condition. For instance, if the Trifecta Labs have been consistently good, and suddenly only the CRP is high, that might be purely because the patient had a recent injury. If only the ESR is high, it could be due to a mild autoimmune reaction, perhaps a recent exposure to gluten. Or maybe LDH is high because the patient just completed a major workout or took a long hike. It's possible for transient events to throw off a person's chemistry. Lab results are clues that must be examined within their greater context.

We never treat a lab; we never treat a target. We support the entire person and treat the entire terrain. Any time we get myopic about one lab looking a little off, it's wise to take a step back and look at that bigger picture. How's this one lab result playing against the entire terrain?

6. D3 levels (25-OH and 1,25-OH)

Vitamin D3 is a powerful nutrient that interacts with almost every terrain component: immune function, mental health, metabolism, inflammation, and circadian rhythm. Vitamin D is so well-researched, so well-known for its diverse health effects that it has its own institute in the NIH: The Vitamin D Council. It's stunning that we know so much about it, even in conventional medicine, and yet tend to downplay it and rarely monitor D levels with any regularity.

The first vitamin D revelation that I share with my patients is the fact that your D levels are NOT fine at 30—that's the cutoff for low-normal, per conventional medicine. Those levels may be normal for the general population, but the general population is not healthy. *I want to see levels above 50 in healthy individuals and 80 to 100 in those who are actively cancering*—as long as their serum calcium levels stay within range (9.5 or lower).[46] The next vitamin D revelation is regarding how to address deficiency. When D levels are low, the best, most effective source is sun exposure (get outside!). The next best source is food. My last resort is supplementation. When supplementing vitamin D, it's crucial to monitor serum calcium levels (through the CMP), and always provide K2 along with D to ensure appropriate balance and absorption.[47,48]

D levels are highly influential on both conventional and integrative treatment success. That includes mistletoe therapy. In my practice, I've noticed that patients with low D3 levels do not have as strong a response on mistletoe as those with normal or optimal levels. Both in practice and in published studies, I've also noticed that patients who are vegan or vegetarian, those who are morbidly obese, and those who take antacids, steroids, or cholesterol lowering medications are all chronically low in D3.[49-52] Given that up to 70 percent of the population is D-depleted (based on true healthy levels, not unhealthy "norms"),[53,54] this is a conversation we need to have before starting VAE therapy or any other treatment. Address vitamin D deficiencies and insufficiencies first! Of course, vitamin D can act like a hormone, so once balanced levels are achieved, switch to maintenance dosing based on test results.

Terrain-labs integration:
Looking at labs from multiple terrain perspectives

As mentioned earlier, I constantly evaluate my patients through the lens of multiple terrain-based body systems. While we don't have room here to evaluate all ten of those terrain components, let's look at how mistletoe particularly interacts with five of them. We'll notice how terrain-based testing can evaluate the patient's baseline and monitor the shifts we want to see through the course of treatment.

Stress and biorhythms

In the integrative oncology world, when we think of mistletoe therapy, we often think of its effects on the immune system, its direct effects on the tumor, and perhaps the secondary effects on mental and emotional health. But I first learned about VAE therapy through an anthroposophic lecture on how mistletoe's primary effect was to *restore rhythm* in the body. In the anthroposophic medicine (AM) world, cancer is regarded first as a *loss of rhythm,* both within the body and between the body and its surrounding environment. That concept challenged me and stuck with me. Rudolf Steiner, the co-founder of AM, once said, "One can ascend to a higher development only by bringing rhythm and repetition into one's life. Rhythm holds sway in all nature." This is a beautiful holistic theory, and it has scientific support. We know now, through multiple studies, that night shift workers with dysregulated circadian rhythm, experience higher incidence of metabolic diseases and cancer.[55-59] In 2017, the Nobel Prize in Physiology/Medicine went to researchers studying circadian rhythm biology and its implications in human health.[60] In recent years, we have also learned that every individual cell maintains a particular rhythm,[61,62] and that the microbiome and our response to *any* therapy is circadian rhythm dependent![63,64] *Rhythm holds sway.*

When evaluating a patient's relationship with natural rhythms and how they process stress, I begin with plenty of biographical inquiry and lifestyle questions. Observational data and a comprehensive patient history are given equal weight with lab work and other quantitative testing. I want to know the patient's career history and relational patterns, along with bedtime routines and average amount of sleep, bowel and appetite patterns, average time spent outdoors, experience of seasonal weather, and typical stress levels and how they process it. I hope to see cycles, *healthy rhythmic patterns*. But if someone is coming to me because of an active cancering process, more often I see areas of zero rhythm: night shift work, chronic sleep deprivation, constant insatiable hunger, artificial light exposure from dawn to bedtime, no time spent outdoors, constant stress, no periods of rest or release.

Once I have a detailed picture of the lifestyle vulnerabilities and the changes that could rebuild natural rhythms for the patient, I begin choosing the lab tests that would shine even more light on their situation. As always, every patient completes a CMP. To me, the metabolic panel reveals both metabolic function and the *inherent rhythms* of those metabolic organs. Metabolic systems are rhythmic systems, constantly rotating through the tasks of producing energy and cleaning up waste byproducts. The CMP can show me where that rhythm has stalled.

I also look at a patient's D3 level for clues about their natural rhythms. Of course, D levels hint at whether they're spending enough time outside without sunscreen. Vitamin D also impacts hundreds of epigenetic factors involved in metabolic function, hormone regulation, and immune response. It influences the very rhythm of our biology and can affect personal biography, too, as low D levels are associated with depression. Specifically, vitamin D appears to be involved in serotonin and dopamine pathways. If a patient's D levels are low, it is a reason for me to ask about all these other QOL and rhythm-oriented factors.[65,66]

After looking at the CMP and D3 levels, we look at a couple of specialty labs directly related to circadian rhythm: The Adrenal Stress Index (ASI) and melatonin levels. The ASI looks at cortisol output at multiple points during a 24-hour period. Cortisol output is not static; it has a rhythm. Many patients today show fairly healthy output during the day, but very low cortisol in the morning and then an uptick in the late evening. That's the opposite of how a cortisol graph should look. Cortisol should be secreted about an hour before we wake up, creating a spike that raises body temperature and blood sugar, making us want to jump out of bed ready for the day. Instead, in chronically stressed patients, cortisol levels are sluggish in the morning and may get even lower during the day. Then at night, the body overcompensates, trying to increase cortisol in preparation for the next morning. All night long the cortisol level is slightly elevated, and the patient never gets deep restful sleep.[67,68] This can be measured with an ASI test. Similarly, we can measure melatonin levels and will often see a complementary dysregulation. Where cortisol is chronically elevated at night, melatonin is often chronically too low.

Healthy sleep–wake rhythms are crucial to healing in any disease state, but especially during cancer treatment. Addressing these issues early in the treatment cycle will affect the efficacy of all other treatments.[69] Thankfully, treating disrupted sleep-wake cycles begins with simple lifestyle choices—from daytime sunlight exposure and melatonin supplementation to removing all electronic devices from the bedroom. We'll discuss some of these integrative treatments and lifestyle choices in chapter 9.

For now, let it suffice to say that all integrative therapies work better when the patient cultivates healthy natural rhythms in daily life. Mistletoe therapy has a unique circular relationship with body rhythms. Its effects are stronger when the patient intentionally reestablishes a healthy circadian rhythm, and mistletoe itself helps enhance biological rhythms. It both fosters rhythmic balance and is enhanced by strengthening circadian rhythm.

Immune function

Similar to evaluating a patient's rhythmic patterns, evaluating immune system function begins with thorough inquiry into the patient's history. I want to know if they get sick often, if they experience fevers frequently, or if they *never* get fevers. All extremes are of interest to me. I'm certainly interested if I hear that someone gets sick all the time. But more often than not, patients come to me saying, "I'm the one who never got sick. Until I got cancer!" This pattern of never getting sick is a red flag in the opposite direction. Healthy immune function involves getting sick occasionally: burning through an infection, experiencing and then resolving a good healthy fever.

Once I've got that broad immune history down, I look at quantitative labs. D3 levels show up here. Vitamin D's association with immune function is well established. Remember, I want to see levels of 80 to 100 for someone who is actively cancering. I also look at the patient's CBC, noting their NLR and combing through all their white blood cell counts. I look for levels that are out of range for an optimally healthy person (not just levels based on population norms). Again, look at appendix F to get those true healthy ranges. There are immune function clues here that you might not see if you were evaluating the CBC using the conventional normal ranges.

Beyond D3 and general CBC white blood cell counts, it's possible to request additional tests to determine specific counts for NK cells (CD56+ cells) and activated T cells (both helper and killer cells). There's a single test by Labcorp (see Resources) that can provide both of those. It's good to acquire the baseline and then monitor these levels during VAE therapy. Labcorp provides reference ranges, but I also keep in mind that VAE therapy affects these cell counts. I expect all of them to be "mid- to high-end normal" during treatment. If they're low, it's a flag that there's a serious underlying health condition that needs to be addressed.

I also evaluate zinc levels, because of that nutrient's key role in supporting immune function. It's important to request a Red Blood Cell (RBC) zinc test, instead of a standard serum zinc level. Serum zinc can occasionally look healthy simply because you hit it at a good moment. RBC zinc essentially provides a three-month average of the mineral status. That's much more accurate. (In fact, any time I measure any mineral status, I ask for the RBC version.) In general, when zinc levels are low, macrophage and NK cell function are compromised.[70] Clinically, I've noticed that if zinc levels are poor, the response to VAE therapy may not be as robust. This is likely due to effects on immune cell quantities and function. Ideally, zinc insufficiency would be corrected before starting immune-modulating therapies.

Inflammation

Chronic systemic inflammation is the driver of cancer metastasis, and it fuels many other metabolic diseases too. This terrain layer is intertwined with blood sugar balance, dysregulated biorhythms, and associated chronic stress. As mentioned earlier, inflammation cycles get "stuck" and refuse to resolve when the terrain is overwhelmed by dietary and lifestyle factors. When it comes to monitoring and determining multiple root causes of chronic inflammation, the Trifecta Labs are key. Those three labs are how we assess whether a patient is maintaining homeostasis in those inflammatory pathways, or whether the inflammatory fires have gotten out of control.

Outside of the Trifecta, other labs that give insight into inflammation include: *fibrinogen activity, uric acid* and, believe it or not, *ferritin*. Fibrinogen activity levels are well known as an indicator of thick sticky blood patterns causing hypercoagulation and chronic systemic inflammation. If CRP is high, fibrinogen activity is likely high, too. It's another test that can shine light on the whole inflammatory picture. Meanwhile, uric acid can show us issues with methylation, poor immune function, oxidative stress from inflammatory processes, acidosis, and mineral imbalances.[71] It can also be an indication that we should ask if the patient is getting enough hydration and enough dietary magnesium, or explore whether they're consuming too many dietary oxalates. Ferritin levels are also informative. There are many types of anemia, and only one is true iron deficient anemia. Practitioners are too often seduced into prescribing iron when they note low RBC, hemoglobin, or hematocrit levels. For patients who have cancer, this can wind up feeding the inflammatory metastatic fire.[72,73] You must make sure ferritin levels are within their sweet zone (see appendix F). If true iron deficiency anemia is diagnosed, consider rebuilding the blood through naturopathic dietary and herbal approaches, instead of iron supplementation.

Mistletoe therapy has a unique relationship to this terrain factor. As mentioned in chapter 2, it is distinctly immunomodulatory in its interaction with inflammatory states. It initially prompts an acute, and highly beneficial, inflammatory response. That acute inflammation and transient cytokine release is helpful for activating the immune system. This "good inflammation" will spike, then resolve in a healthy wave. Meanwhile, other components in VAE can decrease many markers of unhealthy chronic inflammation including: IL-6, CRP, COX-2, NFkB, and VEGF.[74,75]

Mental and emotional health

Similar to evaluating a person's circadian health, evaluating mental and emotional health requires extensive lifestyle and biographical inquiry. Unfortunately, if I began every new patient intake with this terrain focus, I'm pretty sure all my patients would run away! We all have a strong preference for discussing the tangibles. *Let me change my diet, let me take this supplement, I'll even learn Tai Chi, but if you ask me about my childhood, I'm out of here!* And yet this terrain factor is critically important, especially when treating cancer. When I have totally compliant patients who are doing everything right with their diet and lifestyle and treatments, and they're still seeing no treatment response, I know with certainty that this terrain factor is the primary obstacle. This is real. We know now that mental and emotional challenges can affect immune cell counts and activity.[76–80]

If I hit blocks during verbal inquiry, I will often order a few quantitative tests and use that hard data to introduce the topic more obliquely. Yes, there are quantitative tests that can shed light on a patient's mental and emotional health. On a very basic level, blood sugar has a significant impact on emotional wellbeing. Anxiety, depression, and bipolar conditions are very sensitive to the ups and downs of blood sugar.[81,82] Vitamin D3 shows up as an influencer for this terrain factor, as well, with compromised levels manifesting as depression or seasonal affective disorder (SAD).[83] Sometimes these simple lab tests can be conversation starters. I might say, "You know, these ranges are associated with pretty extreme energy swings," or "a level this low typically triggers noticeable depression." Then I can simply ask how that issue has manifested for them. This opens the conversation a little more gently than hitting it head-on during our first encounter.

If I have a patient's epigenetic profile, I can also look for certain genetic SNPs (single-nucleotide polymorphisms) associated with mental health challenges. This includes: MAO, BDNF, COMT, VDR and/or CYP2R1, ADRB2, and MTHFR. Some of these are associated with serious anxiety or rage. Others are associated with personalities that can easily get stuck in life.[84–87] Such conditions respond exceptionally well to low-dose psychotropics, intermittent fasting, meditation, and prayer. When I approach the patient with both a test result and a solution based in solid brain science, it suddenly lets them get curious about mental and emotional health from the entry points of epigenetics and brain health.

Similar to the relationship between VAE therapy and rhythm restoration, there is a circular relationship between VAE and mental health. If a patient has a major challenge in this terrain factor, it can result in lackluster treatment effects across the board. But as soon as the patient takes a small step toward addressing mental and emotional self-care, all other treatments can begin to take root, including mistletoe. Continuing a positive cycle, VAE therapy can further enhance mental health through its ability to enhance beta-endorphin levels.[88] This lesser-known effect of mistletoe may be the reason for a frequently reported side benefit: an enhanced sense of purpose and spiritual clarity.

Metabolic function and blood sugar balance

Choosing and embracing a diet that supports metabolic flexibility is a major key to cancer treatment success. We'll look at a few cancer-fighting dietary choices in chapter 9, but for now it's important to know that the body achieves metabolic flexibility when it no longer needs a steady flow of sugar to feel sane. In short, that means a low- or no-carb diet and eating at strategic times. This approach nourishes healthy cells while causing severe stress for cancer cells—making them more vulnerable to both conventional and integrative treatments.[89]

That said, testing begins with simple inquiry about a patient's dietary habits, then we progress to keeping a dietary journal or using a health and diet and macronutrient monitoring app like Cronometer or MyFitnessPal. These apps provide immediate feedback and help patients discover, on their own, how much sugar they're actually consuming each day.

In terms of quantitative testing, we need to go beyond the patient's fasting blood glucose level. It's possible to simply hit that test on a good day. The HbA1C is much more accurate, as it provides a three-month average. Even then, a patient may be maintaining good blood sugar levels, but cranking out abnormal amounts of insulin to do so. Thus, it's important to check fasting insulin levels, too. It is possible to see a normal fasting blood glucose and a normal HbA1C, along with insulin in the teens, twenties, or higher. That insulin is a driver of cell growth, including cancer cells. It attaches as a ligand to IGF receptors and stimulates cellular replication.[90] If you see high insulin levels, it's wise to test IGF-1 as well.

In addition to blood sugar-oriented testing, the standard CMP and the Trifecta Labs are also key for evaluating metabolic function. The CMP gives me a picture of all those activities associated with metabolism and detoxing the byproducts of normal metabolism. The Trifecta Labs show me what kind of fuel the body is burning in its mitochondrial factories. It shows me whether the metabolic fires are burning cleanly or inefficiently.

Ultimately, metabolic challenges and blood sugar issues can render certain conventional treatments ineffective. This includes radiation, chemotherapy, PARP inhibitors, and other aromatase inhibitors. People who are metabolically flexible (consistently eating lower-carb) see more robust response from all their treatments, both conventional and integrative.[91] Lab tests focused on metabolism and blood sugar can be the motivation that helps patients embrace a cancer-fighting diet.

In my own practice, I've witnessed the power of establishing a foundation of metabolic flexibility and then combining that with VAE therapy. Lower carb intake creates great stress for cancer cells. That leaves the cancer more vulnerable to all treatments, including integrative therapies like mistletoe. In yet another circular relationship, we've also seen mistletoe help mitigate blood sugar and insulin production challenges in animal studies.[92,93] We're still learning which constituents in mistletoe might be responsible for these effects, but it's yet another possible side benefit of VAE therapy.

Final Thoughts on Specialty Tests and Tumor Markers

There are literally hundreds of other lab tests that we can conduct for any patient. We list some of the more common ones in appendix F, and recommended laboratories are noted in the Resources Section. Physicians who want to explore more nuanced testing and learn how to respond effectively to lab findings, especially related to epigenetics, tumor markers, and cytotoxicity screening, should consider further education through the Physicians' Association for Anthroposophic Medicine (PAAM) or the *Metabolic Approach to Cancer, Mastermind Course* through DrNasha, Inc. (see Resources). Ultimately, it's the patient's condition and goals that guide the breadth and depth of testing strategies. When exploring more refined testing options, three good rules of thumb come to mind:

- Not every lab result is cause for concern. It's the practitioner's responsibility to shine light on whether a certain lab finding necessitates treatment action.
- Don't treat an epigenetic SNP unless it's expressing. For example, if a patient has a SNP indicating that they could run chronically low on a certain nutrient, always run an evaluation for that nutrient to confirm they are indeed deficient.
- Tumor markers are useful metrics. But they're not the be-all, end-all evaluation of the cancering process. The Trifecta Labs are often more prognostic than elevated tumor markers. Review all metrics within their larger context.

Ultimately, labs are incredibly impactful when they become tools to motivate empowering change, especially changes related to diet and lifestyle. Discussing significant lab results can be a positive tipping point moment in a patient's journey. It can be a gateway to much deeper personal discoveries. Always remember, we're not here to treat cancer. We're here to support the person and nurture their entire terrain.

PART 3:

HUMAN-CENTERED MEDICINE

"Still, as ambitious cancer researchers study soil as well as seed, one sees the beginnings of a new approach. It would return us to the true meaning of 'holistic': to take the body, the organism, its anatomy, its physiology—this infuriatingly intricate web—as a whole. Such an approach would help us understand the phenomenon in all its vexing diversity; it would help us understand when you have cancer and when cancer has you. It would encourage doctors to ask not just what you have but what you are."

—SIDDHARTHA MUKKHERJEE
("Cancer's Invasion Equation,"
The New Yorker, Sept. 11, 2017)

CHAPTER 6

THE PHYSIOLOGY OF WARMTH

Dr. Adam Blanning, MD

"We must succeed in enveloping the tumor with a mantle of warmth...we must be sure that in every case a preparation of viscum (mistletoe), applied in the way we advise...will generate a mantle of warmth." —RUDOLF STEINER

Steiner's words offer a key insight as to why mistletoe prepara- tions provide unique support in cancer therapy.[1] You do not hear many people talking about being given a prescription for a "mantle of warmth" by their doctor! It sounds unusual, maybe even a little senti- mental, like someone sending you warm greetings or a warm hug—but that would be only a superficial understanding of Rudolf Steiner's indi- cation about mistletoe therapy. It's really an invitation to learn more about what anthroposophy calls our whole *warmth organization*. This is an important bridge toward whole-person healing.

Warmth Organization: The different aspects of heat and warmth in the human being as an organized whole, including distribution of heat within the body, thermosensation and the feeling of physi- cal and emotional warmth.

Oncologic care in the U.S. typically makes distinctions between what are considered standard of care (SOC) medical treatments (like surgery, chemotherapy, and radiation) and then a separate group that includes all the other less-easily controlled or more individualized parts of care. When comparing the two aspects of treatment, objective, physical measures are usually given the greatest priority. Scans and biopsies are "king." This means that the parts of you which can be easily X-rayed, biopsied, or measured with a blood test get the most attention. Those aspects certainly offer important insights, but alone, they provide an incomplete picture. We are more than just the combined sum of our imaging results and tumor markers; more than a machine with broken parts. Healing needs to involve not only physical measures, but also functional, emotional, and spiritual factors. We will describe what that expanded picture can look like and how it contributes to a more holistic view of illness and healing.

To do that, let's go back to our clue in the Steiner quotation above. If warmth is an important part of healing a tumor, then we should look with fresh eyes to see how warmth can be observed and assessed.

When you go to a medical appointment, how do people measure your warmth? The obvious answer is with a thermometer, usually on the head. We can make that measurement very quickly to see if the temperature is normal or abnormal. But if we are experimenting with the idea that warmth can actually be a therapeutic "substance," then we should not only ask whether the temperature is normal, but more broadly, "Does this person have *enough* warmth?" We tend to think about a temperature being abnormal only if it is elevated, since a higher temperature can be a sign of infection or inflammation. But maybe we should also begin to think about the possibility of a *deficit of warmth*.

The definition of a "normal" temperature has been 98.6°F (37°C) for decades, but a surprising study shows us that our warmth is not, in fact, a static measure. That guideline for normal body temperature was set more than a century ago, and it is no longer true. That's because the average body temperature of people living in the United States has been steadily decreasing over the last 150 years. A research study titled "Decreasing human body temperature in the United States since the Industrial Revolution" looked at three very large collections of medical records, gathered from 1860 to 1940, 1971 to 1975, and 2007 to 2017. Through comparing those records, researchers determined that the average body temperature has decreased by about 0.05 degrees Fahrenheit (0.03 degrees Celsius) every ten years, since 1860.[2] The progressive decrease in body temperature has been true for both women and men (though women tend to have a slightly higher average temperature). The decrease is also consistent for both black patients and white patients (the only races observed in the Civil War study). Perhaps the most important finding is that today's average body temperature is now approximately 97.9 Fahrenheit (36.6 Celsius) according to a 2017 British study,[3] far lower than what has, until recently, been considered "normal."

As previously mentioned, most medical care focuses on those aspects of health that can be most easily measured and analyzed with statistics. So, some of the first reactions to this study went along the lines of: "Were their thermometers accurate 150 years ago?" and "Did they really keep good records?" Also, "Did they measure big enough groups of people to really be able to make such generalizations?" Those questions about reproducibility, accuracy, and statistical significance are good ones. We need to make sure that the basic facts are true so that we feel confident in the quality of measurements we use to make decisions.

The researchers who carried out this study looked hard at those factors, considered the accuracy of the type of thermometers used more than a century ago, and determined that the shift in average body temperature does, in fact, seem to be true and accurate. Our warmth has been steadily decreasing, and it is very important to think about that fact if *enhanced warmth* is something we should be using in cancer care.

Now, there is more to this story. The researchers took a second step, an important one. They asked at what time of day the temperatures were taken. Why focus on such a little detail? The answer is because our temperature will actually be different in the evening than it was in the morning, even when we are not sick. Warmth fluctuates throughout the day. Body warmth rises and falls so that our body temperature goes up an average of 1.08 degrees Fahrenheit (0.6 degrees Celsius) from early morning hours (when we are still asleep) to the mid-afternoon, when we are most alert and warmest.[4,5] That fluctuation means that the researchers did need to account for the time of day when a temperature was taken. Indeed, even accounting for that variation, the authors still found that our temperature has been decreasing over the last century. These combined studies show us that warmth is dynamic, shifting not only over the course of a day, but also over the course of multiple generations.

Once we recognize that warmth moves and changes, almost like the rise and fall of tides in the ocean, that can also prompt us to think about fever in a different way. Fever is typically categorized as a symptom of illness. But what if we think about the warmth of fever as potentially also being a healing substance? If that concept were true, then we would expect to find research demonstrating medical benefits from fever. That research is not hard to find. The American Academy of Pediatrics states in their guidelines on *Fever and Antipyretic Use in Children* that: "Many parents administer antipyretics [fever reducers] even when there is minimal or no fever, because they are concerned that the child must maintain a 'normal' temperature. Fever, however, is not the primary illness but is a physiologic mechanism that has beneficial effects in fighting infection."[6] The guidelines describe different ways that fever helps the immune system and maintain that, instead of routinely suppressing fever, allowing the body to produce an elevated temperature actually "retards the growth and reproduction of bacteria and viruses, enhances neutrophil production and T-lymphocyte proliferation... [and] helps the body recover more quickly from viral infections."[7] Suddenly we are gaining evidence that fever, as a warmth tool of the immune system, has direct therapeutic effects.

Anthroposophic practitioners have long worked with and supported the dynamics and effects of warmth when caring for illness. Multiple generations of doctors and patients have confirmed that we may not only passively allow a temperature to rise (as part of the body's immune response to an infection), but that we can also actively *work with* that desired warmth instead of solely fighting it. In the early stages of a fever, when someone looks pale, feels chilled, achy, and uncomfortable, the immune system will soon be working hard to make the whole body warm—from head to feet. If we recognize this pattern, we can aid the process by providing warm clothing and blankets, warm drinks, even putting a hot water bottle on the feet. We don't need to give fever-reducing medicines at this stage; we certainly don't put someone in an ice bath. *Rather we observe what the body is trying to do and actively support it.* Then, once a fever has really built up, and the body is completely warmed through, we can watch for the shift when the body decides it needs to release warmth and move it away from the head. That can be done with simple things like warm compresses of diluted lemon juice placed on the calves. This kind of treatment aids the release of warmth through evaporation, even though the calf compresses are administered underneath blankets.[8] Antipyretics can, of course, still be used when they are needed, but they become more the exception than the rule. Simple, natural tools and a dynamic view of warmth create a whole new field of therapeutic thought.

Does that natural supportive approach work, and is it worthwhile? The answer is yes. A large study of anthroposophic medical treatments for acute respiratory and ear infections (treatment for which also included the prescription of a variety of natural medicines) showed that, for patients receiving conventional medical treatment, about 26 percent were prescribed an antibiotic, whereas patients seeing an anthroposophic physician received an antibiotic prescription only about 5 percent of the time.[9] That is more than an 80 percent reduction in antibiotic use. Not only were fewer antibiotics used, but the patients also needed fewer analgesics (pain reducers) and antipyretics (fever reducers), and patients had a "somewhat quicker short-term resolution" of their symptoms—meaning they felt better slightly sooner than patients receiving conventional care.

Expanding our understanding of warmth organization by defining the "fourfold human being"

The studies we've just looked at show that we can, with practical steps, enlarge our concept of medical care. That kind of enlarged therapeutic toolbox doesn't hurt. It doesn't compromise medical decision-making. Far from it—it helps. But to include these factors we have to start thinking more flexibly, more dynamically. In conventional care, we often look at warmth as a value that should be kept within a fixed range. Instead, we could think about tides and transitions of warming and cooling. We need to move from relying solely on "facts" to also considering "flow."

That kind of thinking might feel revolutionary, but it has actually been part of medicine for thousands of years. The ancient Greeks spoke about medicine on four levels, the first two being "earth" and "water." While we tend to dismiss their observations as simplistic and naive, they taught about a kind of medical thinking that can consider both measurements and *dynamics*. We are less adept at that now. We need to strengthen our capacities for observing how our physiology moves and changes in time, and how working in harmony with those dynamics can enhance our regeneration and recovery.

Flow	When?	Dynamics of Change	Fluidity	Plant	Time/Recovery Forces
Facts	What?	Measurements	Anatomy	Mineral	Physical/Structural Forces

Table 6.1: Developing a more dynamic medical view—facts vs. flow

The study discussed at the end of the previous section did not achieve such a dramatic shift in antibiotic prescriptions simply because physicians allowed a fever to rise and fall. Doctors also used a number of natural medicines, understanding that many of the processes that happen in the human body also find a related kind of expression in the natural world. In terms of warmth, our body moves back and forth between building and holding warmth, then distributing and releasing warmth. The natural world, in contrast, shows examples where just one part of that process finds very strong expression. As an example, some plants love warmth. They grow most joyfully in warm climates where there is lots of sun and heat over a long growing season. These plants take in as much warmth as they can; they are wide open to it and actually do not thrive in colder climates because they are so wide open to the environment. We are familiar with many of these plants because of the fragrant oils they produce, often used as spices and natural remedies. This is a task these plants excel at: taking in the heat of sunshine and internalizing that energy within a dense oil. Biochemically, oils are calorie-dense; they help us create our own warmth when we need it. A good example of this kind of heat-loving plant is rosemary (*Rosmarinus officinalis*).

Yet, there are other plants that thrive in very different conditions, plants that grow and survive for many years in cold, wet, chilled conditions. Those plants have a different task. They cannot rely on outer sunshine for all the warmth that they need. They must somehow protect themselves from the outside and create an inner space that will not be overwhelmed by surrounding conditions. They must create and hold their own, inner, stable warmth. A good example of that kind of plant is peat moss (*Solum uliginosum*), which grows on the cold and rainy moors in Scotland. Peat moss works with warmth in a very different way from rosemary.

Each of these plants does, in fact, have a special relationship to warmth. They produce specific phytochemicals and develop unique botanical structures as part of their work to collect or maintain warmth. The sum total of these constituents and structures reveals a kind of signature, a unique gesture, displaying that plant's attitude and interaction with warmth. Let's look at some examples of how this kind of thinking can be applied therapeutically.

In the medical condition known as Raynaud's phenomenon, people get very cold extremities because their arteries tend to clamp down and spasm. Blood flow becomes limited. Raynaud's is particularly common in people who have scleroderma, a chronic connective tissue disease with an overall hardening of tissues in the body. But when an oil containing rosemary extract gets massaged over such a person's arm, circulation immediately improves. The clamped-down arteries relax, and you can see how warmth flows through the hands and fingers. You can actually see it occur when you take thermal images![10] So, when someone needs warmth to fill a part of the body that has become too hardened or too fixed—when they need a process of filling, opening warmth—rosemary can be helpful.

But what about when someone is having pain and inflammation, maybe pain that is strongly influenced by outside shifts like the change in barometric pressure that happens before a storm? There we need something different. We don't want to add more warmth if things are already painful and inflamed. Rosemary would be too much, too aggressive. In this case, we would instead make use of peat moss, *Solum*, which does, indeed, prove to be very helpful. Massage with *Solum* oil has been shown to reduce chronic pain.[11] *Solum* helps provide a sheathing, protecting kind of warmth.

Many medical traditions have been doing this for millennia— observing a gesture or archetype of a plant and then using it for an associated therapeutic benefit. In the conventional mindset, we often regard such thinking as imprecise and primitive. But time and again, modern science finds that such early scientific hypotheses were not far off. We learn that a heat-loving plant does indeed contain active components that produce a warmth response in the human organism.

These gestures, or archetypes of a particular kind of process, not only occur in the body, they also happen in our feelings, in our soul life. Sometimes we need a wave of warmth to fill us, loosen us, and relax and open up what has become stuck and hardened. Other times, we just need gentle sheltering; we don't want anything more from the outside. We need to be able to hold and protect what is our own. As part of whole-person cancer support, we can think about rosemary being helpful for tissue that has become scarred, feels wooden-like, or is numbed and cooled as a side effect from chemotherapy; we can think about *Solum* as being helpful for pain or difficulty in regulating one's own warmth after radiation.

Now, it's important to notice that we have just taken a step into a third realm, a realm of differentiated qualities and gestures. This third level is not something we easily X-ray or measure on a blood test. It is also not something we will understand just by watching how things change over time. To enter the realm of "qualities" we have to know something about a person's experience—how do you feel? We have to look for parallel expressions of process and understand how an activity in the human body finds its companion in the natural world. We might ask: Is something happening in the body that has a parallel in the patient's soul life? We begin to regularly observe how these differentiated processes show up on both a physiologic level (such as a blunted dynamic of circulation and warmth) and an emotional level (like a loss of trust or a stuck social dynamic that won't budge).

The ancient Greek physicians talked about this level as the element of "air." This makes a certain sense because we find this third aspect of combined physiologic and emotional expression in creatures that actively breath in and out. Let's make that very concrete: a stone has physical shape, density, size, color—measurable aspects, but no awareness, no breath. It does not have the third element of "air." A plant is a little more complex. Plants also have physical shape, density, color, and size, but they also grow and change in time. They sprout, flower, and reproduce, through cycles of life. Certainly, a plant has something more than a stone, but still not the same "wakefulness" as a creature that freely moves and quickly reacts. To find that level of awareness we must look to the animal world. Animals have all three: shape/size/color, growth/dynamics/change in time, and wakefulness/respiration/emotion. Human beings have these three levels too (plus one more, which we will consider next). Anthroposophic medicine (AM) recognizes that we can see the difference between these three levels by observing:

Measurable, physical qualities and structures: We can see this
    isolated level in a human (free from any of the other aspects)
    only in a corpse.
Growing, healing, regenerative capacities: These work quietly
    when we are in a deep sleep, without movement or awareness.

The wakeful processes of breath, emotion, and interaction: This
is the realm of many of our basic activities of day-to-day life.

Qualities	How?	Gestures & Archetypes	Awareness	Animal	A wakeful person
Flow	When?	Dynamics of Change	Fluidity	Plant	A sleeping person
Facts	What?	Measurements	Anatomy	Mineral	A corpse

Table 6.2: A third layer of dynamism—facts, flow, and qualities

To get to the fourth quality we have to really expand our mind
and our heart. We need to look at all parts of our humanity. How is a
human different from an animal? Animals sense, move, and react with
instinctive wisdom. They exemplify specialized skills: a hawk flies, a
dolphin swims, a badger digs, and a lion hunts. That is what they do,
and they excel at it. Humans have learned to do all those things too
but aided by developing techniques and tools. A human being is not
specialized for any of those tasks, yet can choose to participate in all
of them. People choose and refine their activities in the world, through
contemplation, self-reflection, and evaluation. There is a fourth level
of medical care that relates to these higher states of meaning, morality,
and self-identity, which is not fixed but continuously evolves.

Rudolf Steiner, PhD, the Austrian philosopher, scientist, and
teacher—who spoke about that "mantle of warmth" that mistletoe
therapy creates around a tumor—really challenged the medical community to embrace this fourth realm. He pointed out how it needs
to be part of all our medical thinking, not just an afterthought. We
should develop ways of thinking and observing so that we can move
between physical measures and spiritual meaning, between temperature warmth and warmth of heart. If we can do that, then we will
develop a relationship to what is best described as a whole "warmth
organization." He spoke to a group of young medical students about
this in the following way:

> You find a great gulf within you, over which you must find the
> bridge. You must find the bridge from the medical-scientific to the
> moral, to the loving. You see, when I speak, for example, of what

I call the warmth organization of the human being, for you it is initially an abstraction. But you must find the bridge to experience this warmth organization in such a way that you find your way from the experience of the warmth differentiations of the individual organs to moral warmth.

You will have to experience what is called 'heart warmth' in such a way that you will feel this warm heart right into the physical. You will have to find the way from the scientific-physiological to the spiritual-moral, and from the spiritual-moral to the physiological-anatomical.[12]

That process, of bridging "spiritual-moral" to "physiological–anatomical" feels like a lofty goal, but again, if we look carefully, it is not so far away. Let's look at some more published studies.

An intriguing examination of warmth involved college students on several campuses who were asked to evaluate the personality of another person (someone who had been videotaped during an interview).[13] What the students did not know is that the research aspect already began when they were greeted in the lobby of the building by a study coordinator, who escorted them on an elevator up to the place where the interviews were being held. Here is their fascinating study method: while riding the elevator, the study coordinator always asked the student to hold the coordinator's coffee cup, which was predetermined to be either hot coffee or iced coffee. *Holding a cup of hot or iced coffee during a short elevator ride*—that was the study intervention. The rest of the process was exactly the same. What they found was that "people who had briefly held the hot coffee cup perceived the target person as being significantly [interpersonally] warmer." A second part of the research asked study participants to examine and rate either a hot or cool therapeutic pad. Then, at the end of the session, participants were offered an immediate gift for themselves (a beverage) or a coupon to later "treat a friend" to some ice cream. Those who had examined the warm therapeutic pads were more likely to choose the gift coupon for a friend. Experiences of physical warmth and cold influence how much we see the good in another person and how generously we act. This shows a real bridge between "physical warmth" and a "warm heart." We can perceive another person differently through the activity of our personal "warmth organization."

We are aided in that process by experiences of outside warmth, but we also change our own warmth organization when we become more interested in another person, when we are "fired" by enthusiasm, when we "warmly invite" someone into greater social connection. Such warmth changes may be subtle (hard to measure with a simple thermometer check), but they are real. Self-directed, self-engendered warmth supports us on a path of deeper connection and understanding of the outside world.

We can know ourselves better, too, through self-engendered warmth. The importance of warmth as a tool of the immune system has already been described. Our bodies create fever because better warmth fosters better immune function. But warmth also plays a developmental role. We will look at one more study to round out our survey of warmth.

A study of children with autism spectrum disorders found that, during fever, these children exhibited "fewer aberrant behaviors...on the Aberrant Behavior Checklist subscales of irritability, hyperactivity, stereotypy, and inappropriate speech compared with control subjects."[14] This was true not only while the children had an elevated temperature, but also when behaviors were rated again by the child's parents seven days after the fever had finished. Children with an autism spectrum disorder usually become more irritable and hyperactive when they are uncomfortable and turn to anchoring behaviors like hand flapping or repetitive speech patterns as a way to orient and anchor themselves. This study suggests that with an experience of very strong warmth (fever), the children felt different. We can hypothesize that the reason they behaved differently was because they felt more comfortable in themselves, felt more comfortable in their bodies.

This fourth level of warmth has not only to do with morality (seeing goodness in others), and with self-awareness (how do I sense and feel myself), but also core aspects of meaning. It's a level of growth and development—not physical growth and regeneration, but spiritual change. It is not surprising that the Greeks referred to this level as the element of fire. This is the level where we learn to better know ourselves and gain a greater, truer sense of self.

Meaning	Why?	Development	Self-Awareness	Human	A self-actualizing person
Qualities	How?	Gestures	Awareness	Animal	A wakeful person
Flow	When?	Dynamics	Fluidity	Plant	A sleeping person
Facts	What?	Measurements	Anatomy	Mineral	A corpse

Table 6.3: A Fourth and culminating reality

There is always a little bit of mystery with this fourth level, as the spiritual is so completely individual. In AM, that aspect is known simply as the "I" because we can really say "I" only about ourselves; we cannot say it, or easily know it, for another person. This level, and the three preceding levels, are not so easy to describe in everyday language. So, within the practice of AM, four unique terms are used to designate these four levels of being. Drawing from the table that we've developed so far, the anthroposophic version would look like this:

"I"	Self-awareness. Formative forces of the human **spirit**.	Why/Who?
Astral	Emotion and sensation. Formative **soul** forces.	How?
Etheric	Growth and Regeneration. Formative **life** forces.	When?
Physical	Physical properties. **Substance** and measure.	What?

Table 6.4: The anthroposophic fourfold human being

If physical factors are answered with the question "What?" and dynamic, etheric forces with the question "When?" then astral and "I" aspects come into view with the qualitative question of "How?" and, finally, the meaning-oriented questions: "Why is this happening?" as well as "Who am I trying to become?"

A core part of our human experience is our capacity to be self-reflective. We question if we are doing the right thing. We want goodness and kindness to be part of our healing path. A doctor can't, however, write you a prescription for this fourth level. There are no "milligram" designations for meaning and morality because they need to be sensed and developed from the inside. This is the realm of self-engendered activity, of self-engendered warmth, of self-engendered change. It cannot be quantitatively prescribed, but having this aspect acknowledged, supported, and companioned by those around us makes the pathway easier and more meaningful.

Mistletoe and the fourfold human:
Beginning to understand the multilevel effects

These four "organizations" offer a comprehensive, yet individualized pathway for healing. It may not seem possible to address these diverse aspects of our humanity all at once, in one snapshot, one PET scan, one visit—because we can't. This is not about just following a standard protocol. Working to make lasting transformations takes time. Here are four major ingredients we need to focus on:

1. We must affirm that we are more than a diagnosis, more than a biopsy, more than a tumor marker level. We are more than just the physical measurements of disease.

2. Just as our temperature rises and falls each day, we also need to work in a rhythmic, breathing manner to stimulate healthy warmth. Mistletoe treatments help tremendously with that process, stimulating us to build up strong warmth, then letting it balance out—stimulating inflammation, then letting it resolve. Each "in-breath" and "out-breath" of cyclic warmth brings change. We need to appreciate and work with etheric dynamics of warmth and see that they are, in fact, part of a living process.

3. Just as there are many types of illness, so too there are many kinds of healing support. A multi-dimensional toolbox should be encouraged, simply because it works better. We build a comprehensive view: Where are we out of balance, where do we find stuck patterns, and how can we reeducate those patterns? Physiology and emotion flow into one another, which means we can heal from both sides (physical health makes us feel better, feeling better makes us healthier with stronger immunity). We can and should heal from both

sides, body and soul. We can address this astral realm of healing gestures with natural medicines, artistic therapies, body therapies, nursing treatments, counselling—a whole community of support. These aspects not only enrich our therapeutic toolbox, they also allow us to participate, in an active way, in our own healing process.

4. Maybe this really should be first: we must consider who is on this journey. Am I a diagnosis (such as "triple-negative breast cancer") with a name, or am I a unique human being going through the process of living with a cancer? How have I changed in this process? Who am I now? What is my truth? Even when someone goes into remission and is told to go back to "normal" life, that is an illusion based only on the world of facts and physical measures. For while life might outwardly look the same, inwardly it will be quite different. To preserve this fourth level, we need to not give away too much of ourselves. We need to not give away too much of our warmth to fear. Fear takes away warmth. Gratitude, trust, and love are its antidote.

By looking at all these research studies, we can see that working with a tumor should involve cultivation of our whole "warmth organism." Building a "mantle of warmth" around a tumor is not just about a temperature measurement. It is not just a kind sentiment. It is about whole person healing that supports us on the levels of facts, flow, qualities, and meaning; on the levels of the physical, etheric, astral, and "I"-organizations.

A cancer develops because some part of our body has fallen out of the whole. Tissue that no longer follows healthy physiologic patterns begins to grow. It manages to evade the attention and intervention of the immune system. When tumors grow, they are *in* us, but no longer truly part *of* us. Warmth—on physical, functional, emotional, and developmental levels—aids reintegration. It is no coincidence that we've seen a decrease in average body temperature over the same time period that we've seen increasing cancer rates. *They are two expressions of a common shift, a kind of splintering of health.* They stem from an increasingly disorganized immune response and distracted sense of self, of "I." Both are strengthened through support of the *warmth organization*. Mistletoe, as a warming therapy, enhances immune activity around the tumor, while also enhancing a level of spiritual warmth and "I" organization. It's one of the unique side benefits of mistletoe therapy. Patients often express an inexplicable increase in their sense of purpose and spiritual clarity, part of an overall improvement in quality of life. This is a sign of VAE enhancing and modulating warmth cycles, on the etheric, astral, and "I" levels. The next chapter will unfold and explore the nuances of these complex whole-person effects.

CHAPTER 7

WHAT IS "CONSTITUTIONAL CARE" IN THE ANTHROPOSOPHIC WORLD?

Seeing the Whole Person, the Whole Human Organism, before Providing Care

Dr. Peter Hinderberger, MD

"One will understand the human body only if one sees it as an expression of the soul and spirit. If it is seen only as a physical body, it will remain incomprehensible." —RUDOLF STEINER

First, a story: Robert grew up in a family of teachers. His father's parents were teachers, and his older sister had become a teacher, too. It was the family tradition. So young Robert felt a significant expectation that he would become a teacher. He set out on that path without giving it a whole lot of thought. Then, as he finished University, Robert's mother said to him, "You know how much you like Susan, and the two of you were such pals when you grew up next door to each other. Why haven't you proposed to her yet?" Robert couldn't deny that he did like Susan very much, even considered her his closest friend. So, he married her.

Then, when Robert was in his forties, he got terrible news. He had colon cancer. Not only was the illness deeply troubling, but the whole situation set him into a whirl of deep self-reflection. He realized that he really hadn't chosen his current life. He was married and had two children and was well into his academic career. Sometimes that career was exceedingly stressful, and university politics wore on him. But in all honesty, he'd never wanted to be a teacher. He really wanted to be a carpenter. He was married to Susan, but he'd never been sure that he was even attracted to women. He was in great crisis from his illness, and an even greater crisis of personal identity and purpose. Sometimes it felt like the cancer had entered his life story in order to interrupt and uproot everything. It felt strange, but he began to see his cancer journey as an opportunity to discover who he really was.

Why is this such a common theme among people who have cancer? The phenomenon is so common, it was the focus of Lawrence LeShan's book, *Cancer as a Turning Point.* We know that cancer diagnosis often triggers deep soul-searching.[1] But why is that? Why does this disease in particular become a doorway to refining one's own purpose and identity?

In this chapter, we'll wrestle with those questions. We will look at the anthroposophic description of cancer development and how spirit and soul interact with the physical and functional realities in the body. We'll see that today's physical risk factors for cancer (such as toxin exposure and unhealthy foods) are real and influential, but they are not the only factors involved for people who have cancer. As many of my own patients have discovered through their healing journey, there are other factors related to the soul and spirit, which are equally influential. Mistletoe, so well-known for its measurable immunological effects, has surprising gifts to share with the soul and spirit as well. With these deeper understandings, we can see how to address root causes and care more effectively for the whole person.

Understanding the human being's layers: Fourfold and threefold aspects

In the previous chapter, Dr. Blanning described the concept of the fourfold human. Let's briefly review that model. Then we'll look at one other anthroposophic model and explore both in terms of cancer development.

Physical: We each live in a physical body that is, without any other forces present, only a composite of minerals and elements arranged as organs and structures in a human shape. Without life force, the body is merely a corpse.

Etheric: The physical is enlivened by life forces, which anthroposophic practitioners refer to as the etheric body or etheric forces. In Asian medical traditions, this is known as *chi,* or *qi.* Etheric qualities include the person's age and general vitality. Are they frail or sturdy? Do they have energetic reserves, or are they exceptionally fatigued? At the most basic, the physical and the etheric together indicate that a body is alive. Etheric forces are pure life forces. They require structure and organization to grow and create in healthy ways.

Astral: A level above the etheric, we find the astral forces, which are more commonly referred to as the soul. These forces encompass a person's emotions, character, and temperament. Astral forces are highly involved in all daily activities, decisions, and interactions. They also interact with the physical and etheric to bring structure and balance to those realities. Astral forces influence and direct motion and emotion.

The "I": At a level even higher (and potentially more unifying), we find the "I" or the spirit—the person's truest self. Ideally, the "I" is in touch with all three other aspects of the fourfold human. The I cannot be damaged or traumatized like the astral forces (soul) can be. The "I" *is*—it does not change. However, the "I" is *cut off* far too often from the other members (the astral, etheric, and physical). In a moment, we'll see how that cutting-off, or disassociation, can affect the physical body and etheric forces.[2]

Anthroposophic medicine (AM) practitioners often refer to soul and spirit as the higher members of the human being and physical and etheric as the lower members. How these higher members and lower members connect—or fail to connect—is key to how well the immune system functions.[3]

It's fairly easy to recognize the *physical*. That's what we perceive with our eyes. That's the part of us that can be observed and quantified by physical, analytical means. The difference between the other three levels can feel a little more challenging. I think of it this way: The *spirit (the "I")* connects us to the Divine. It is unchanging, and it is what makes us truly unique and individual. How the spirit experiences daily life is connected to the *soul* (the *astral forces*). Through our senses, we are constantly exposed to stimuli when we are awake. Initially we react to these stimuli through the astral forces. The initial reaction is instinctual, either sympathy or antipathy. Only through our "I" can we modify these impressions and make them specifically personal. The *etheric forces* are pure, unbridled growth, like yeast. Etheric life forces are not formative or structural on their own. Their tendency is to expand, to multiply. Although they give structure to organelles (intracellular "organs" like nuclei, mitochondria, and ribosomes) and cell membranes, they depend on astral forces and the *"I"-organization* to create boundaries, structure, and specialization.

That concept of *"I"-organization* requires some description. The "I," on its own, is eternal. It exists, with or without a body. But once the "I" is incarnated in a body, it needs a tool, an instrument, with which it can dive down and bring structure and boundaries into the astral and etheric forces and all the way down to the physical cellular level. That instrument is the *"I"-organization*. Throughout childhood and early adulthood, the "I" uses the *"I"-organization* to individualize the body and all its systems fully, including the immune response. The "I"-organization is what directly encounters the astral forces and the lower members, serving as an organizing and supervising entity.[4]

In AM, in addition to this fourfold human paradigm, we have one more lens through which we view and assess a patient. The threefold human refers to three energetic–functional systems that are at work throughout the body all the time. The nerve–sense system, the metabolic system, and the rhythmic system are each associated with certain organ groups, but they are actually present and active in every cell of the body.[5]

Metabolic system: Focused on creating movement and change. It is associated with anabolic processes (making complex molecules), warmth, activity, and has a centrifugal (outward, expanding) tendency. This system is centered under the diaphragm (digestive tract, liver) and in muscles. It governs the metabolic processes of every living cell.

Nerve–sense system: Focused on taking in and processing stimuli. It is associated with catabolic processes (breaking down complex molecules), coolness and stillness, and has a centripetal (inward, contracting) tendency. This system is centered in the brain and CNS, but is active throughout the body, wherever sensory cells take in and processes stimuli.

Rhythmic system: Balances the activities of the metabolic and nerve–sense systems. The regulator between those polar opposites, the rhythmic system maintains balance and harmony between all body systems. It is strongly associated with the rhythmic activity of the lungs (inspiration–expiration) and heart (diastole/systole), but this sense of rhythm is clearly active in every biological process in the body. Every cell has cycles of activity (expansion) and receptivity (contraction), movement and stillness.

The Energetic/Functional Systems of the Threefold Human

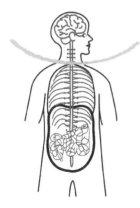
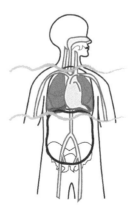
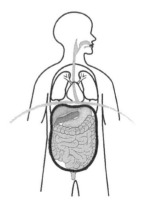

A. The sensory-nervous system

B. The rhythmic system

C. The metabolic system

Looking at the threefold human, we see the organism as fluid, wave-form, and rhythmic. The systems are associated with certain organs, but all three systems work synergistically and parallel in every cell, in all organs and tissues. These are not reductionist binaries, rather they are energetic systems that are healthiest when there is a sense of balance and flow. Harmony of these systems equals life and vitality.

When AM practitioners talk about "constitutional polarity," they're referring to the nerve–sense system and the metabolic system working at opposite poles. The rhythmic system is the balancing center. Any of these three systems can be imbalanced (over- or underactive), resulting in a host of symptoms that might appear unrelated at the surface. AM practitioners constantly evaluate their patients through both the threefold and fourfold paradigms. This is a framework through which we evaluate a patient's constitution—their overall condition in terms of energy, temperature, and rhythmic balance. Disparate presenting symptoms begin to reveal their common connections when we look at the whole person from this layered and systemic viewpoint.[6]

Threefold and fourfold principles in modern life: A perfect storm for cancer development

As far as the threefold human, the most common imbalance that I see today is overstimulation of the nerve–sense system. We are constantly in our heads, feeling overwhelmed, overworked, and overloaded with minute-by-minute news cycles. Work and life stress command our days. The body was not made for excessive exposure to electronic devices and relentless chronic stress. The human being is designed for slow processing, metabolizing, and maturing—both food and ideas! When presented with a new idea, the human being would prefer to have time to digest it and warm up to it. A new thought often will not impress us at first. But with time and digestion, we modify the information, merge it with our own thoughts, and synthesize something new. Eventually, we share the new information with someone else, completing our learning process.

Today, we rarely make time for that healthy processing. We let sound bites hit us rapid-fire, never digesting them, and feeling the stress of only the initial reception of a new and abrasive thought. We tend to be force-fed far too much stressful information each day—sometimes every hour! We now know that high-stress lifestyles are associated with accelerated cancer progression.[7] There are multiple energetic reasons for that, as we'll see after looking at how modern life affects the other two spheres of the threefold human.

Threefold dysregulation and cancer risk factors

Along with an overstimulated nerve–sense system, the standard Western lifestyle tends to include a diet of many processed foods as well as a lack of exercise and time outdoors. The metabolic system struggles under the stress of low-quality fuel and a lack of healthy movement. Simultaneously, the rhythmic system is confused and dysregulated by our loss of day-night rhythm. Electric light and electronic devices force our bodies to stay wakeful and alert all the way up to bedtime, which may be much later than is healthy.

Both integrative and conventional medicine have begun to take these risk factors seriously, recognizing the existence of Metabolic Syndrome. The associated diseases (heart disease, pre-diabetes, diabetes, fatty liver) respond beautifully to lifestyle transformation. But, left unchecked, such conditions can become cancer risk factors themselves.[8] Some conventional practitioners have also begun to acknowledge the seriousness of rhythmic system dysregulation. They refer to this more commonly as circadian disruption. Dysregulation in the rhythmic system is associated with certain cancers. Multiple studies have found that night shift workers have higher cancer rates.[9] This holds true regardless of the individual's socioeconomic status.[10]

What is happening here? From a threefold human perspective, our modern lifestyles predispose us for *dominance of the nerve–sense system*. Meanwhile, the *metabolic system is weakened* by poor lifestyle choices, and *the rhythmic system is weakened* by an arrhythmic schedule and artificial day and night rhythm. It is painfully common to live in a body where all three of these energetic systems are imbalanced. This threefold dysregulation often first manifests as a chronic feeling of cold, especially cold hands and feet, and as a lack of feverish diseases. The imbalance can also appear as inexplicable fatigue. Conventional medicine has few answers for someone who merely feels tired and not-their-best most of the time. Often standard lab work seems to indicate they are healthy.[11]

So many of my patients come to me saying, "I was never the person who got sick. But now I have cancer!" This is always a clue to me that a deep threefold imbalance was developing long before the cancer diagnosis. When I ask such a patient when they last had a strong fever, they say that it was in childhood, if they've ever had a significant fever at all. Here is where we see the first vivid connection between an imbalanced threefold system and the cancer development process. The body's ability to dance back and forth between nerve–sense and metabolic system activities is deeply connected to immune function. Warmth is a sign of immune system activity as much as it is an indicator of heightened metabolism. When AM practitioners say that "we lack warmth today," this is what they are talking about. The immune system has been slowed, muted.[12,13]

As much as we need stillness and coolness to properly sense and process new information, we need warmth and activity for healthy growth, repair, and immunity. Nerve–sense system activities are inwardly focused; metabolic system activities look outward. The rhythmic system balances and coordinates the two poles. In anthroposophic care, we often witness how much we can improve any patient's general condition simply by increasing warmth and nurturing healthy rhythm—particularly by bringing warmth to the limbs and supporting the heart. The body needs all three systems functioning in harmony in order to be well. Just as the stress of an overstimulated nerve–sense system can compromise immune cell numbers and activity,[14] we've also seen exercise and meditation practices improve immune cell counts and function.[15,16]

Fourfold imbalance and cancer development

We've seen how imbalance in the threefold human can set the stage for the immune dysregulation that is present when cancer takes root. Let's look through the fourfold lens as well. There are even more clues here regarding how the immune response begins to lose its ability to monitor and address cancerous cells.

Cancer cannot be compared to any other illness like diabetes, hypertension, arthritis, and son on. Once a person is diagnosed with cancer, the patient feels like there is a foreign entity in their body. For the rest of their lives, they will not forget that they have cancer. Every event, every decision is shared with the cancer: "How would my cancer react, how does this influence my cancer?" Cancer is seen like an unwanted guest or a bully.

People who have survived a major childhood trauma have a higher incidence of cancer as adults.[17-19] Though profoundly unfair, this is also a clue, and neuro-immunological clues can be empowering once you are aware of them. From an AM perspective, we view both "shock trauma" (single, highly impactful incidents) and "chronic trauma" (many micro-traumas over the years) as significant risk factors for cancer. The person who survives an earthquake as a child, and the person who is worn down by decades spent in an unhealthy workplace, can both experience damage to their immune system function.

From a fourfold human perspective, the trauma, or traumas, trigger a disassociating chain reaction, in which soul (astral) and spirit (I) begin to pull back from the physical body and its etheric life processes. The stages and progression of cancer are caused by a dysregulation of the fourfold principle. The physiological breakdown develops like this[20]:

Initial overwhelming and disassociation

1. The sensory system (stress) overwhelms the metabolic system. This arhythmic, catabolic dominance weakens the etheric life forces. This leaves an area in the physical body bare of life.

This is a "void" in the physical, which we refer to as *locus minoris resistentiae.*

Proliferation

2. Cells in that area start to divide and proliferate of their own accord in a disorderly fashion leading to autonomous proliferation or dysplasia.

3. Tumor cells impose and use their own etheric forces for growth, leading to localized (*in situ*) carcinoma.

Invasive movement

4. Cancer cells impose and use their own astral forces for movement (astral forces are the basis for motion), leading to *invasive cancer.*

5. Cancer cells impose and use their own I-organization leading to *metastasis.*

Metastatic cancer

6. Cancer cells establish their own "personality" and overwhelm their host, leading to *Stage IV advanced cancer* and *cachexia.*

By the end of this process, the spirit ("I") is quite cut off from the soul (astral) and lower members. Rudolf Steiner hypothesized that the "void" in the physical (mentioned in step 1) is the beginning of cancer.[21] Eventually, if the cancer progresses unchecked, the tumor imposes its own "I" or character on its host. Thankfully, there are many moments earlier in the process when this cascade can be checked.

Undifferentiated cells are a primary feature of this process. For many patients swept up in this experience, there is also a sense of *poor psychological differentiation.* Remember the spirit (the "I") is never traumatized; it is the truest self and is always connected to the Divine. But the soul (astral) can be profoundly traumatized, to the point that the spirit cannot take hold of the soul and the lower members. The spirit can be cut off from the other fourfold members. This is how wounds in the soul can manifest in the physical. A person's soul formation, their *psychological differentiation*, can influence *cellular differentiation*. Poor cellular differentiation is associated with cancer development.[22]

When the spirit is cut off from the physical, the immune system is also affected. The primary task of immune cells is to differentiate between self and non-self. When the "I" (the truest expression of self) cannot connect with the immune system, that core purpose of recognizing self and non-self becomes confused. Yet, this is the essence of what the immune system must do in the presence of cancer. It needs to clearly recognize cancer cells as unhealthy—they are no longer an expression of the healthy self.

Threefold and fourfold understandings in tandem

Taken together, the threefold and fourfold perspectives show us a picture of modern life as a perfect storm of cancer risk factors. In conventional medicine, when we discuss cancer risk factors, we are usually referring to environmental toxin exposure, smoking, or genetic issues. These are legitimate and powerful risks. But they are rarely the only factors involved. Psychological, spiritual, and circadian disruptions are just as influential from an AM point of view.[23-25] Indeed, when we look at geographic regions where cancer rates are higher, such as the Mississippi delta area, we see a concentration of carcinogenic toxins (waterborne agricultural chemicals and oil refinery pollution) paired with the inherent stress of severe poverty.[26-28] Both physical and spiritual risk categories must be addressed to bring lasting healing.

Remember the story of Robert at the beginning of this chapter. From a threefold and fourfold standpoint, modern people are keenly at risk of living someone else's life (fourfold disruption), while also chronically dysregulating their core energy systems (threefold dysregulation). This alone fosters a spiritual terrain that is especially vulnerable to an active cancer process.

All these ideas are philosophical and spiritual, and yet there are clear quantitative findings associated with them. Whether we look at cancer incidence among night shift workers or among trauma survivors, we can't deny the connections. The book *Radical Remission* by oncology researcher Kelly Turner is also compelling. When Turner interviewed over 1,000 cancer survivors who had experienced inexplicable spontaneous remissions, she identified nine lifestyle and treatment choices that all the survivors had in common. Only three pertained to common integrative treatment strategies: significant dietary change, using herbs and supplements, and taking leadership in one's healing. The other six factors were related to the individual's soul and spirit care, including: trauma resolution, cultivating healthy relationships, and purpose-finding.[29]

From an AM perspective, these remission cases are radical but not inexplicable. Turner's intensive research interviews happened upon principles that AM practitioners have applied for over one hundred years. We regard soul and spirit care as equally efficacious therapeutic modalities, alongside any other anthroposophic, integrative, or conventional treatments. *Self-care, purpose-discovery, decreasing electronics exposure, increasing exercise and time outside, switching to a less stressful job, cultivating empowering friendships, trying artistic therapies, and fostering healthier sleep patterns*—from an AM perspective, these are medicinal therapies.

Acute versus chronic inflammation: The body's early warning flags before cancer appears

Throughout this book, we've looked at inflammation as it relates to assessing a patient's immune system. Anthroposophic practitioners often express concern about the lack of feverish diseases and a dominant cold constitution among most of our patients today.[30,31] Now that we understand a little more about how modern life affects the threefold and fourfold human organism, perhaps this concern about inflammation makes more sense.

Again, as my colleagues have already noted, we often see signs of unhealthy *chronic inflammation* among our patients. Chronic joint and soft tissue pain, injuries that heal poorly, gut health issues, and even cognitive problems can all be signs of a chronic inflammatory state. This type of inflammation, believe it or not, is associated with a *cold constitutional tendency.* It is not a healing inflammatory response; it is inflammation that has gotten stuck in a damaging cycle. Chronic inflammation hardly ever causes fever and can even be accompanied by below-normal temperature. Instead of serving the healthy purpose of clearing out a pathogen, it forms deposits and leads to hardening processes like atherosclerosis, osteophytes, and cirrhosis of the liver.[32,33] This is an inward, focusing, centripetal process. The end result is tissue hardening and energy stagnation. We feel worse than before.

Conversely, healthy inflammation is associated with a heightened and healthy immune response. A strong fever is a sign of healthy immune activity. It is transient; after it resolves, the body is stronger than before. When people have an acute fever all they want is to rest, fast and drink fluids. Those are good instincts, and the end result is healing. Similarly, heightened immune activity at the site of a wound or injury is uncomfortable, but not a bad thing. Good inflammation is defined by its wave form—it rises, flushes out the problem, then subsides.

Symptom	Acute Inflammation	Chronic Inflammation
Fever	HIGH	None, though occasionally LOW
Energy	Severe sudden lethargy	Chronic tiredness
Thirst	Dramatically increased	No change
Appetite	None	No change, though occasionally intense cravings
Direction	Centrifugal – Moving outward	Centripetal – Moving toward center, concentrating
End Result	Healing – Feeling better than before	Hardening – Wearing out

Table 7.1: Acute vs. chronic inflammation

As we learned in chapter 5, monitoring markers of chronic inflammation can be highly empowering for patients. When we see the immune system swing back toward a chronic inflammation profile, we know it's time to provide focused support to bring the patient back into balance. Chronic inflammation is an early warning that lets us know the immune system is not in a place where it can effectively deal with existing cancer or ward off potential recurrence.[34]

In AM care plans, we look for ways to come alongside the body and support a healthy inflammatory rhythm. This is the case for any of our patients, but especially so for those with cancer. Part of the reason VAE provides such surprising effects is that it helps with this core task: reestablishing healthy warmth cycles. Our therapies are often focused on helping the immune system remember how to cycle through times of heightened inflammation and then progress through to optimal resolution. Mistletoe, as a warming therapy, is an especially effective adjuvant.

Mistletoe's mysteries: Applying fourfold and threefold principles to reverse course and restore health

Mystery is mistletoe's standard. We've studied mistletoe's effects and its active constituents extensively, but many of the plant's characteristics remain inexplicable: its strange orb-like symmetry, its metabolic activity in winter, its parasitic quality that somehow doesn't kill its host. Even mistletoe's leaves are a mystery. The leaf surface is identical on both sides; there is no definable top or bottom as we would see in any other leafy plant. This indicates that mistletoe is an exceedingly primitive plant—predating all the tree species we know of today. But if that's the case, how did mistletoe first survive on this planet without any host trees? These are touch points that thrill the souls of those who are interested in the gesture and character of botanical medicines.

As an anthroposophic physician, I look even more closely at specific mistletoe gestures that compare and contrast with the gesture of cancer. Constitutionally, one might regard cancer as "freedom in the wrong place." Similarly, mistletoe has a kind of displaced freedom; it does not follow seasons, it has no typical root system, and it is evergreen, though it does lose its leaves every seven years. Cancer is comprised of "primitive cells" that have, in a sense, forgotten their differentiated purpose, and mistletoe has a highly primitive plant structure. Both cancer and mistletoe have abundant life forces and strong creative energy.

The two entities differ significantly too. Cancer is similar to pathogenic parasites, in its capacity to steal energy from and eventually kill its host. Mistletoe is a *hemiparasite*; it needs a host tree, but it does not kill its host. Rather, it preserves its host. In a sense it has overcome its own parasitic identity. Cancer and mistletoe appear to be polar opposites in several other categories, with cancer typically described as chaotic and fast-growing, while mistletoe is highly structured and slow-growing. Instinctively we associate cancer as a dark entity. Mistletoe has a remarkably interesting relationship to light: it prefers dark over light but contains chlorophyll in its root system (the sinker root). Chlorophyll depends on light. How chlorophyll can thrive in the sinker root is still a mystery!

All these energetic signatures are important. From an anthroposophic perspective, mistletoe conveys these unique gestures when we use VAE as a remedy. Let's look at how mistletoe interacts energetically with the threefold and fourfold human.

Cancer	Mistletoe
Displaced – Freedom in the wrong place, undirected growth	Incongruous – Freedom in areas that are usually well-bounded
Abundant life forces	Abundant life forces
Primitive cells – Undifferentiated	Primitive plant structure
Parasitic Qualities – Can destroy its host	Hemiparasite – Doesn't destroy its host
Earth-oriented	Cosmic plant
Chaotic	Structured
Fast-growing	Slow-growing
Prefers darkness – Little magnesium, anaerobic (low-oxygen) metabolism	Balanced between light and dark

Table 7.2: Comparative gestures of cancer and mistletoe

Using mistletoe to restore both systemic harmony and personal purpose

Mistletoe is well researched for its quantifiable effects on the immune system. We've identified mistletoe lectins and viscotoxins and determined many of their specific activities (chapter 2). Researchers are continuing to identify the actions of other compounds in VAE. From a threefold and fourfold perspective, those researched *quantitative* effects harmonize with broader *constitutional* shifts.

Through the threefold lens, mistletoe restores rhythm. It certainly warms the metabolic system. Whether observing the reaction at the subcutaneous injection site or heightened body temperature during fever therapy, mistletoe clearly warms the body. Mistletoe practitioners also observe its ability to reset the rhythmic system. This is equally valuable. Mistletoe seems to restore rhythm to the dance between nerve–sense and metabolic systems, thereby restoring coordination between all body systems. This is still a clinical observation only, but researchers are starting to explore the possible methods of action.[35] We often pair mistletoe intentionally with cooling therapies to further reeducate the body in its ability to complete and resolve cycles of warm and cool (see chapters 8 and 9).

From the fourfold perspective, warmth enhancement is again central. According to AM, warming the immune system and warming the soul and spirit are synonymous. Throughout published case studies, one finds stories of mistletoe's most fascinating side benefit. During mistletoe fever therapy, some patients find that old traumas are stirred up and organically resolve themselves (see chapter 3).[36] There are spiritual shifts, that we regard as deeply intertwined with the health of the immune system. The immune response is, at its essence, a defense system commissioned to discern between self and non-self. The "I" is the essential self. The immune system is an expression of the "I"; it reflects the person's degree of "I"-organization. Cut off the spirit from the physical and etheric, and the immune response becomes inefficient and confused. Restore that connection, and the immune response clarifies. These are philosophical and spiritual ideas, and yet quantitative research supports them. Depression (often a kind of loss of connection to one's truest self and purpose) affects immune cell counts.[37–39] Unresolved trauma can influence cancer risk.[40–43]

With that in mind, maybe "improved sense of purpose" isn't a random side benefit of VAE therapy. Rather, it stems straight from the underlying healing mechanism. Mistletoe's warming effect restores the "I"-organization. The "I" (spirit) is able to plunge downward to the etheric and physical to restore order among cells and the immune response.

Healthy formative forces can finally lay hold of the unbounded life forces that allowed cancer to take root. Mistletoe seems to convey its gesture—all its symmetry and structure—during VAE therapy. It centers the spirit and soul, and out of that essential shift, formative and organizing forces can reach the body and its immune system.

Researchers point to mistletoe's ability to increase beta-endorphin levels.[44] It's true this effect likely helps with overall outlook. Patients feel more positive and, in some cases, experience mild pain-relief, too.[45] However, there is a deeper reinvigoration of the soul and greater sense of connection to the spirit, which seem beyond the reach of an endorphin boost. It's worth noting that these spiritual "side effects" are common among all warming therapies. There's something spiritually powerful about physical warmth.

Anthroposophic care for the whole human organism

When someone has cancer, it is like a house is on fire. You wouldn't go after a massive house fire with a handheld extinguisher. Instead, you call professionals who come in, and then it gets ugly. The firefighters break the windows, and they flood the house, and they get the job done. They are effective. Mission accomplished. The fire is out, but the house is not livable anymore! Now, you wouldn't call the firefighters the next day and ask them to rebuild your house. They would say, "This is not in our job description!"

Metaphorically, that is where anthroposophic and integrative oncologists come in. But we can actually get involved before the house is completely ruined. Thankfully, the body is different from a house. We can support the body during chemotherapy and radiation and surgery. In the best situations, our therapies can mitigate side effects of conventional care and even enhance the desired effects of the conventional treatments.

Conventional oncology aims to destroy the cancer, and it is very good at this objective. *Integrative oncology* seeks to optimize the patient's inner terrain in order to starve the cancer and help the human organism fight the cancer. *Therapy and pastoral counseling* help the patient fight the cancer on an emotional and spiritual level. *Anthroposophic oncology* includes all the above and adds artistic therapies to enhance the patient's creative resources, as well as distinctly anthroposophic remedies that encourage normal form and function. The world would be a better, more healing place for people who have cancer if all these practitioners began to speak with each other and care for each patient as a team.

Ultimately, we could strive for what Rudolf Steiner called "spiritual science."[46] Particularly with cancer, we cannot limit ourselves to the physical reductionist sphere only. If a patient comes to me and they have hypertension, the reason is often quite obvious. With cancer, the "why" is rarely obvious. Spiritual factors are involved. Analytical science looks solely for molecular answers. Spiritual science looks at the whole being. It is no coincidence that most spiritual paths encourage people to think with their hearts and feel with their minds. If we combine the two like that, we develop a *holistic consciousness*. When we take action from within that holistic consciousness, we create sustainably. There is a moral quality to our action that is not self-righteous, but compassionate. When I treat the whole person, transformation can take place, for both my patient and myself. Patient and doctor work together to develop the treatment and care plan.

Nature is synergy. So, we treat the whole person, acknowledging that all factors (threefold and fourfold) matter equally. AM practitioners also tend to use whole plant extracts, acknowledging that all components of the plant matter in its ability to convey helpful effects. With mistletoe, we recognize that all its activities—immunologic, anti-tumor, warmth-enhancing, "I"-organizing, soul-centering—all these effects taken together, convey the benefit of improved quality of life.

Begin with balancing constitutional polarities

Almost every medical practice on the planet understands that the physical manifestation of disease is the last manifestation of an imbalance on the non-physical level. Only conventional Western medicine fully divorces its diagnostics and treatments from any spiritual awareness. The threefold and fourfold models are *constitutional frameworks* through which we can restore awareness of both physical and non-physical realities.

An anthroposophic practitioner begins with looking for imbalances in the polar nerve–sense and metabolic systems. We look at the rhythmic system and assess its function as the balancing center for those two poles. Observing the fourfold human, we look for weak life forces (etheric) and any sense that the soul (astral) or the spirit (the "I") are pulled back from the physical and etheric. We look for the energies that are dominant and those that are weakened or cut off. Patient care stems from this assessment, rather than a list of physical symptoms only.[47]

Cancer is not solely a genetic or physical problem. An individual patient may have genetic and physical risk factors. Yet, there are non-physical factors involved too. With all cancers, we want to empower the immune response. Understanding that the immune response is an expression of the patient's spirit (the "I"), the anthroposophic practitioner's goal is to bridge any disconnection in the fourfold human and to bring the "I"-organization and its warmth downward, back into the physical and etheric. This is why we use warming therapies like mistletoe.

Involve patients in their own care

Anthroposophic care involves the patient actively, and appropriate VAE therapy is an excellent example of this foundational principle. As practitioners, we can provide a remedy, even mistletoe, in a way that is not empowering. The patient may passively take the remedy and hope for the best. This takes freedom and power away from the patient; they are dependent on their physician and the drug. Instead, if I describe a few changes that the patient could make, and let them choose, this is empowering. I might say, "Just try this way of eating. Try it for three weeks; that's all." They try it, and they come back and say, "That was very hard. But I feel so much better." That experience is *em-powering*; it puts power back in the patient's hands.

The anthroposophic practitioner does not interfere with the patient's freedom. Serious disease often gives us an opportunity to change, but we have a choice in the matter. Among all modern diseases, cancer is unique in its ability to prompt major personal transformation. It is not like arthritis or heart disease. Cancer is so individual and intimate. So, it often becomes a major turning point.

Mistletoe therapy, when provided appropriately, is empowering for the patient. Finding the appropriate dosage, administering the subcutaneous injections, self-monitoring, and reporting on injection site reactions—these are all the patient's responsibility. Particularly when VAE therapy is paired with appropriate and personalized dietary change, I see patients become true leaders in their own health and treatment plan. This further strengthens their will. VAE therapy can be hard work, and a patient must actively choose it. Dr. Marion Debus said:

> Patients tend to think of doctors as the ones who will get them out of their crisis. But with cancer, because of the stuck-ness and the coldness, we actually have to get them into a *stronger crisis*. The therapy is not meant to be gentle; it's meant to put the person into a new crisis so that the "I" is able to take hold of the warmth organism in a new way.[48]

This refers to the heightened acute inflammation that comes from awakening the immune system. This is not a comfortable process, and a patient must be aware of this, understand the ultimate benefits, and choose from a place of resolve and commitment.

In anthroposophic care, developing the treatment plan is highly collaborative and personalized. I regard every patient encounter as a karmic event in which I will learn as much as the patient. As we journey together I, too, learn more about the importance of reinvigorating the "I"-organization and restoring the rhythmic system in its balance between the metabolic pole and the nerve–sense pole. In today's imbalanced world, we spend so much time in a cool, analytical space inside our heads. We all benefit from providing ourselves with more focused care for our metabolic systems, through enhancing warmth and physical movement. We all benefit from incorporating more natural rhythms into our lives. You cannot go wrong with increasing warmth and restoring rhythm! It's these lifestyle choices that allow the body to return to a state of self-regulation and harmony.

Other adjuvants alongside mistletoe

Mistletoe is itself a powerful adjuvant to conventional cancer care. Similarly, there are other anthroposophic and integrative therapies that serves as effective adjuvants to mistletoe. Dr. Steven Johnson will discuss other anthroposophic remedies next. He'll focus especially on *Helleborus niger*, which is often provided to enhance the rhythmic effects of mistletoe. Anthroposophic remedies tend to focus on caring for the etheric, astral, and "I" levels. They also encourage threefold balance and rhythm. After learning about some of the more common anthroposophic remedies, Dr. Nasha Winters will comment on well-vetted integrative therapies that are safe and particularly helpful along-side mistletoe. Through all these recommendations, I hope you notice the personalized nature of anthroposophic and integrative oncology. I hope you see the degree to which every aspect of the human organism is respected and valued for its involvement in the healing process.

CASE STORY ONE: JANE

Singing My Own Healthy Song				
Physician: Dr. Peter Hinderberger	**Patient**: Jane	**First seen**: 2011, cancer diagnosis Nov. 2015.	**Age:** 57 (first visit)	**Sex:** Female
Cancer Type & Stage:	Invasive ductal ER- PR-, HER2-negative, Stage III right breast cancer			
Risk Factors:	Stressful homelife, multiple metabolic health challenges, food sensitivities, and chronic fatigue			

Jane was my patient for a few years before she had cancer, but she came to me with many other health challenges. She was in her fifties, and she was struggling with serious chronic fatigue. She described herself as "feeling drained to near collapse." At the time, Jane was 5'6" and weighed 211 pounds. She also had several food sensitivities (milk, wheat, tomatoes, nuts), chronic diarrhea, menopausal complaints (hot flashes), hypertension and hyperlipid-emia (high cholesterol), heart palpitations, euthyroid multinodular goiter (meaning her thyroid was still functioning well), tinnitus, beginning cataracts, and fibrocystic breast disease. That last concern was a flag, but there were so many other challenges we needed to work on just so she could face each day with any energy at all.

Jane was alone at her initial visit with me. Her husband did come with her to at least one appointment, but he was not especially engaged. He seemed quite stoic. He wanted to know my recommendations, but there was not much active compassion coming from him. He and Jane were raising two adopted daughters, who were teenagers and had begun to present some intense parenting challenges. Both daughters were depressed and had suicidal ideations. So, Jane's homelife was not easy or necessarily supportive in the face of her own health issues.

Whenever I spoke with her, I saw a woman who was completely worn out. She needed to be cared for. She asked me to be her Primary Care Physician, and I began to coordinate her care. I referred her to a cardiologist, endocrinologist, and gynecologist, and I recommended a few supplements, dietary changes, an exercise program, and calcarea carbonica (a homeopathic remedy appropriate for her constitution).

Over the next four years, Jane began to proactively care for herself. She became interested in nutrition and lost 36 pounds on a diet that was gluten-free, dairy-free, and avoided processed carbohydrates. She put herself on a brisk walking program. Jane felt physically and emotionally lighter, even though her children continued to struggle in life, and they still weighed on her.

Then, in 2015, Jane was diagnosed with a 2.5 cm area of poorly differentiated invasive ductal Stage III right breast cancer. Initially it was assessed as ER+ PR+, HER2-negative. But then her oncotype score came in at 53 and showed that she was actually triple negative (ER- PR-, HER2-negative). This was concerning as this typically implies a fast-growing cancer that is more likely to recur.

Oncotype scores don't always mean much, but a score of 53 is high and was indicative that Jane would benefit from chemotherapy. This was an aggressive cancer, so she had a lumpectomy (six out of six lymph nodes were negative) and began what was supposed to be seven cycles of Taxotere and Cytoxan. Jane did not tolerate chemotherapy well, and she stopped after four cycles. She did continue with twenty fractions of radiation therapy over 28 days.

Alongside her conventional care, I treated Jane with *Viscum Mali* Series 1. She was able to build up to 50 mg for her subcutaneous (SC) injections. She remained at 50 mg of *Viscum Mali*, three times per week, for three years. She also took pregnenolone, along with calcium D-glucarate and DIM, as an alternative to an aromatase inhibitor (a strategy also described in Mary's case story, see chapter 4). She took vitamin D for general wellness and an herbal anti-inflammatory product.

At three years out, Jane still showed No Evidence of Disease (NED). This was fantastic news for someone who'd had a Stage III diagnosis. We dropped the SC injections down to twice per week. With all my patients who have survived breast cancer, I recommend this minimum twice-per-week VAE schedule for ongoing preventive care.

From 2016 to 2018, I saw more than just physical changes in Jane. She let me know that she had been exploring reiki, working with crystal therapy and chanting exercises, and taking tai chi classes. Her daughters were grown and had moved out. They continued to struggle in adulthood, but Jane was making powerful choices to nurture herself. Her own self-care had evolved from avoiding poor dietary habits to building her health proactively in a positive form.

Jane attended programs at her community's nonprofit support center for cancer survivors and began meeting with a psychologist. Going to therapy was especially transformative for her. As she put it, this helped her better cope with " ... my body, life's griefs, and environment." Jane read Dr. Kelly Turner's book *Radical Hope: 10 Key Healing Factors from Exceptional Survivors of Cancer and Other Diseases*. This was inspiring for her. Soon Jane was describing a whole lifestyle of spirit and soul nourishment. She began barefoot walking in the woods, went to a massage therapist regularly, and began playing a musical instrument. She intentionally made time for relaxation. She said she was getting rid of physical and emotional clutter and had learned to "sing my own healthy song."

There is nothing more encouraging, more heartening than watching someone face cancer head-on and then seize the time for greater personal change. This is when the deepest astral (soul) healing can occur. As of January 2021, Jane had been cancer-free for over five years and was dismissed from her oncologist's care. She continues on mistletoe and her supplement protocol, and she's in an incredibly positive space now.

CASE STORY 2: RACHEL

Small Community, Giant Creative Spirit				
Physician: Dr. Peter Hinderberger	**Patient**: Rachel	**First seen**: Nov. 1995; first cancer diagnosis July 2006	**Age**: 73 (58 at dx)	**Sex:** Female
Cancer Type & Stage:	Poorly differentiated (grade3) endometrial cancer; all four lymph nodes found negative upon total hysterectomy. Two small, unspecified nodules in the lungs.			
Risk Factors:	Metabolic and cardiovascular health challenges; history of basal cell cancers			

Rachel was in her mid-forties when I first met her in 2012. She had a history of basal cell cancers but was coming to me for several other health concerns. At the time of her new patient exam, she was 5'6" and 188 pounds with high-normal blood pressure and a systolic murmur (3/6). She also had uterine fibroids and IBS, along with significant anxiety. Her main anxieties were about her family and friends. And cancer. She was worried about some form of cancer appearing again. She wanted to make her own health a more significant priority.

Rachel was married and had four children. She was a Licensed Clinical Social Worker (LCSW) specializing in family therapy. An Orthodox Jew, she worked at a Jewish community center known for its incredible services for the unemployed and people with disabilities. I got the impression there was significant pressure for her to maintain incredibly high-quality client care. She was composed, thoughtful, attentive, and a good listener. I could see more of the therapist than the mother in her. I could also tell she had a comfort level with listening to others—far more than expressing herself.

A nutritionist helped Rachel with some dietary changes, probiotics, and digestive enzymes that helped her gut issues. I recommended some herbal tinctures, vitamin E, and prescribed calcarea carbonica (a homeopathic remedy appropriate for her constitution). Rachel continued to come to my clinic, on and off for the next 12 years. I helped her through some perimenopausal ups and downs and back pain.

Unfortunately, Rachel's earlier anxiety became a reality when she was diagnosed with poorly differentiated endometrial cancer at age 58. She had a total hysterectomy, and all four removed lymph nodes were negative. One oncologist recommended five weeks of daily radiation. Another oncologist recommended chemotherapy, because the cancer consisted of poorly differentiated cells and extensive lymphovascular invasion (only four lymph nodes were harvested). Indeed, a CT scan showed two small, unspecified nodules in her lungs. Rachel said she felt like there was a "ticking clock" inside her.

She opted for chemotherapy: six cycles of Abraxane and Carboplatin. She completed chemotherapy, the CT scan was repeated, and the scan was clear! This news was "a powerful emotional, religious experience" for her and motivated her to "work on preventive measures for the future." This is when something really clicked for her in terms of soul (astral) and spirit ("I") care. She declared that she had decided "to become more differentiated... pursue my needs as an individual, less driven by my expectations of others, the need to please, the need for approval." In short, she wanted "to focus on healing me." She took a sabbatical from her work and set aside that time for her own healing.

Rachel started on an alkaline diet. She began taking curcumin, LDN, and vitamin D, and began SC *Viscum Mali.* But the dietary shifts, supplements, and mistletoe therapy were small adjustments compared to the personal transformation that unfolded.

To some degree, as rich and beautiful as her Orthodox community was, I'd often sensed that Rachel's experience there was keeping her small. She remained in that community, but she began to drastically alter the tone and expectations of all her relationships. She even rewrote her *ketubah* (a Jewish marriage agreement) and managed to stay married to her husband through that process! She wrote a book about rising above disease and, in it, quoted both Rabbis and leaders from other traditions. Rachel's life began to be characterized by a sense of expansiveness. Her own children were grown by now and starting families of their own. She became more active in the lives of her grandchildren and began learning a musical instrument. This was a time of true personal renaissance.

As of 2021, Rachel has now gone 15 years with no evidence of disease (NED). That is to be celebrated. Her personal transformation is equally worth celebrating. She has come into her own. Rachel is a woman who treated cancer as a wake-up call instead of a punishment. She laid hold of this season in her life and bloomed, without concern about where she was planted or how others might perceive her. It's been a transformative experience for her and all her loved ones.

Chapter 8

Pairing AM Adjuvants

Helleborus and Other Anthroposophic Remedies Provided alongside Mistletoe Therapy

Dr. Steven Johnson, DO

"The greatest mistake in the treatment of diseases is that there are physicians for the body and physicians for the soul, although the two cannot be separated." —Plato

"One can ascend to a higher development only by bringing rhythm and repetition into one's life. Rhythm holds sway in all nature." —Rudolf Steiner

Mistletoe both facilitates and is synergistic with other treatments, often enhancing their effects or mitigating side effects. In the next two chapters we'll look at therapies often paired with mistletoe, beginning with a focus on anthroposophic preparations that both treat cancer and support the many physical and emotional symptoms that appear with cancer.

Of the many anthroposophic medicine (AM) remedies that we use alongside mistletoe, perhaps one of the most striking is *Helleborus niger*. Mistletoe and *Helleborus niger* have several intriguing similarities and differences when the two are compared. The helleborus plant is a winter-blooming perennial evergreen. It grows in northern climates and presents with dark green pedate leaves (fanned outward from a common center). The leaf stalks grow low to the ground and look almost tropical. The plant is eye-catching, and yet holds such a low profile that you might miss it if you weren't looking for it. The large white or pink bell-shaped flowers bloom early in spring, often when snow is still present. In climates that don't experience heavy snowfall, the blooms can appear in November or December, resulting in the plant's common name: the Christmas Rose.

Helleborus niger, like mistletoe, follows its own natural rhythm, blooming in the winter or very early spring. They have that independent quality in common, but the two plants also have some intriguing polarities (contrasts). Those polarities become more apparent when looking at them as anthroposophic remedies. Mistletoe and helleborus are well-suited adjuvants (additional supportive therapies). They tend to balance each other, with mistletoe containing more inflammatory constituents and helleborus containing more anti-inflammatory properties. In this chapter, we'll look closely at *Helleborus niger,* then we'll define several other anthroposophic therapies commonly used alongside mistletoe.

Introduction to Helleborus niger: The most common AM adjuvant paired with mistletoe therapy

Helleborus has a vast herbal medicine history and was already known at the time of Hippocrates (460–370 BCE) as a remedy for certain psychiatric conditions.[1] It was used throughout early Greek, Roman, and European medical traditions for such conditions and to treat seizures, dementia, and inflammation.[2] Roman politicians used *Helleborus niger* for cognitive enhancement, to "stimulate quick-witted thinking" before debates and speeches.[3] Through the centuries, early physicians often noted the importance of dosage when administering helleborus. Like any powerful medicine, small amounts could have profoundly beneficial effects, but too much could aggravate the original condition or cause toxicity.[4,5]

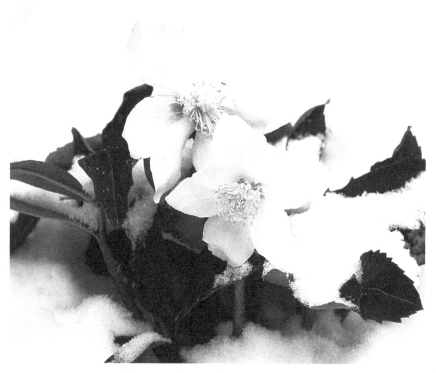

*Helleborus is known for its unique quality
of blooming in the winter months.*

Administering helleborus in cancer care dates back to the Middle Ages in Europe.[6,7] It can also be found in traditional Islamic medicine.[8,9] Samuel Hahnemann (1755–1843), the founder of homeopathy, focused on *Helleborus niger* for his postdoctoral thesis in 1812,[10] summarizing its many historic uses. Rudolf Steiner, the co-founder of anthroposophic medicine, would have been aware of the history of helleborus when he recommended it as a complement to mistletoe therapy.[11]

As noted earlier, *Helleborus niger* and mistletoe possess several interesting similarities and differences. Both are metabolically active in the wintertime, with helleborus blooming and mistletoe fruiting in winter. This striking independent nature is referred to as *temporal autonomy*. These two plants are independent from common flowering and fruiting rhythms in nature. Both plants develop slowly, coming back year after year as long-lived perennials. When AM practitioners see sturdy, independent, well-centered plants like this, they regard them as potentially strong remedies for both immune and physiological regulation (see chapters 6 and 7). Such plants enhance self-regulation within the body.[12,13] This intuitively forecasted benefit has scientific support. *Helleborus niger,* like mistletoe, has been found to contain substances that positively affect cognitive and mental health, improve focus, and encourage a sense of wellbeing.[14]

The contrasts between helleborus and mistletoe speak to their therapeutic qualities. Most plants have a clear earth-to-sun orientation, but mistletoe forms a sphere, which is not oriented toward gravity or the sun. In contrast, helleborus has strong roots with a normal relationship to gravity, the sun, and upward growth. The lectin content (a strong anti-cancer substance) is high in mistletoe, while there are few to no lectins in helleborus. Mistletoe is well-known for its strong warming or inflammatory effect (cytokine release). Meanwhile, *Helleborus niger* is anti-inflammatory, containing compounds known to decrease cytokine levels.[15,16] So both remedies are immunomodulatory, but in different polarities. It could be said that while mistletoe enhances healthy inflammation and immune activity, helleborus brings structure to that activity.

In cancer care, we most often administer helleborus as a complement to mistletoe. Because of their contrasting polarities, they are most often administered at different times of the day or on different days altogether. Then they are free to complement, instead of negate, each other's effects. There are also situations, such as leukemia or complex brain tumors, in which *Helleborus niger* is used in lieu of mistletoe.

Lab research: Helleborus actives and effects

Early anthroposophic uses of helleborus relied more on careful observation, case studies, and herbal traditions. Currently, the research on *Helleborus niger* is growing but still limited. There are several compelling studies that have identified key actions and immune system effects. Its constituents include beta-ecdysones,

	Mistletoe	Helleborus
Similarities	Temporal autonomy (winter blooming)	
	Slow development, long lifespan	
	Suppressed vitality	
Differences – Botanical	Roots and plant not oriented toward gravity or light	Roots and plant oriented toward gravity and sun
	Centripetal (inward) orientation	Centrifugal (outward) orientation
	Leaves undifferentiated (same on top and bottom)	Leaves with normal differentiation
	Fruit is the most therapeutic plant part	Flower and leaves are the most therapeutic plant part
	Warmth oriented	Light oriented
Differences – Therapeutic Effects	Warming, metabolism-boosting, fever-inducing	Cooling, forming, anti-inflammatory effects(19)
	Promotes initial cytokine release (prompts healthy acute inflammation)(17)	Decreases pro-inflammatory substances (mitigates chronic inflammation)(20)
	Lectins (in very high doses) cause hemagglutination (clumping, centripetal action)(18)	Saponins (in very high doses) cause hemolysis (centrifugal dispersal)(21)
Differences – Homeopathic Principles(22)	Dominant Phosphorus Principle	Dominant Sal Principle
	Connection with organs in the lower part of body	Connection with upper organs (lungs, brain)
	Glycoproteins connect with the I-organization	Saponins (i.e. steroids) connect with astral forces (soul, consciousness)
	Addresses sclerotic (hardening) conditions	Addresses chronic inflammatory conditions

Table 8.1: Viscum album *and* Helleborus niger: *Similarities and differences (Compiled by Dr. Steven Johnson, based on manufacturer materials, general anthroposophic principles, and clinical observation)*

which appear to induce *apoptosis* (normal cell death) in lymphoma cells and are cytotoxic to Molt4-leukemia cells.[23] These beta-ecdysones are also likely responsible for anti-epileptic effects and cognitive health benefits.[24] Other compounds appear to convey additional cytotoxic effects in cancer cells.[25,26] Yet more benefits include diuretic and expectorant effects,[27] which are beneficial to mitigate common side effects of some cancers.

Small studies have found that *Helleborus niger* can increase healthy lymphocyte proliferation.[28] It also conveys a dose-dependent suppression of TH-1-associated pro-inflammatory cytokines (an anti-inflammatory effect).[29] It does not alter the activity of CD cells or alter the activity of neutrophils.[30] Again, it's immunomodulatory, but generally modulating in a different direction from mistletoe.

Studies have looked specifically at *Helleborus niger*-induced apoptosis of lymphoma cells and have found a dose-dependent response— the greater the dose, the greater the cell death in the cancer cells.[31] In 2010, Filderklinik in Germany looked more closely at this effect and found that while apoptosis increased in cancerous cells, healthy lymphocytes were not affected.[32] So, at least in small *in vitro* studies, it seems that *Helleborus niger* can induce apoptosis in cancer cells, while not harming healthy immune cells. These studies are too small to fully evaluate *Helleborus niger* as a remedy. One hopes more studies will appear in the future.

We use *Helleborus niger* in many different homeopathic potencies and strengths, depending on the medical condition. These potencies are often alternated according to the intention of the practicing clinician. *Helleborus niger* is available in ampules and oral forms. There are also several combination helleborus remedies, which I formulated and are now offered by Uriel Pharmacy (see table 8.4, page 174). These "Comps" combine *Helleborus niger* with other adjuvant remedies that are supportive for specific stages of cancer and symptoms commonly encountered. I formulated these comp remedies based on common anthroposophic treatment principals in 2019, and early reports are encouraging.

Most common Helleborus niger indications in anthroposophic cancer care

When discussing clinical observations with my European colleagues, I find that *Helleborus niger* is used most frequently in cases of lymphoma, leukemia, myeloma, sarcoma, and prostate cancer. We tend to recommend helleborus in a broader range of cancers when there are metastatic complications such as edema of the legs, lungs, or brain.

Helleborus Consideration	Findings
Observed clinical effects	Anti-inflammatory, antioedematous (edema preventive), diuretic, immunomodulatory, psychologic stabilization, roboration (general strengthening), tumor inhibition
	Via inhalation therapy: broncho-spasmolytic, inhibition of hemoptysis, mitigation of tickling in throat, mucolytic
Contraindications	None, apart from avoidance during pregnancy or lactation.
Adverse drug reactions	Rarely transient redness at subcutaneous injection site, sometimes accompanied by slight itching/burning
Helleborus Constituents	**Pharmacological Effects**
β-Ecdysone (structurally related to plant steroids, androgens, sitosterone)	Cytotoxicity toward Molt4-leukemia cells
	Apoptosis induction in lymphoma cells
	Differentiation, regeneration of nerve and glia cells
	Antiepileptic
	Anxiolytic (anxiety mitigation)(34)
Macranthoside 1 (steroidal saponin)	Diuretic, expectorant
	Anti-inflammatory
	Emmenagogic (promotes menstruation)
Protoanemonin	Cytotoxic (inhibits mitosis) toward cancer cells(35,36)
Total aqueous extract	Immunomodulation (proliferation of lymphocytes, suppression of Th1-associated cytokines)(37)
	Anti-inflammatory, anti-rheumatic(38)

Table 8.2: Considerations and botanical constituents of Helleborus niger[33]

Helleborus Indication	Potency	Administration Method
Advanced cancer with marked inflammation	D12 – D3	1 ampule (amp) subcutaneous (SC), 3x/week
Anxiety, agitated depression in patients with cancer	D6	1 amp SC, 3x/week
Brain tumors or metastases	D12 – D3	1 amp SC or IV infusion (in 100 ml physiol. saline), 3x/week
Cachexia, tumor fever	D12 – D6	1 amp SC or IV, 3x/week
Dry cough (in lung cancer or metastases)	D6 – D3	Inhalation therapy, 1x/day (or IV* 3x/week to up to 1x/day)
Edema (brain), effusions	D12 – D3	1 amp SC or IV, 3x/week (up to 1x/day)
Impaired memory/concentration after brain irradiation	D4 – D3	1 amp SC, 3x/week
Kaposi's sarcoma	D6 – D3	1 amp peritumorally, 2-3x/week
Malignant lymphoma, multiple myeloma	D12 – D6	1 amp SC or IV, 3x/week
Prostate cancer	D6 – D3	1 amp SC, 3x/week

Table 8.3: Common applications of Helleborus niger
*(clinical guidance adapted from observations
published by Debus*[39] *and Schnürer*[40]*)*

Because of the cognitive and mental health benefits, it's also used with any cancer patient who is struggling with significant anxiety or depression or is dealing with "chemo-brain," which manifests as problems with concentration and mental focus after treatment. Such brain fog can also happen after radiation or hormone treatments. *Helleborus niger* is a well tolerated, gentle adjuvant with few to no contraindications, apart from avoiding it during pregnancy and lactation. When used in a potency below D3, careful clinical observation is needed. Remember, the lower the homeopathic potency number, the higher the concentration of botanical compounds. Most clinical observations regarding *Helleborus niger* come from European cancer clinics.

Lymphoma

With all lymphoma treatment strategies, *Helleborus niger* may be used either alone or with mistletoe. It is a good alternative to mistletoe therapy when the patient may be too weak or sensitive to handle the inflammatory effects of mistletoe. When *Helleborus niger* is paired with mistletoe to address the effects of lymphoma, typically Helixor® A or P, Iscador® P, or AbnobaViscum® Fraxini are used. These are the most researched mistletoe options in this situation. Lymphoma is a common condition in which *Helleborus niger* has proven itself useful (see chapter 10).[41]

Helleborus niger may be used at D3, D4, D6 to D12 potencies, as daily subcutaneous (SC) injections for a few weeks, and then dropped down to two or three times per week. My European colleagues have found this safe and beneficial during CHOP chemotherapy protocols, including immunotherapy with Rituxan. Often, we hold off on mistletoe therapy while a patient is on Rituxan or provide it only in very low doses while observing the effect on cell counts. In some of the established European clinics high-dose fever-inducing mistletoe has been used, but this is experimental and requires a well-controlled hospital or in-patient clinical setting.

For patients who have lymphoma, there are many anthroposophic homeopathic remedies that have been found to be clinically useful in European hospitals and private practice. A few examples include homeopathic Plumbum, Stibium, or Vitis Stibium tablets (available through Uriel and Weleda Pharmacy). Such remedies send a modulating signal to the body, which dampens cell proliferation and metastasis, while strengthening immune function.[42] Archangelica ointment applied to lymph nodes several times per day can also be comforting and supportive for sore or congested lymphatics. Usually, these natural substances are integrated with conventional treatments and other natural remedies. These remedies are just a sampling of what anthroposophic practices regularly apply.

One of the most beneficial integrative treatments that I've seen in lymphoma cases is *medical hyperthermia*.[43] This is approved only in Europe right now, with the exception of a medical trial. Several clinics have demonstrated positive results. Hyperthermia has a long history of exploration with many positive outcomes, but it has yet to be seriously studied.

Brain tumors and brain edema

European practitioners have noted that *Helleborus niger* can be useful in caring for patients who have brain cancer and brain metastasis. It may help with edema.[44] These physicians find that boswellia, along with *Helleborus niger*, potentially mitigates mild brain edema (swelling). More studies are needed to explore this possibility. These two substances can be provided alongside mistletoe to lessen mistletoe's potential inflammatory effects. This strategy can lessen the potential for brain edema (see chapter 10). This is not always effective, and steroids are often still needed.[45]

When mistletoe is used for brain tumors, usually Helixor A is the safest way to initiate therapy, and then other host trees may be considered based on the clinician's training and expertise. However, it's important to note that, in cases of severe brain edema, mistletoe therapy may not be indicated. A monotherapy of *Helleborus niger* may be considered instead. Anthroposophic care is always individualized. In the hands of a well-trained clinician, treatment will often impart a sense of wellbeing and resistance to common complications.

Lung cancer

Currently there is some case study evidence of non-small cell lung cancer (NSCLC) responding to *Helleborus niger* and mistletoe combination therapy. A case study of malignant pleural mesothelioma (MPM) was also recently published, in which SC and IV mistletoe were alternated with *Helleborus niger* injections, resulting in a 38-month partial regression and 56 months survival.[46] This is an extremely aggressive cancer and, in this situation, the patient had refused all other conventional therapies.

A few anthroposophic hospitals provide nebulized *Helleborus niger* as an experimental therapy for *hemoptysis* (coughing up blood) and shortness of breath. Early reports are positive, but we are still awaiting published case reports or clinical studies for this off label use.[47] *Helleborus niger* D12 or D6 is added to a nebulizer (diluted with 0.9 percent sodium chloride and filled to 5 mL) and inhaled for 15 minutes, one to three times daily. I have seen this provide significant relief for mucous plugging, as well as for hemoptysis (coughing up blood), in patients who are challenged with *pleural effusion* (water on the lungs), and in cases of severe congestion. The earlier this is started the better, and the results are improved with adjuvant treatments. At this point, this therapeutic technique is based on clinical observation only.

Concomitant (associated) conditions

Managing lymphatic congestion can be a major issue with many cancers. Any time there's a need to enhance lymphatic drainage, helleborus can be provided along with other common natural remedies including diuretic teas, dandelion, nettles, green tea, and borage. These are good adjuvants to lymphatic massage. Lymphatic edema may be addressed with Uriel's Borago Venous Leg Gel. The Venous Leg Gel ingredients include borage, witch hazel, horse chestnut, and several other botanicals.[48] This is gently massaged into the affected area several times a day. My patients have found the combination of *Helleborus niger* and this topical product to be effective.

Helleborus is also beneficial in providing mild mental health benefits.[49] When patients are dealing with serious anxiety, I will start them with one ampule daily of *Helleborus niger* D6 or D12, depending on symptom severity. Helleborus Comp E, available through Uriel Pharmacy, is also a good possibility. I often pair *Helleborus niger* with other common natural remedies such as valerian, passionflower, melatonin, L-theanine, L-tryptophan or 5-HTP, St. John's wort, and SAM-e, as indicated by their metabolic type and tolerances. This requires a solid educational background in metabolic or functional medicine to make appropriate recommendations. In the future, genomic testing may also help with making these selections.

Helleborus niger also works well with other anthroposophic homeopathic remedies for depression and anxiety. In anthroposophic clinics, a small sample of common remedies are:

- Magnesium Phosphoricum (4x to 30x)
- Bryophyllum argentum (3x, 2x)
- Bryophyllum (1%, 5%, and 10%)
- Alternating low- and high-dose phosphorus (6x and 30x).

St. John's Wort, also referred to as *Hypericum* (a primary active in St. John's Wort), is commonly provided as an anthroposophic medical therapy. There are several specially prepared pharmaceutical preparations of St. John's Wort, alone and in combinations, which we find very helpful. Again, this is just a sampling of possible approaches. This type of care is highly personalized and requires a diagnosis from a well-trained physician.

Many European clinicians are experimenting with providing *Helleborus niger* for its anti-inflammatory properties in arthritis and autoimmune conditions. They typically provide SC injections of *Helleborus niger* D3 to D6. I have had some similar success in providing *Helleborus niger* as a treatment for Lyme disease symptoms, specifically after the disease has progressed into its chronic autoimmune phase. These situations are not directly related to cancer care, but we do see an increase in autoimmune disorders (such as RA) in patients who have cancer or are cancer survivors. It is helpful to know that the immuno-modulatory effects of *Helleborus niger* can potentially provide support both during an active cancer process and for autoimmune conditions too. The anti-inflammatory and immune-modulating quality of *Helleborus niger* makes it especially appropriate for cancer patients who are at risk for autoimmunity.[50]

Tumor types and patient constitution:
Evaluating indications from an anthroposophic perspective

While it's useful to provide a straightforward list of *Helleborus niger* indications, it's even more empowering to evaluate helleborus with a constitutional lens—looking at the gesture of the medicine and then matching that gesture to certain disease processes or the constitutional typology of an individual patient. This helps both patients and practitioners come to a deeper appreciation of the treatment and how it might be applied in situations not covered in this book. Similar to Ayurvedic and traditional Chinese medicine, anthroposophic medicine is not oriented only toward a clinical diagnosis, but also toward individual qualities, constitutional typologies, and tendencies we observe in people on physical, mental, and spiritual–creative levels.

In general, *Helleborus niger* is recommended in cancer cases where there is a strong *centrifugal* (spreading) tendency such as acute leukemia and lymphoma.[51] It's also used when a patient has myeloma or any cancers connected with the reproductive organs, lungs, or brain. We use *Helleborus niger* when tumor cells are metastasizing. Because of its cooling anti-inflammatory quality, *Helleborus niger* is especially valuable for advanced stages of cancer or when there are concerns about recurrence.[52]

When matching a patient's constitution to helleborus, there are certain qualities we observe. On a constitutional level, we look for signs of inflammation such as swollen or warm joints, fever, edema, or other signs mentioned throughout this chapter already. Helleborus patients often struggle with an agitated depression. They can be very anxious and might even be in a state of persistent shock and disassociation. This may be from the trauma of facing their illness or from a residual longstanding past trauma, or both. Trouble concentrating and scattered thoughts are other possible indications.[53] Helleborus also speaks strongly to the male constitution and has connections to the human reproductive organs. When the constitution of a patient reveals these signs, we often see stronger therapeutic responses to *Helleborus niger*. This is the art of medicine often lost in modern cancer care. There are strong connections between nature and the human being, and if we listen, many insights reveal themselves and can later find correlation through scientific evaluation.

Other common adjuvants in AM cancer care

Integrative–anthroposophic cancer care providers often recommend several other botanicals and remedies. The following will not provide an exhaustive list and shouldn't be regarded as treatment guidance. Rather the goal is to share a holistic paradigm shift, viewing multiple adjuvant treatments as an extension of conventional oncology. The goal of anthroposophic and integrative health should never be to antagonize modern medicine, *but rather to extend and humanize it.* The two branches need to become one approach to health. Like deciding on mistletoe host trees, selection of adjuvant treatments can be informed by an anthroposophic-holistic picture of the human being, as well as the scientific evaluation of chemical constituents.

AM practitioners often provide other natural remedies that would be familiar to naturopathic doctors and integrative physicians. Dr. Winters will touch on some of them in the next chapter on integrative oncology. But there are also several uniquely anthroposophic remedies that probably aren't as familiar to anyone outside the AM world. Let's learn more about those.

Anthroposophic homeopathy

Anthroposophic practitioners use unique homeopathic plant and mineral preparations. Generally speaking, anthroposophic homeopathy uses lower potencies than those found in classical homeopathy. Each AM remedy is prescribed based on an understanding of how the substance relates to particular organs and physiological processes, as well as the threefold and fourfold understandings of the human organism (see chapters 6 and 7). To be clear, mistletoe therapy may be used alongside classical homeopathy or AM homeopathy.

Below I will present just a few examples of the more common AM remedies I like to use, to show how we might begin extending modern medicine and integrative oncology. Again, these medical traditions are at their best when they work alongside each other. Anthroposophic medicine is a highly individualized practice requiring extensive training and experience. Different remedies take on a different level of importance and application, depending on the clinical and biographical situation of the patient. Refer to the "Resources" section for more anthroposophic texts.

> *Astragalus Formica:* Astragalus supports immune function and has also been studied for anti-tumor effects and its ability to mitigate fatigue.[54] Formica supports excretion (detoxification) and ultimately promotes rejuvenation.[55] Both these remedies are often used in combination with other synergistic remedies.

> *Aurum (Homeopathic Gold):* Aurum supports regulation of the autonomic nervous system (ANS) and can be stabilizing for depressed mood and sadness.[56] It can be helpful in cancer treatment, because it strengthens the "I"-organization, a key to health in AM. I often regard it as useful for encouraging personal growth and helping a person step toward a new life situation. Aurum is used in many combination remedies. I particularly recommend Uriel Pharmacy's Aurum Lavender Rose cream. This provides Aurum with rose oil, and other botanicals, including frankincense and myrrh. It is calming, relieving anxiety and nervousness. A company called Weleda also makes a wonderful

remedy called Aurum/Cardiodoron, which is very helpful to support circulation during times of stress.

Bryophyllum (Mother of Thousands): When patients have symptoms of anxiety or nervousness, I often suggest bryophyllum. Commonly known as Mother-of-Thousands, this succulent plant grows hundreds of tiny new plants around the rim of each of its adult leaves. It conveys this strong regenerative process when taken as a remedy. It's also useful when a patient is severely traumatized, perhaps to the point of exhaustion. Bryophyllum comes in many combination forms and is fairly unique to AM.[57]

Carbo Betulae or Carbo Chamomilla: Carbo *Betulae* is helpful for addressing GI issues, including mucosal inflammation, diarrhea, and sugar cravings.[58] Often chemotherapy, radiation and the stress of illness can weaken or inflame the lining of the GI tract. In my own clinical practice, Carbo *Chamomilla* has been helpful with addressing heartburn, leaky-gut, colitis, or irritable bowel, which often occur during chronic illness. From an AM perspective, Carbo *Betulae* also supports the "inner breathing process," strengthening the internal breathing rhythm needed for inner stability.

Hepatodoron and Vitis Stibium: Crafted from grape and wild strawberry leaves, it is a longstanding observation of AM physicians that Hepatodoron (Weleda) and Vitis Stibium (Uriel Pharmacy) help with liver support and healthy sugar and glycogen metabolism. They also encourage healthy sleep cycles, which are vital to regain self-regulation in the body. From an AM perspective, homeopathic stibium brings a formative element into the metabolism, which is helpful to encourage stability and prevent the cellular proliferation seen in tumor growth.

Borago Venous Leg Gel: A topically applied, borage-based gel, especially effective for leg edema (and general lymphedema).[59] This is appreciated especially by many patients with varicosities or poor lymph drainage. It is so important to stimulate venous return, in order to support whole health. This remedy brings form to "fluid" or "vital" processes. Those Etheric Processes (see chapters 6 and 7) need to be contained and are part of the constitutional cancer picture in AM.

Anthroposophic organ preparations, homeopathic metals, and comps

In the world of AM cancer care, physicians have historically pre-scribed homeopathic organ preparations and homeopathic metals. Most AM physicians still recommend potentized organ preparations associated with the organ of tumor origin. For instance, we would pre-scribe Prostata GI 8X for prostate cancer. We may also provide organ preparations for any organ where metastasis has occurred or is likely to occur. In addition to organ preparations, there is a long history of providing specific homeopathic metals along with mistletoe therapy. Some preparations of Iscador mistletoe are provided with the metals already added to the extract. Some AM physicians still provide one of the four traditionally added homeopathic metals alongside mistletoe therapy: *mercurius vivus* (mercury), *argentum* (silver), *cuprum* (cop-per), *or stannum* (tin). The metal used depends on the organ of tumor origin. As homeopathic remedies, actual concentrations of these metals are so low that toxicity is not an issue. Rather the homeopathic dosage encourages or "signals" the body toward a particular balance. All these principals are taught within anthroposophic medicine training.[60,61]

Helleborus Comp	Condition	Homeopathic Constituents
Helleborus Comp A	Chronic lymphoma and leukemia	Ampules: Helleborus 2X, Arsenicum alb. 17X, Plumbum silicium 20X, Argentum met. 8X, Stibium 6X, Phosphorus 12X, and Formica 6X.
Helleborus Comp B	Acute lymphoma and leukemia	Ampules: Helleborus 4x, Argentum met 17X, Phosphorus 30X, Formica 20X, Lien 8X, Plumbum met. 30X, Colchicum planta tot. 4X, Equesetum 20X
Helleborus Comp C	Solid tumors with metastases	Ampules: Helleborus 12X, Lien 8X, Plumbum met. 30X, Formica 6X, Stibium 12X, Argentum 20X, Cheledonium pt.

Table 8.4: Helleborus niger compound products (comps)
(data courtesy Uriel Pharmacy, 2020)

Uriel Pharmacy provides five "Helleborus Comps" formulated with specific conditions in mind. The three comps in table 8.4 combine *Helleborus niger* with other appropriate adjuvant homeopathic remedies, many of which we have discussed in this chapter. They are provided in ampules, which may be administered via subcutaneous injection or taken as an oral sublingual, held under the tongue.

AM care for the individual soul and spirit

In the U.S., looking at the human being as having a spirit, soul, and physical body is too often relegated to a realm of "nice but not scientific or practical." The word *spiritual* has become taboo for many modern people. These misunderstandings are unfortunate. Some clarification seems necessary. The word *soul* refers to our capacity for different levels of consciousness and feeling. Healing of the spirit refers to recognizing the individual person—their creativity, potential, and goals. Having goals and inspirations can be key to overcoming cancer and coping with it. Read any cancer survivor's story, or reflect on you own, and the importance of acknowledging the "whole person" becomes self-evident.

In European anthroposophic care, therapies which support the soul and spirit are regularly integrated with conventional treatments, herbal and nutritional remedies, and homeopathy. In some cancer clinics, special nursing care and creative therapies such as eurythmy (movement therapy), art therapy, speech therapy, and biography work are seen as pivotal for the overall success of a treatment program. Indeed, how can a cancer survivor begin the hard work of reinventing their lives if they have not nourished their soul and spirit to gain new inspiration for the future? AM cancer care prescribes these soul- and spirit-nurturing therapies as part of a complete and humanizing treatment strategy.[62]

> *Art and Music Therapies:* Focused on deep abstract expression through basic forms and colors or simple melodies and harmonic sound (as opposed to classes on specific painting or musical techniques). Helps the patient enliven their astral forces and empowers their creativity and trouble-shooting abilities.

> *Biography Work:* Asks patients to write about key moments in their life stories. Focused on pattern- and purpose-finding, as well as therapeutic expression. Helps patients rediscover their current situation as one moment within a larger, whole narrative.

Eurythmy: Supports the etheric body through therapeutic, rhythmic movements. Helps restore the body's sense of rhythm in all its processes. Qigong and tai chi are practices with similar benefits.

Therapeutic Speech: Differs from conventional definition of "speech therapy." Anthroposophic therapeutic speech focuses specifically on the power of language, using the spoken word in an artistic way. Highly effective for patients who do not feel grounded, helps them come back inside themselves.

Rhythmical Massage: Provided by rhythmical massage therapists and anthroposophic nurses to increase circulation and warmth, as well as retrain the body to inhabit its own sense of rhythm. Similar to gentle lymphatic massage, which is commonly provided for patients with cancer in the U.S.

In addition to artistic therapies, specially trained anthroposophic nurses provide warming compresses and special body treatments. They work very consciously with specific soul gestures for comfort and healing. Compresses and nursing treatments enhance warmth and a sense of wellbeing, often reducing pain and stress. Anthroposophic nursing holds to the tenet that patient care is an art. When a person experiences true loving care it awakens their potential to heal. The holistic nurse is often the person who recognizes what is the most important need for the patient in any given moment.[63]

Wise remedy selection: Allowing the patient lead the treatment

After the shock of initial diagnosis, patients often experience the secondary shock of learning about the entire field of treatment options, both conventional and integrative. The list of recommendations can become an additional burden. For patients, when choosing to include holistic treatment options, it is important to find a knowledgeable practitioner who can assist as a guide, discerning which modalities are best.

I have had patients come to me so excited about mistletoe, that they commit to using mistletoe therapy alone. They don't always get the same results as those who use mistletoe in wise combination with other adjuvants or the insights of metabolic medicine, like that practiced by Dr. Winters (see chapters 5 and 9). Of course, there are exceptions, and I have seen good results with an appropriate diet, conventional therapy, and mistletoe alone in motivated patients who find and cultivate their own *salutogenic* (health-building) approach.

I've heard a saying that a house can be built well and made beautifully, and yet be built with many different techniques to achieve the same goal. I think this applies to integrative and metabolic medicine as well. We have such wide-ranging therapeutic tools today. Thankfully we also have the ability to evaluate and choose the best methods for each patient. Anthroposophic and integrative practitioners can learn a lot from modern medicine, and conventional practitioners can glean much from our practices, too. There is a balance to be found that is unique to each person, in terms of nutrition, lab evaluation, diagnostic techniques, natural and conventional treatments, and other therapeutic interventions. The secret and sign of a good practitioner is that they are always seeking out this balance for each patient as an individual. The best practitioners recognize that comprehensive healing is that which takes place on the level of spirit, soul, and body.

CASE STORY ONE: DEBRA

Caring for Anxiety, Opening Treatment Doors				
Physician: Dr. Steven Johnson	**Patient**: Debra	**First seen**: Sept. 2019	**Age:** 58	**Sex:** Female
Cancer Type & Stage:	Stage III, right-sided breast cancer (ER+ PR+, HER2-negative). Severe anxiety and panic attacks, reducing ability to complete both conventional and integrative/anthroposophic treatment plans.			

Debra was a 58-year-old woman who frequently experienced anxiety and panic attacks during IV chemotherapy, mistletoe injections, or any minor invasive procedure. Any time such a procedure began, she would sweat, her hands shook, she experienced heart palpitations, and she had a severe sense of doom and foreboding. Debra had fainted in the recent past during a routine blood draw, which led to a hypoxic seizure.

This challenge with her panic attacks became so extreme that it affected her treatment choices. Debra told me she had refused further IV chemotherapy because of her severe symptoms. She certainly questioned whether she could administer the subcutaneous mistletoe injections that I had recommended. It was clear her anxiety had become life-limiting. We had to address this before she could continue any other treatment options for her breast cancer.

First, I recommended an anthroposophic remedy called bryophyllum (5% liquid), advising her to take it three times daily on days that she was scheduled for an anxiety-triggering procedure. One of those doses would be in the morning and another timed thirty minutes before the procedure. Bryophyllum is a unique remedy that is used in Ayurvedic medicine as well. It is very helpful for fresh traumatic anxiety. It also helps patients change repeated patterns of anxiety and panic. I taught Debra some deep breathing exercises, and we worked on meditations intended to help her center herself and become more in control of her behaviors and reactions to situations that scared or traumatized her.

Debra felt empowered enough that she decided to try this approach in an attempt to resume chemotherapy. She always took the Bryophyllum 5% Liquid a few minutes before her IV chemotherapy, as well as taking the remedy three times daily on non-IV days. Her IV nurse also allowed her to bring a tube of Aurum Lavender Rose Cream (Uriel Pharmacy), which she rubbed onto her chest before and during the IV. This cream contains many essential oils, including lavender, rose, and geranium. It also contains homeopathic gold, boswellia, myrrh, peat moss, and Saint John's Wort. Debra was also given a warm hot water bottle and a flannel sheet to wrap over her chest over the application of the cream. Debra repeated this calming cream application and mild warming therapy at home when self-administering her mistletoe injections. She practiced her breathing and centering meditations prior to her procedures.

Debra reported to me that her symptoms and anxiety gradually reduced over one week. She was able to complete her course of chemotherapy for her breast cancer and continued with the self-administered mistletoe injections. The fainting spells and severe panic reactions ceased entirely. As she repeated these procedures successfully, her confidence grew. Over time, all her remaining panic symptoms became less of an issue. Her anxiety in general also lessened dramatically. Debra is currently doing well, and her cancer is in remission.

CASE STORY TWO: BOB

Multiple Adjuvant Synergies for Treatment-failed Lung Cancer (NSCL)				
Physician: Dr. Steven Johnson	**Patient:** Bob	**First seen:** June 2017	**Age:** 54	**Sex:** Male
Cancer Type & Stage:	Non-small cell lung cancer. Stage IV, adenocarcinoma of the lung (pT4N2M1a), EGFR/RAS/ALK negative. Failed standard of care (SOC) chemotherapy.			
Risk Factors:	Smoker and poor diet primarily consisting of fast food and processed foods. No prior inclination toward preventive health.			

When Bob came to me, he'd already completed five cycles of chemotherapy (carboplatin/taxol x3, then carboplatin/pemetrexed x2) for his Stage IV, non-small cell lung cancer (NSCLC). Unfortunately, scans showed continued progression. Remissions are rare in NSCLC. Bob made an informed decision to stop further chemotherapy and initiated complementary medical care options.

Bob had no prior knowledge of, or affinity for, natural or holistic medicine. His diet was horrible, primarily fast food and processed foods. He didn't significantly change his diet during his treatment, despite many well-intentioned efforts. However, Bob believed strongly that he could get better, and he was fully dedicated to all the other components of his integrative treatment plan.

I recommended high-dose intravenous vitamin C (IVC 75 g, three times per week) and subcutaneous (SC) mistletoe injections every other day. The IVC was administered over a cycle of eight weeks, followed by a protocol of IV mistletoe twice weekly for eight weeks. This cycle was repeated twice before my colleagues and I reported on the case. Bob was also closely followed by his conventional oncologist during the entirety of the process.

I provided several other supportive nutritional supplements and anthroposophic remedies along with the primary SC and IV treatments. This included homeopathic stibium, plumbum, formica, and liver remedies. Bob also took several naturopathic supplements including boswellia, quercetin, and green tea extract, which he took consistently throughout his therapy course.

Because his case was advanced, Bob also struggled with a severe cough, shortness of breath, severely reduced exercise tolerance, and frequent hemoptysis (coughing up blood). He agreed to an experimental protocol with nebulized *Helleborus niger* D12, daily for eight weeks. Bob's cough, wheezing, and hemoptysis resolved over six weeks. After eight weeks, he transitioned from the nebulized treatment to continued oral *Helleborus niger*.

It was not fully clear if the *Helleborus niger* treatment contributed to Bob's overall remission, so it was not reported in the originally published version of this case study. However, for my colleagues and me, it was our impression that it played a significant role.

Six months into this non-standard therapy, PET and CT scans showed that Bob had experienced full remission by RECIST (Response Evaluation Criteria in Solid Tumors) standards. There was evidence of decreased FDG activity in the biopsy-proven primary and metastatic sites. A year after being diagnosed with advanced NSCLC, Bob still felt healthy and well.

Bob did not continue follow-up therapy after his remission. He ceased the IV therapies, SC mistletoe, and the other herbal and anthroposophic therapies. We can only assume that his poor diet remained the same. His conventional oncologist reported that Bob was in continued remission for about six months, and then a small recurrence was found.

Regardless, as the original published case study noted, "Whether the initial remission and the surprisingly long PFS [progression-free survival] is due to IV ascorbic acid and/or mistletoe is unknown. A review of the literature reveals reports of similar astonishing clinical results after treatment with either agent."[64] Clinically, I have found there is reliable synergy when IVC, mistletoe, and *Helleborus niger* are provided in strategic rhythms. I continue to use a similar approach for patients with similar cancers. Ideally, they continue ongoing maintenance therapies and sustain their remissions for far longer time periods.

CHAPTER 9

BUILDING THE BRIDGE BETWEEN MISTLETOE AND OTHER INTEGRATIVE THERAPIES

Dr. Nasha Winters, ND, FABNO

Special thanks to Dr. Paul Faust and Dr. Mark Hancock for their contributions to this chapter

"We can all influence the life force. The tools and strategies of healing are so innate, so much a part of a common human birthright, that we believers in technology pay very little attention to them. But they have lost none of their power."
—RACHEL NAOMI REMEN, *Kitchen Table Wisdom*

"Our biological rhythms are the symphony of the cosmos, music embedded deep within us to which we dance, even when we can't name the tune."   —DEEPAK CHOPRA

As we've often mentioned, mistletoe is not typically a stand-alone therapy. It works particularly well when paired with conventional care and other anthroposophic or integrative therapies. The following won't be a comprehensive description of all integrative cancer care modalities. There are many other excellent books that have already tackled that expansive topic; several are listed in the Resources section. Rather, we'll focus on six treatment categories that are both well vetted for cancer care and work exceptionally well alongside mistletoe. When developing this list, we also homed in on therapies that do not negatively affect standard of care (SOC) treatments when administered appropriately. If anything, these therapies enhance SOC and mitigate SOC side effects so that patients can stay the course of their conventional treatment programs.

Let's look first at the current landscape of complementary medicine practices, from which we draw these therapies. Then we'll discuss the therapies themselves and review two detailed case stories. These are patients who especially benefited from the unique synergy that stems from pairing mistletoe with multiple integrative and conventional treatments. The body terrain is multi-faceted, and so successful treatment selection always touches multiple terrain points.

Many streams, one river:
Patients thrive when practitioners work together

In the world of integrative and holistic medicine, practitioners often speak of the "silo-ing" that happens in conventional care. Specialists focus on one body system or one disease niche, and the hundreds of specialists rarely get to speak with each other. It's not their fault; it's just the nature of our current medical system. In contrast, integrative and complementary practitioners strive to observe the whole body and all its intertwined systems before diagnosing and choosing supportive therapies. We have that sense of holism at our core. But even natural health practitioners can become siloed within their own traditions. We shouldn't be so separated. It would be healthier to view all our rich healing traditions as petals on the same lotus flower.

It's very hard on patients when they feel they must keep their care providers away from each other or hide some of their chosen therapies from their conventional practitioners. Indeed, in the U.S., about 80 percent of patients with cancer utilize some form of natural or alternative cancer care each year.[1] Depending on the study, only 30 to 40 percent of these patients tell their conventional oncologist.[2] This is both

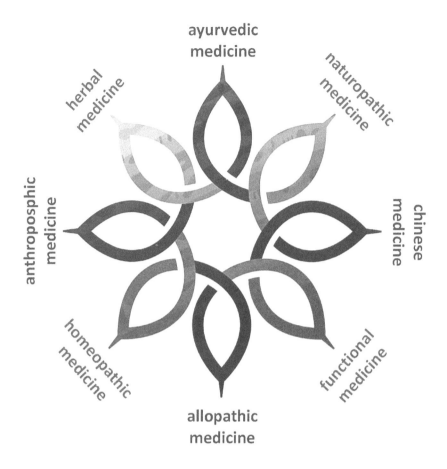

ayurvedic
medicine

naturopathic
medicine

herbal
medicine

anthroposphic
medicine

chinese
medicine

homeopathic
medicine

functional
medicine

allopathic
medicine

stressful and risky. When we all talk to each other, therapies can be timed better for both optimal effects and safety.

Ideally, true integrative oncology draws from all traditions, including SOC, choosing the best treatment options for the specific patient and situation. All our healing arts have something to offer the complex *body-ecosystem.* Just as the body is an ecosystem, where inputs in one space inevitably affect the whole organism, the multiple healing traditions make up a *healthcare ecosystem.* A healthy ecosystem is defined by strong connections between all its components—whether that's a natural landscape or the human body or the entire field of medical arts. Restorative treatment focuses on rebuilding connections. Optimal healthcare (care that *restores health,* as much as it addresses disease) builds and nurtures strong connections, both inside the human body and between multiple healing disciplines and treatment modalities. It's all useful, it's all needed.

Along the way, there's a deep need for all of us to shed war metaphor from our discussions of all diseases, but especially in cancer care. A war on cancer can only become a war on the human body. When we rely solely on a scorched earth treatment approach, it destroys internal body–ecosystem connections. Perhaps, as we replace the war-on-cancer metaphor with a new language of *ecosystem restoration*, we will organically begin to see more interaction between all practitioners of all disciplines.

Mistletoe's companions:
Identifying and defining diverse integrative treatments

If you're a practitioner, depending on your medical art, some of these therapies will be familiar. Some might be new. Some require deep observation and testing before prescribing them for a specific patient. Two of them—*metabolically flexible diets* and *circadian rhythm restoration*—are universal in their application. Implementing some form of both will significantly increase the efficacy of all other therapies, including conventional care and mistletoe. In fact, I consider both to be foundational with all my patients. Without metabolic flexibility and without an intact circadian rhythm, a patient's immune profile will be characterized by systemic chronic inflammation, and that immune profile translates into treatment failure. With my patients, I often refer my own version of the "CDC," which I define as Circadian Rhythm, Diet, and Community. I regard these as foundational cancer care therapies, not just helpful extras.

1. Dietary transformation:
Low-carb, high-fat diets and metabolic flexibility

There are far too many magic-bullet cancer diets! In reality, there are many paths to Rome, and any of these low-carb variations can

Quick Definition	Low- to no-carb eating, emphasizing vegetables and healthy fats. Triggers the body to begin burning fat instead of glucose as its primary energy source.
Best Contexts	ALL patients with cancer (or any other disease state). Foundational prerequisite dietary therapy. Enhances efficacy of all other therapies.
Contraindications or Considerations	No contraindications. A ketogenic diet should be considered therapeutic, followed for a fixed duration of time and under the guidance of a practitioner skilled in teaching its principles and monitoring its effects.
Monitor These Labs	Insulin (preferably under 3), Hemoglobin A1C (under 5), IGF-1 (near 100). *If any of these are elevated, you aren't metabolically flexible yet.* Also track organic acids profiles; diet diaries and macronutrient counters; and blood, urine, and breath ketone levels.
Affects these Terrain Elements	ALL, but especially Metabolic Function, Inflammation and Hormone Balance

be successful: low-carb vegetarian, ketogenic (high-fat, some protein, no carbs), paleo (veggies, fruit, eggs, and meat), carnivore (all protein), and intermittent fasting. Yes, all of us benefit from incorporating way more vegetables into our diets—ideally at least half of every meal should be non-starchy veggies. We also need some animal-derived proteins, even if they qualify as vegetarian (pastured organic eggs; high-quality, organic, full-fat dairy). In the simplest terms, the best diet is, most importantly, the one that the patient will follow! Plus, it needs to:

Consist primarily of vegetables and healthy fats
Qualify as low- or no-carb
Meet the individual needs and constitution of the patient
Respect that when you eat may be just as important as what you
    eat (see the next section on Time Restricted Eating)

What do the successful anti-cancer diets have in common? They all help the body become what's called *metabolically flexible*, or able to burn fat for energy in lieu of glucose.[3] Today, in Western culture especially, we eat a carbohydrate-dominant diet. This has turned us *metabolically inflexible*; we are addicted to fast-burning carbohydrates and have trouble restoring our ancestral fat-burning metabolism. Very few Americans are metabolically flexible anymore—only about 12 percent. That means at least 88 percent of people who have cancer (more likely all!) are metabolically broken.[4]

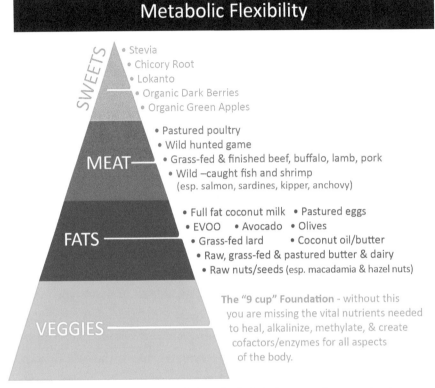

Metabolic Flexibility

SWEETS
- Stevia
- Chicory Root
- Lokanto
- Organic Dark Berries
- Organic Green Apples

MEAT
- Pastured poultry
- Wild hunted game
- Grass-fed & finished beef, buffalo, lamb, pork
- Wild –caught fish and shrimp
(esp. salmon, sardines, kipper, anchovy)

FATS
- Full fat coconut milk • Pastured eggs
- EVOO   • Avocado   • Olives
- Grass-fed lard   • Coconut oil/butter
- Raw, grass-fed & pastured butter & dairy
- Raw nuts/seeds (esp. macadamia & hazel nuts)

VEGGIES

The "9 cup" Foundation - without this you are missing the vital nutrients needed to heal, alkalinize, methylate, & create cofactors/enzymes for all aspects of the body.

3 cups leafy greens: spinach, chard, kale, collards, bok choy, romaine, arugula, etc.
3 cups colorful veggies: onions, garlic, leeks, mushrooms, asparagus, beets, artichokes, etc.
3 cups cruciferous veggies: broccoli, cauliflower, Brussels sprouts, collards, cabbage, kale, etc.
Also, Spices & Herbs: turmeric, garlic, onions, cinnamon, basil, thyme, oregano, coriander, cumin, cayenne, mint, etc.

Thanks to Dr. Terry Wahl's for coining the 9-cup foundation

A revised food pyramid: The best anti-cancer diets begin with removing grains from the foundation of the food pyramid and emphasize non-starchy vegetables and healthy fats instead.

We were all told in school that grains and starch (bread, pasta, rice, potatoes) formed the base of our food pyramid. Just eat healthy whole grains and you're fine, right? Actually, no. This dietary advice, inspired mostly by an emerging grain-based industrial agriculture initiated in the mid 1800's, has turned our bodies into carb-dependent junkies. For nearly 200,000 years, humans were hunter gatherers. Sugary foods (fruit and honey) were an absolute rarity. It was only 10,000 years ago that we became Neolithic farmers, and though we increased our carbo-hydrate intake, we expended a lot of energy to plant, cultivate, harvest, and prepare our foods compared to modern agriculture practices and lifestyles.

Today, even though our lives and environments are massively altered, our bodies haven't changed much. That ancestral diet still matches our cellular metabolism. Our cells know how to thrive on that fuel.[5] Modern foods abound with white sugar and flour, industrial sweeteners, and carbohydrates that break down into yet more sugar. Our cells have turned into hyperactive sugar-burners. This glucose-rich environment is also super friendly to cancer.[6] Our ancestral metabolism prefers to burn fat instead of sugar, but we cannot access that state of *metabolic flexibility* if there is easier-to-burn glucose present in our systems. That's why drastically reducing carbohydrates is the first and primary step toward metabolic flexibility. Turn off the carb faucet, and the body remembers how to burn fat for energy.

You have likely heard of the therapeutic *ketogenic diet*. The ketogenic diet has been found to improve the survival odds in brain cancer. At the time of this book's publication, there were over fifty other clinical trials underway looking at the effects of the therapeutic ketogenic diet on glioblastoma (brain cancer) and several other cancer types.[7,8] Unfortunately, thanks to a swell of misuse and poor description of ketogenic principles in the mass media, there is now a great deal of confusion about what true ketosis is and how to harness it effectively. "Keto" is not an Atkins diet, the focus of which is low-carb, high-protein. Rather, ketogenic eating involves low- to no-carbohydrate eating, with a strong emphasis on *healthy fats*, and not as much emphasis on protein. This diet typically restricts carbohydrates to 20 grams per day and protein to 0.8 grams per kilogram of body weight per day, while fat (healthy, non-inflammatory fats!) makes up over 80 percent of caloric intake. This diet is not easy to follow and takes extensive training and meal planning to do well. However, it is very powerful.

A successful ketogenic diet achieves *ketosis*—the state in which the body is burning fat molecules (ketones) as its primary fuel, instead of sugar. In true ketosis, the body thrives in this state; it is neither in shock nor desperate for a sugar hit. Ketosis, in turn, creates a microenvironment that is neutralizing to aggressive cancers.[9] Ketosis induces several effects simultaneously on immune, metabolic, and genetic aspects of the cancering process:

1. Reduces glucose and insulin
2. Modulates oxidative stress
3. Reduces inflammation
4. Enhances anti-tumor immunity
5. Alters gene expression
6. Sensitizes tumors to SOC treatments and other adjuvant (supportive) therapies[10]

A therapeutic ketogenic diet should be guided by a practitioner specifically trained in implementing and monitoring this medical therapy. It is a challenging therapeutic choice, but transformative in certain cancering processes.

As mentioned earlier, this is not the only dietary path that can restore metabolic flexibility. Really, any diet that keeps carbs below 50 grams per day can guide the body toward ketosis. (We call that low-carb now, but historically 50 grams was normal!) Pairing low-carb with high-fat is even more effective. Low-carb eating paired with a 70 percent good-fat intake will push the body in the direction of the ketogenic diet and its associated benefits. Whatever the specifics of your dietary approach, it is transformative to replace the carbohydrate foundation with a mix of vegetables and healthy fats.

Time-restricted eating as another powerful metabolic tool

It's important to note that time-restricted eating (TRE) can also help the body achieve ketosis. TRE can be as simple as extending your nighttime non-eating period. In fact, simply *not eating for 13 hours or more* on a daily basis is associated with decreased breast cancer recurrence.[11] TRE means, for example, ceasing to consume anything other than water after 7:00 p.m. each night and then eating breakfast at 8:00

a.m. That's it. TRE is powerful because it requires the body to dip into ketosis every day, particularly during some of the most reparative deep sleep time periods in the night. Too many of us snack all the way up till bedtime, resulting in continued overactive glucose-burning throughout the night. The body never gets to enter a deep reparative state. TRE is, by far, one of the easiest dietary and lifestyle choices with quantitative benefit for patients who have cancer. In my own clinical experience, I've seen it enhance the effects of SOC treatments and other integrative therapies alike. If you are a patient who is limited in how many therapies you can pursue, mistletoe therapy and fasting are an especially effective and simple combination.[12]

Whatever the dietary path, restoring metabolic flexibility is crucial. I no longer work with patients if they want to use mistletoe but continue eating from the drive-through. It's that important. You can have all the firefighting therapies in the world, but if you're still pouring gasoline on the fire, the blaze will only grow. Conversely, when you cut off cancer's favorite fuel, while simultaneously *enhancing the resiliency of your healthy cells*, absolutely every integrative therapy and SOC treatment will be more effective.

2. Therapeutic warmth:
Medical hyperthermia and other heat therapies

Quick Definition	External heat therapy. Raises body temperature enough to achieve immunomodulating effects or, at high enough temperatures, directly cytotoxic, tumor-damaging effects.
Best Contexts	Especially beneficial for highly aggressive cancers. Medical hyperthermia is often administered alongside conventional cancer care in several European clinics.
Contraindications or Considerations	All heat therapies can enhance detoxification processes. This can be stressful if patients are in a weakened state. Use binders (explained below). True medical hyperthermia is only available in Europe at this time.
Monitor These Labs	VEGF, CRP, ESR, LDH, pulse oximetry, tumor reduction seen on imaging, and self-reports regarding QOL and pain
Affects these Terrain Elements	Immune Function, Inflammation, Angiogenesis (changes microcirculation, improves oxygen perfusion)

While conventional oncology in the U.S. has been aware of medical hyperthermia for decades, and several hospitals are even equipped to provide it, the therapy has been mostly forgotten here. Occasionally, we will hear of its use alongside radiation for conditions such as sarcoma, head and neck cancers, and cervical cancer.[13] But even these uses have essentially stopped outside of a few locations. That's unfortunate because it is transformative in many cancer scenarios. For now, medical hyperthermia is widely available in Europe, Southeast Asia, and Canada, in a variety of treatment settings. In those regions, it is used as an adjuvant to radiation, chemotherapy, mistletoe, and IV vitamin C.

To clarify, true medical hyperthermia is not a sauna or hot bath. High heat medical hyperthermia is completed only in a hospital setting. The patient is sedated, and they are constantly monitored with multiple thermometers, supported with infusions of sodium bicarbonate to prevent acidosis, and the head is raised and cooled. In this highly monitored and supported state, the body temperature is slowly raised to 107.6 degrees Fahrenheit (42.0 Celsius). At that high temperature, the heat can convey direct cytotoxic effects and damage tumor cells.[14] Patients with highly aggressive, complex, and treatment-resistant cancers can be served very well by this approach. In Europe, this form of hyperthermia is rarely used as a sole treatment. They use it more like a Trojan Horse to drive the primary treatment of choice into the cancer cells to induce cell death. The therapy appears to help overcome drug resistance.[15] It activates NK cells, accentuating that effect that we also see with mistletoe therapy.[16] It ultimately lowers markers of chronic inflammation and enhances perfusion in organs and tissues.[17,18] My colleagues and I have found that hyperthermia is especially effective in complex sarcoma cases (see chapter 10) and in lymphoma. When I have a patient for whom medical hyperthermia could be course-altering, I do send them to Europe to receive this invaluable therapy.

All that said, there are more moderate forms of hyperthermia that are available in North America. They do not warm the body all the way up to that cytotoxic target of 107.6 degrees Fahrenheit (42.0 Celsius). While not directly *cytotoxic*, these therapies can be *immunomodulatory*, and that is valuable as well. Moderate hyperthermia includes warming therapies such as FAR infrared sauna and lower-heat local or regional hyperthermia, or it can be as simple as a hot bath or hot compress. Such applications can result in a mild *abscopal effect*. That means the tumor cells in one local area become stressed, and immune cells are drawn to the site. If the immune cells manage to breach the tumor's microenvironment, they will "learn" about the tumor and hopefully take that information to other tumor sites in the body.[19] (We'll learn more about this phenomenon in the next chapter.) All intense heat therapies have at least some potential for this abscopal effect.

Perfusion hyperthermia as a potential new tool in the U.S.

In the U.S., there have been trials for something called *perfusion hyperthermia*. This involves placing the patient on, essentially, a dialysis machine. All their blood is cycled through, heated to 107.6 degrees Fahrenheit (42.0 Celsius), filtered, and returned to the body. I had several of my patients with Stage IV ovarian cancer (failed by multiple lines of therapy), take part in such a trial. It greatly extended both quality and quantity of life.[20,21] The researchers in this trial also discovered, by accident, that this particular hyperthermia treatment managed to clear preexisting Lyme disease, Epstein-Barr, and Hepatitis B infections. Temperatures that high could certainly kill off those infections, and the filtration process likely prevented a massive cytokine release in response to the sudden pathogen die-off. This elimination and removal of a background pathogen burden can only benefit the overly stressed immune system in patients who have cancer.

Detoxification considerations

All forms of hyperthermia can heighten the body's detoxification processes. This can be stressful if patients are already in a weakened state. Often, I recommend waiting on detoxifying therapies (including sauna and other home-based heat therapies) until after an SOC treatment program is complete. But sometimes hyperthermia stands out as the most effective option for a patient, even during SOC. Whatever the timing, it's crucial to increase hydration and take binders during detoxifying therapies like hyperthermia.[22,23] Binders are molecules that literally bind to toxins, neutralizing them and helping the body flush them out efficiently. Otherwise, newly liberated toxins can cause havoc on their way out or head into circulation and get stuck in some other part of the body. Effective binders include bentonite clay, activated charcoal, and humic or fulvic acid. There are several other anthroposophic, homeopathic, and herbal remedies that promote excretion, and each doctor has their own toolbox.

3. Nutrient therapies: IV vitamin C and other therapeutic vitamins

Quick Definition	High dose (greater than 25 grams) of vitamin C, administered via IV.
Best Contexts	Typically beneficial for all patients with cancer, especially during chemotherapy
Contraindications or Considerations	All IVC patients must be screened for their G6-PD levels prior to treatment; contraindicated for patients with a genetic G6-PD deficiency. Some studies suggest vitamin C can negate the effects of radiation, but that concern should be focused on oral vitamin C. See Further Considerations at end of this therapy description. IVC and VAE should be administered separately, ideally on different days. Glucose monitors cannot differentiate between vitamin C and glucose; readings may spike as high as 550. This is *not* a glucose spike; do NOT treat it with insulin.
Monitor These Labs	CRP (under 1), ESR (under 10), LDH (under 175 or 450, depending on the lab range), CBC focusing on platelets (should normalize to 175-250), NLR (2-to-1), also VEGF (IVC can inhibit VEGF: less than 50 plasma or less than 350 serum)
Affects these Terrain Elements	Immune Function, Inflammation, and Angiogenesis

We refer to IV vitamin C (IVC) as a cooling therapy, somewhat like *Helleborus niger* as described in chapter 8. This is an important distinction to make if we're also providing a warming therapy like mistletoe. Because of these differences, we recommend providing IVC and mistletoe on separate days. Ideally, after VAE therapy, the patient's body temperature should have a chance to naturally come down to normal. Then begin the IVC therapy. It's not that the chemical constituents have poor interactions. It's simply that IVC is cooling enough systemically, that it can compromise some of the warmth-induction from the mistletoe. That warmth is valuable and needs to be protected. The cooling nature of IVC is beneficial, too, but in a different way. We want the body to receive the full benefits of both therapies, to cycle fully through the warmth of mistletoe, to the cooling of IVC.[24,25] The philosophy is very similar to that used in alternating mistletoe and *Helleborus niger*. The cooling nature of IVC can be quite noteworthy in some patients. They may feel cold and might need a blanket during their IVC treatment.

At high enough levels, IVC has been found to be directly cytotoxic to cancer cells.[26] When administered via IV, we can reach vitamin C plasma concentrations that are 70 times higher than those reached through oral ascorbate.[27] These high concentrations ultimately yield some extracellular H_2O_2, which healthy cells can address, but cancer cells can't (they have no ability to clear it). IVC also provides powerful mitigation of common chemotherapy side effects by protecting stomach cells (nausea prevention)[28] and protecting hair follicles (mitigation of hair loss).[29] Yet it does not hinder the desired effects of the chemotherapy treatment.[30] These dramatic SOC-supporting effects are often prominent enough that they catch the attention of conventional oncology teams. IVC often starts conversation and builds bridges with the conventional care world, because of its noteworthy effects during chemotherapy. Not only does it minimize weight loss and hair loss; it also generally improves QOL[31] and provides immunomodulating[32] and anti-angiogenic effects.[33,34]

To achieve these benefits, we need to hit vitamin C tissue saturation. Do not guess at a correct dosage for a specific patient. Tissue saturation can be measured using a glucose monitor, because glucose monitors cannot differentiate between glucose and vitamin C. (Both patients and their conventional providers must be aware of this issue, so they don't accidentally treat a "glucose spike" that isn't from glucose!) Vitamin C tissue saturation is reached when a glucose monitor reads 350 to 450 after IVC treatment. The Riordan Clinic (www.RiordanClinic. org) provides a fantastic IVC protocol guide, which is a free download on their website.

Further considerations: Concerns about G6-PD,
oral vitamin C support, and vitamin C during radiation treatment

All patients considering high-dose IVC therapy must be screened for G6-PD levels prior to initiating treatment. G6-PD is an enzyme that patients must have at a healthy level before they can receive this therapy. There is a genetic mutation that can result in chronically low levels of G6-PD (which would disqualify the patient for IVC therapy). If a patient is missing this enzyme and takes high-dose vitamin C, it can result in hemolysis (RBC breakdown), which can be fatal. It is also important to note that even in patients without that mutation, chemotherapy can induce a temporary G6-PD deficiency. The deficiency may last for days or weeks, depending on the chemotherapy drug used, the patient's genetic single nucleotide polymorphisms (SNP), and their liver function. Retesting is crucial. With your chemotherapy patients, always rerun their test before initiating or re-initiating IVC. Years old tests do not count if the patient is going through or recently had chemotherapy.[35]

Ideally, patients should be supported with oral vitamin C between IVC treatments. This is to help maintain tissue saturation and extend its positive benefits. I prefer a whole food sourced liposomal (non-ascorbic acid) form of vitamin C at a dosage of 2 to 4 grams per day.

Some studies suggest vitamin C can negate the effects of radiation, but that confusion lies in the difference between oral and IV administration. Oral dosing has more of the antioxidant effect, which does suggest contraindication with radiation. In contrast, IVC in high dose has a *pro-oxidant* effect and is possibly synergistic with radiation.[36] It is best to discuss this with your trained high-dose IVC practitioner to determine whether this therapy combination is appropriate for you.

Other nutrient therapies common alongside mistletoe

Again, we don't have the space in this context to provide a comprehensive list of nutrient therapies, and many other books have covered this ground extensively. But there are three more nutrients that we rely on heavily when providing mistletoe therapy. As mentioned in chapter 5, maintaining healthy vitamin D levels is pivotal to the success of mistletoe therapy. Macrophages must be bound to vitamin D to be activated.[37] When we're vitamin D deficient or insufficient, our macrophages are not working efficiently. Numerous studies have also found a correlation between low vitamin D levels and higher cancer risk.[38,39] If we're about to embark on an immunomodulating therapy like mistletoe, we want to make sure the immune cells have all they need to function at their best. So, it's ideal to address low vitamin D levels before starting mistletoe.

The same goes for Omega-3 status. Poor Omega-3 levels can compromise the effects of mistletoe.[40] Omega-3, especially the Omega-3 to -6 ratio, can throw off the inflammatory balance in the body. Too much Omega-6 (a common theme if you're eating the Standard American Diet) can send chronic inflammation into overdrive.[41] This is another issue to address before starting mistletoe therapy if you want to achieve optimal benefits.

Vitamin A is crucially important as well, but for a different reason. Vitamin A induces cell differentiation. Cancer is always trying to *dedifferentiate*.[42] It's trying to go back to that stem cell state because, in that state, it can do what it wants and continue evading the immune system. If there is a breast cancer cell sitting over in a bone, the immune system can identify it and say "you don't belong there." But if a cancer cell de-differentiates, it doesn't look like a cancer cell, and the immune system will miss it. Supplemental vitamin A can help restore cell differentiation, making cancer cells more visible.[43] Again, if we're going to start an immunomodulating therapy like mistletoe, we want to equip the immune system with its most basic building blocks. It's always wise to test nutrient levels like vitamin A before supplementing, since vitamin A is fat-soluble. Unlike water-soluble vitamins, excess cannot be flushed out in the urine. If a vitamin A deficiency or insufficiency is found, we supplement only with retinol, *not* beta-carotene. This molecular form is crucial for successfully reversing deficiency.

4. Botanical medicines:
Cannabis and the endocannabinoid system

Quick Definition	Cannabis provided in a variety of forms to improve endocannabinoid function, mitigate pain and nausea, promote immune function, restore sleep, and increase appetite.
Best Contexts	Benefits most patients if they have no SNPs that may negatively affect their experience of cannabis.
Contraindications or Considerations	No contraindications. However, do not recommend cannabis for patients with CYP2C9*3 or FAAH associated SNPs, as described later in this section.
Monitor These Labs	CRP (under 1), ESR (under 10), LDH (under 175 or 450, depending on lab range), as well as CBC, NLR, organic acids testing. Also, self-reported changes in QOL.
Affects these Terrain Elements	Immune Function, Inflammation, Stress & Biorhythms, Mental and Emotional Health, Microbiome & Digestive Function (appetite and nausea).

Medicinal cannabis use continues to grow as more patients hear about success stories. For practitioners, it's important to cut through the hype and base our clinical recommendations on science—thankfully there is a growing research base now. We can also empower ourselves with an understanding of the genetic SNPs that can influence a person's experience of cannabis, quickly ruling out those who would likely have a bad encounter with this powerful herbal medicine. We'll discuss that nuance at length in a moment.

Human use of cannabis as medicine has been noted for over 10,000 years. More recently, an Irish physician, Sir William Brooke O'Shaughnessy, was known for studying cannabis while working in India, validating its medicinal uses, and introducing it to Western medicine.[44] U.S. physicians were the main opponents when the Treasury Department introduced a Marijuana Tax Act in 1937. Despite the opinions of physicians who often witnessed the clinical benefits of wise cannabis use, it was removed from the U.S. Pharmacopoeia in 1942. By 1970, it was classified as a Schedule 1 drug (as bad as heroin) and was wrongly described as having no medical benefit.[45,46] Cannabis is finally being rediscovered and recognized for its genuine therapeutic benefits.

To understand its wise use, we first need to understand the endocannabinoid system (ECS). We are still learning so much about cannabinoid receptors, but here's what we do know. In simplest terms, the ECS can be thought of as lipids, which are produced by all mammals and interact with and modulate the nervous system and receptors throughout the body. This system is key in how we process pain and anxiety and how we self-calm and resolve intense stimuli. It's also deeply involved in maintaining circadian regulation.

As investigative journalist Martin A. Lee put it, "Cannabinoid receptors function as subtle sensing devices, tiny vibrating scanners perpetually primed to pick up biochemical cues that flow through fluids surrounding each cell."[47] The ECS is involved in how nerve cells signal to each other, how those cells decide to fire again, and when they decide to stop firing. That process is deeply involved in chronic pain challenges, in which nerves begin to fire a pain-related signal and then get stuck transmitting that information again and again. The cannabinoids in cannabis aren't foreign to our bodies. They look and act like molecules that our bodies recognize and naturally make to keep the ECS working properly.

We have two main categories of cannabinoid receptors and two naturally occurring compounds in the body that illicit similar effects to cannabis when interacting with these receptors:

> *CB1:* Associated with the brain, central nervous system (CNS) and organ function. This is primarily neuromodulating.[48] It interacts with the body's naturally occurring compound anandamide (AKA the "bliss molecule"), and it also interacts with the THC in marijuana.
>
> *CB2:* Associated more with immune cells and pain management receptors outside of our brain and spinal column.[49] These reach into the periphery, involving the body's more distal tissues and extremities.

Everyone's ECS is unique. You could say that we each have an endocannabinoid (ECB) fingerprint. This includes a few genetic SNPs that can affect ECS constitutional tendencies and how people experience cannabis. Too many regard cannabis as a magic-bullet therapy: *it's good for everyone!* But when you talk to patients, you begin to run into fairly extreme responses. They either say they've had a terrible reaction, or they feel it's been completely transformative. SNPs are coming into play here. *Patients need to know their SNPs before they try cannabis.* There are several testing companies that elucidate these epigenetic SNPs related to the patient's ECB fingerprint. This helps us learn whether THC is friend or foe. This, along with patient's symptoms, can further specify appropriate *chemovar profiles* (referring to specific terpenoid content of cannabis varieties), which help the individual choose the right cannabis product for their specific health goals.[50–52]

When reviewing a patient's SNPs, those with CYP2C9*3 SNPs should exercise caution with THC. These individuals have trouble breaking down THC, so it stays in their bodies longer and makes them feel crazy! Another SNP that can affect cannabis response is related to the FAAH (fatty acid amide hydrolase) gene. The FAAH gene, or bliss gene, is involved in how we metabolize anandamide (the bliss molecule) into arachidonic acid. A genetic SNP here can result in a temperament that struggles with achieving bliss and contentment. Interpersonally, this individual might be described as a "Debbie-downer." On a clinical level, this person has a downregulated ECS. These patients don't tolerate medicinal marijuana well. The THC can make them more depressed or anxious. With them, pure CBD is a much better and useful option.[53]

Once a patient has been properly screened and deemed a good candidate for trying cannabis, the potential benefits of this medicinal plant are extensive. Cannabis is another true poly-pharmacy plant (like mistletoe), so its benefits are diverse:

Appears to improve metabolic flexibility and the ability to adapt to changing environments (both key functions of a healthy ECS)
Mitigates pain, particularly chronic pain challenges involving a stressed nervous system
Provides anti-emetic (anti-nausea) effects and stimulates appetite
Soothes anxiety and depression, and promotes healthy sleep[54,55]

Those pain, nervous system, and mood benefits are fairly well-known. International researchers are looking at more direct anti-cancer benefits, too. Medicinal marijuana contains compounds that appear to convey anti-angiogenic effects as VEGF inhibitors and direct cytotoxicity for some cancers.[56] These effects convey whether smoked or ingested (though ingested cannabis, of course, takes longer to convey its benefits).[57]

Just as we see plenty of nutrient deficiencies in our patients who have cancer, we can also clinically diagnose a more subtle *endocannabinoid deficiency.* This deficiency can compromise the effects of other therapies, including mistletoe. All the following are associated with lower levels of anandamide, which is at the heart of ECS deficiency: inexplicable pain, musculoskeletal complaints, nausea, IBS and gut issues in general, migraines, and low seizure threshold.[58] If you see these symptoms clustering in a patient, and they have no concerning ECS-related SNPs, they are prime candidates for therapeutic cannabis. When mistletoe therapy and cannabis are combined, we often view mistletoe as resetting the body's inner rhythms. Simultaneously, cannabis increases the body's ability to adapt to new stimuli that might jar that rhythm. It helps the body roll with the punches and then return to its own rhythm (homeostasis) once more.

5. Well-vetted OLDU therapies: Low-dose Naltrexone (LDN)

Quick Definition	An opiate antagonist that indirectly increases the body's production of its own endorphins.
Best Contexts	Immunomodulatory and mood stabilizing for most patients. Good alternative for patients who opt against cannabis.
Contraindications or Considerations	None, except for when using opiate therapies (may negate their effects).
Monitor These Labs	Vitamin D, immune panels, eosinophils, CRP (under 1), ESR (under 10), LDH (under 175 or 450, depending on lab range), hormones (thyroid, adrenal, and sex hormones). Self-report on stress management, sense of well-being, and pain levels.
Affects these Terrain Elements	Epigenetics (affects gene expression), Immune Function, Microbiome & Digestive Function (can lessen IBS symptoms), Inflammation, Hormone Balance, Stress & Biorhythm, Mental & Emotional Health

Just as we frequently see patients with endocannabinoid deficiency, we also see a similar *endorphin deficiency syndrome* as well. These two deficiency states are like twins. They are similar in how they work and in the systems they affect, even if the signaling pathways involved are different. Endorphins are the body's own naturally produced, feel-good chemicals. People with endorphin deficiency often struggle with depressed mood, poor energy, and a lack of enthusiasm—not unlike those with endocannabinoid deficiency.[59] Of course, a recent cancer diagnosis only aggravates this baseline state.

Naltrexone, a pharmaceutical drug better known for its labeled use in preventing relapse in serious opiate addiction cases, conveys a different set of benefits when micro-dosed. Low-dose Naltrexone (LDN) serves as an opiate antagonist that temporarily blocks endorphins from entering cells. This triggers a signal to the pituitary to produce more endorphins. LDN seals off the receptors for a few hours, then releases. Then the body experiences its own heightened endorphin production.[60,61]

LDN is considered a legitimate Off-label Drug Use (OLDU) of Naltrexone. There are a lot of other OLDU options being discussed in various books and cancer-related social media forums, and I even offer a course for physicians on the topic. In all honesty, I'm not enamored with the hype surrounding OLDU pharmaceuticals. Typically, the molecular pathway that these drugs target can be hit just as easily with a natural therapy, but with far fewer side effects. In my own clinical practice, I find LDN to be the exception to that rule. It has a long history of safe use with few to no side effects for most patients. Meanwhile, its benefits are quite diverse.[62,63]

The heightened endorphin-production is the most studied benefit, and it cascades into many improvements in mood, energy, and pain-perception. Other benefits that are being researched include:

Immunomodulatory effects: Increases T-lymphocytes, while calming overzealous immune response (balances TH-1 and TH-2 activity)[64–66]

Adjuvant support: Calms side effects of conventional immunotherapies[67]

General adaptogenic effects: Helps restore circadian regulation and improves QOL[68]

My colleagues and I sometimes experience patient resistance to cannabis use, even among people who would be good candidates. Some simply don't want to have to go to a marijuana dispensary. When this is the case, LDN is an ideal inexpensive and accessible alternative. In my clinical experience, as far as OLDU options, LDN is also the most synergistic with mistletoe therapy.

6. Circadian rhythm restoration: Acknowledging ourselves as part of nature

Quick Definition	Lifestyle choices and some supplements that help restore natural cycles of physical activity, mental states, and behavioral and physiological changes, under the influence of light and darkness, as well as temperature and the seasons.
Best Contexts	All patients. Foundational prerequisite lifestyle choices.
Contraindications or Considerations	None
Monitor These Labs	D3, melatonin, Adrenal Stress Index (ASI), immune profile, and gut microbiome tests. Self-report of QOL and daily patterns/choices.
Affects these Terrain Elements	ALL, with emphasis on Stress & Biorhythms, Immune Function, Microbiome & Digestive Function

Modern humans appeared on Earth about 200,000 years ago. Civilization, including familiar forms of agriculture, settlement, and governance, began about 6,000 to 10,000 years ago. Up until very recently, as a species, our lives were defined by the hard work of food-finding and survival. We lived like that for tens of thousands of years. For most of our existence, even in early agrarian times, our daily schedules were governed by the sun. We worked during the day. We slept at night. Yearly activities were guided by the seasons. We worked hard during growing seasons, we rested and huddled to keep warm during winter or rainy seasons, we made significant migrations to follow food supplies, and we ate foods according to seasonal and geographic availability.

Human lifestyles just 200 years ago are almost unrecognizable compared to how we live today. On an evolutionary timescale, within a few generations, we have fully upended the circadian rhythms that our bodies depend on for optimal health. We stay up well past dark, working under electric light and looking at screens emitting EMF radiation and endocrine-disrupting blue light. We eat the same carbohydrate-rich foods year-round. We live in temperature-stable indoor environ-ments—night and day, regardless of season.

Most people understand that modern life has disrupted circadian rhythm in terms of day-night cycles. Sure, we're all a little sleep deprived. But circadian rhythm refers to, and is involved in, all those other natu-ral rhythms, too: heat and cold, seasonal food availability, amount of time spent outdoors in each season, and seasonal rhythms in how we move (types of exercise) and to what intensity. These rhythms, in turn, affect every other aspect of our inner terrain, but are especially influ-ential as far as immune response, stress response, and the microbiome.

Cancer research is finally catching up with what anthroposophic practitioners, naturopathic doctors, and many other natural health tra-ditions have known for generations. Our loss of connection to natural rhythms of all kinds is making us sick. Indeed, in 2007 one of the better-known circadian rhythm studies put night shift work on the list of known carcinogens.[69,70] Another study questioned the impact of night shift work on breast cancer, since there seemed to be confound-ing factors: people who work graveyard shifts are often poor, the poor often struggle with access to high-quality food, and their lives are also high-stress. Was "working at night" really the primary risk factor?[71]

Point taken. But researchers since then have pried away at that question even further.[72] A more recent study corrected for the socio-economic influences by looking solely at women who were flight atten-dants—half who flew at night, half who flew during the day. Sure enough, those who flew the red eye flights for years had a higher risk of breast cancer.[73]

Another study went on to postulate that the effect might be coming from compromised melatonin levels. Researchers looked at women who had breast cancer, versus age-matched controls. The women with breast cancer had consistently lower melatonin levels.[74] This raised the next logical question: Is melatonin active for cancer? In a 2017 animal study, mice with cancer were injected with melato-nin, and a clear anti-cancer benefit was seen.[75] Since then, an Italian research group has been looking at various cancer types, beginning with breast cancer, then progressing to prostate, lung, and colon cancers. In every cancer they've looked at, patients have severely compromised melatonin levels, and supplementing with it seems to lead to significant anti-cancer benefit.[76]

Circadian dysregulation has major impacts on our immune system rhythms. We're still learning the molecular "how," but the relationship is definitely there. Yes, melatonin has been a powerful adjuvant for many of my patients and is especially effective in working alongside mistletoe to reset deep internal body rhythms. Melatonin supplementation is neither a quick fix, nor can it replace major lifestyle choices to better honor our natural rhythms. But it can be a powerful turning-point helper as patients begin the transition to a healthier way of life. Not only does melatonin get them sleeping again, it appears to have definite antioxidant, DNA-protective, and even anti-angiogenic effects. It is not only the body's "sleep hormone," but also the repair-worker, too.[77]

Therapeutic melatonin dosages during cancer care are much higher than those you may be familiar with. If someone has an active cancering process, I typically recommend 40 mg per day at bedtime. If it's a hormonally mediated cancer (prostate, ovarian, or breast cancer), I recommend up to 180 mg daily for a few months and then reassess. For a patient with a hormonally driven cancer with metastasis to the bones and rapid progression, I might even increase the dose with an additional 60 mg three times daily to slow the process. This strategy has been proven beneficial clinically.[78] Once a patient is in remission, I let them drop down to 20 mg for maintenance, and most tend to remain at that dosage for life. It is interesting that doses like this would be expected to cause daytime drowsiness. Yet, we don't find that to be the case. Low doses of melatonin (0.5 to 5 mg at bedtime) can have profound impact on inducing sleepiness and supporting healthy sleep patterns. However, at the higher doses, we see a paradoxical effect: It is no longer so helpful for sleep, and instead optimizes other physiological effects, as noted above. We also don't see problems titrating up rapidly or stopping cold turkey as one might expect. Still, these are very high doses, and they need to be managed by an anthroposophic or integrative provider trained in therapeutic melatonin administration. For patients with highly dysregulated circadian systems (that's most people today), melatonin supplementation is only an initial, rhythm-resetting step. Cancer diagnosis, unlike any other disease, demands lifestyle reinvention. I work with my patients to educate them about the power of their daily and seasonal life rhythms and their boundaries regarding exposure to electronics and screen time. Some of the most impactful anti-cancer lifestyle choices include:

Pairing melatonin with a consistent bedtime close to sunset!

Keeping electronics out of the bedroom and sleeping in full dark

Minimizing all screen time: Setting time limits on computer and device use and wearing "blue light blockers"

Incorporating high-intensity interval training (HIIT) or similar exercise two to three times per week

Taking daily walks out in nature, experiencing the elements

Trying simple cold exposure therapies: Ending every shower with cold water, intentionally experiencing cold temperatures outdoors, or even more high-tech interventions with cryotherapy (two to three sessions per week can encourage mitogenesis)[79]

Essentially, sleep in a dark, cool room and get outside way more! Also, "sitting" really is the new "smoking." Combining sedentary work postures with hours of EMF and screen time exposure makes for an especially dysregulated life. Get up. Take breaks. Exercise outdoors whenever possible. HIIT-style exercise is especially powerful for people who have cancer, once they're at a point in their recovery when they can tolerate the exertion. The same goes for occasional cold exposure. Both high intensity movement and cold therapies make us more adaptable to stress in day-to-day life, enhance metabolic flexibility, and even enhance immune function. All that makes our internal microenvironment less friendly to cancer. In the end, that's really our goal. It's not so much that we're fighting cancer. We're creating an environment where it can't even take root.

OTHER WELL-VETTED THERAPIES:
Well-researched options that play well with mistletoe

Artemisinin
Boswellia
Curcumin
Fractionated radiation (repurposed SOC treatment)
Green tea extract
Medicinal mushrooms (AHCC, chaga, cordyceps, lion's mane, reishi, turkey tail)
Mental health therapies: Support groups, meditation, trauma resolution work and guided psychedelic therapies
Metformin/berberine: To lower insulin growth factor (IGF-1)
Metronomic chemotherapy (repurposed SOC treatment)
Modified citrus pectin: To lower Galectin-3
Oxygen therapies: Hyperbaric oxygen therapy (HBOT), ozone therapy
Photodynamic therapy and UVBI
Poly-MVA (form of ALA)
Pulsed electromagnetic field therapy (PEMF)

A Note to Patients: Like the featured therapies in this chapter, the therapies above have been selected particularly for their ability to complement, and not interfere with, mistletoe therapy. They are also the least likely to cause any unwanted interactions with SOC treatments. Of course, your anthroposophic or integrative provider should still guide you in incorporating any of these remedies. To learn more about any of them, read:

Outside the Box Cancer Therapies by Dr. Mark Stengler and Dr. Paul Anderson,
Naturopathic Oncology: An Encyclopedic Guide for Patients and Physicians by Dr. Neil McKinney
Textbook of Naturopathic Oncology: A Desktop Guide of Integrative Cancer Care by Dr. Gurdev Parmar (Dr. Tina Kaczor, ed.)

All three of these books are excellent resources that explore well-researched natural and alternative cancer therapies.

CASE STORY ONE: ELLEN

Power of IV Mistletoe in Clear Cell Endometrial Cancer				
Physician: Dr. Nasha Winters	Patient: Ellen	**First seen:** Oct 2013; diagnosis May 2013	**Age:** 65 (at dx)	**Sex:** Female
Cancer Type & Stage:	Diagnosed May 2013 with Stage IV clear cell carcinoma of the endometrium. Metastasis to vaginal cuff, colon, peritoneal cavity, and lung.			
Risk Factors:	Toxic Burden: History of multiple root canals and mercury filling Hormone Balance: HRT following years of OCP use, paired with COMT, CYP1B1, CYP1A1, GST and VDR SNPs Stress & Biorhythm: Prone to anxiety and caregiver for her ailing husband			
Significant Labs:	Low protein/albumin (cachexia). Diabetic with A1C of 6.2, IGF-1 237, insulin 13. Elevated estrone, estradiol levels, high 4-OH, and poor 2:16 estrogen ratios. Trifecta (LDH, ESR, CRP) all elevated. Elevated CEA and CA 125 (cancer markers).			

I first met Ellen in late 2013 after she was failed by her first line of treatment: chemotherapy (Carbo/Taxol) and TAHBSO (total abdominal hysterectomy with bilateral salpingo-oophorectomy and omentectomy). She found her way to one of my cancer retreats for women, which I was facilitating back then. Ellen was desperate to find other options. She'd been offered palliative radiation and more chemotherapy, but since her first round of chemotherapy took her to the brink of extinction, she was hesitant to dive back in.

Diving into her personal and medical history, Ellen noted an enormous amount of stress, including a traumatic childhood, racism (she came from a mixed ethnic background), a nasty divorce, and several years of caring for her current ailing husband. It was difficult for her to say no. Even in her depleted state, she still ruminated with an intense anxiety about everything. Her constitution reminded me of a hummingbird. Despite all that, she was no stranger to integrative medicine and had been an anthroposophic-trained nurse decades before, when she lived in Europe. But over the years, she'd drifted from that ideology.

At the time of our initial consult, Ellen was on daily NSAIDS, Dexamethasone, Zofran, and opiates. Her pain remained unchanged, and she was severely cachectic. She had rapid disease progression in her bowel, causing obstruction. She'd had numerous GI issues her whole life, only to have them worsened by surgery and subsequent chemotherapy.

Ellen also had an autoimmune history of Hashimoto's and Raynaud's. She was a self-professed sugar junkie, and rice was a staple in her diet. She was simultaneously extremely anxious and fearful about what to eat. She went through cycles of avoiding food all together and then, when she got hungry enough, she'd binge on carbohydrate laden foods.

Though Ellen was given less than three months to live, we managed to spend the next nine months restoring her terrain and general nutrition. We focused on a very low-glycemic diet, which also lowered her estrogen dominance load. We weaned her off the steroids and opiates and enrolled her in a Mindfulness Based Stress Reduction (MBSR) course. She began using those tools daily to change up her stress response.

Ellen's initial transformation really began at the women's retreat that she attended. At registration, she was extremely anxious and fearful. She was so cachectic, in such a very painful place physically, it almost seemed the anxiety was keeping her going. One of the major goals of these retreats was to speak frankly with each other about both life and death, in a safe space of like-hearted women. We focused on replacing fear with hope. Ellen responded deeply to this. In a matter of days, she became more rooted, grounded, and embodied. I really believe she had to address this spiritual shift before we could be successful with any other therapies.

After the retreat, we instituted all those dietary therapies and kept in touch via telemedicine. She was originally planning on going straight from the retreat to radiation treatments. I was deeply concerned about this and told her. She was so frail, and her insulin was high. Radiation does not work well if insulin or VEGF are high. My impression was that radiation would provide her little benefit and only stress her system more. "Would you be willing to work on your metabolic issues first?" I asked. "You could get your insulin under control, then reconsider radiation." Surprisingly, she was open to trying this approach.

I always check my patients' monthly CBC, Trifecta Labs (see chapter 5), and cancer markers till they're 100 percent within my limits. Over those first nine months of care, Ellen saw progressive improvement, particularly for her metabolic health (A1C, IGF-1, insulin). Her quality of life (QOL), energy levels, and general out-look radically improved.

Despite her QOL improvements and improving labs, Ellen's scans still showed metastasis in the colon, vaginal cuff, and lungs along with carcinomatosis (metastases throughout the body) and peritoneal implants (tumor deposits). Her oncologists continued to push for more systemic treatments: chemotherapy and local radi-ation. Ellen was still too traumatized from her previous experi-ence to consent immediately. But she eventually succumbed to the pressures and opted for radiation. Unfortunately, this devastated all the progress she had made over the previous months and sent her spiraling back into rapid disease progression and loss of QOL, including daily rectal and vaginal bleeding and excruciating pain.

Because of her condition and the prognosis offered by her pal-liative care team, Ellen decided to make one last trip to say her goodbyes to family members who still lived in Europe. But she was so ill and weak and in so much pain, we knew the two-week trip would be impossible without support. I found an anthroposophic hospital near her family home that could help with supportive care. The doctor who reviewed her records noted they could offer pal-liative support only, but they were willing to care for Ellen while she was there.

I recall getting a call from Ellen only about a week into her care with this hospital. She sounded brighter and more hopeful than ever. She had been receiving daily escalating doses of IV mistle-toe therapy (fraxini) and SC Iscador® Mali, along with *Helleborus niger*. She also received whole body and local regional hyperther-mia, hydration IVs, eurythmy, hydrotherapy, and art therapy. She felt a sense of homecoming on so many levels—seeing one side of her family of origin and being at peace with them, as well as accessing healing methods that she remembered from many years before. Ellen finally had a space where *she* was the one being cared for and not the one doing all the caring. She experienced a com-plete shift in her pain, her QOL, and her outlook.

Once Ellen returned home, her AM physician and I encouraged her to continue the fraxini mistletoe, along with her low-carbo-hydrate diet, and stress reduction practices. Now that she was off the opiates, we added LDN to her treatment program. I was new to providing IV mistletoe, but embraced learning how, especially after seeing Ellen's transformation.

Ellen continued to feel better and gain strength. By the time she had returned from Europe, she could no longer palpate the vaginal or abdominal masses. Her labs, over the next two months, reflected this transformation as well, with her Trifecta Labs near perfect (only a slightly elevated CRP), and the lowest CEA and CA125 we had seen in our work together. Ellen was no longer cachectic, and her A1C was 5.3, near normal range. Her insulin was 4 and her IGF-1 was elevated at 167, but this was still an improvement and was likely in relation to her still having somewhat poor sleep and her estrogen-dominance patterns.

She had a scan at one month after her return from Europe. *All metastasis had resolved,* outside of one residual spot on her colon. Her conventional oncology team chose to focus entirely on that one spot, telling her she was still expected to be dead soon and that she needed palliative chemotherapy. Ellen was devastated and reached out to me. I was devastated that her team overlooked the miracle of her health and the improvements in the rest of her terrain, and instead focused on one tiny spot. None of us expected her to survive, but we certainly expected at least curiosity about her improvements and some willingness to celebrate any victory, big or small.

I encouraged her to contact the doctor back in Germany. His response: "Continue your current protocol, and come back in two months for one more round of anthroposophic treatment."

Ellen had a major choice to make at that moment: to give in to fear or to choose to continue the path that was clearly working for her body. She chose. She didn't let fear dictate her decisions from then on. In September of 2014, she returned to the European hospital and received another series of IV mistletoe and hyperthermia. A month after returning home, she had a follow-up scan. It showed no evidence of disease (NED)! Despite that news, her team at a well-known cancer center insisted that it wouldn't hold, and her prognosis was the same.

Ellen continues to be cancer-free today. I have lost touch with her in recent years, but we check in periodically, and I keep finding her thriving. It was thanks to her that I learned how to apply

IV mistletoe therapy here in the U.S. That led to consulting with a team of researchers at Johns Hopkins Hospital on how to incorporate this protocol into their current clinical trial. I remain grateful for what Ellen's cancer journey taught me. Her experience has blessed hundreds, if not thousands, of others.

CASE STORY 2: GEORGE

Many Roads to Melanoma				
Physician: Dr. Nasha Winters	**Patient**: George	**First seen**: Spring 2011; third diagnosis Dec 2016	**Age:** 56 in 2011	**Sex:** Male
Cancer Type & Stage:	Initially undisclosed previous diagnosis: 2005 Stage I, fully excised, right arm melanoma. 2011 biopsy confirmed prostate cancer Gleason 7 2016 metastasis of the 2005 melanoma; in colon, lungs, and nodes in right armpit.			
Risk Factors:	Toxic Burden: Alcoholism. Immune Function & Biorhythm: Low Vitamin D3 levels, high stress from corporate world. Metabolic & Digestive Function: Diet of highly processed foods, heavy red meat, no vegetables.			
Significant Labs:	High trifecta (CRP/ESR/LDH), high ferritin, high RDW and serum calcium, high fibrinogen, and high homocysteine. Autoimmune thyroiditis. HbA1C, insulin, and IGF-1 showed he was diabetic. *During Stage IV Melanoma:* CRP 14.7, ESR 56, and LDH 629 (after SOC). LDH served as tumor marker to monitor therapy response.			

George sought my care regarding adjuvant support during prostate cancer treatment in 2011. He came to me thanks to the urging of his wife—he was *very* skeptical of all I had to offer and questioned me relentlessly. (Later that became my favorite thing about him, as he pushed me to be ready with answers to such scrutinizing questions.) George was from a very conservative background with great trust in the SOC model. But he was also concerned about losing sexual function if he followed the treatment recommendations of his medical team. This prompted him to consider other options.

George had been watching his rising PSAs for years, with negative findings on his digital rectal exams (DRE). But he finally submitted to a biopsy, which revealed an adenocarcinoma diagnosis and Gleason score of 7. He refused the SOC interventions of prostatectomy, local radiation, and androgen deprivation therapy.

For decades, George's diet and lifestyle were characterized by excess alcohol, red meat, processed foods, late-night business meetings, international travel, hours of sitting, no exercise, and obesity. All of it had finally caught up with him. He knew it too. Just before meeting with me, he'd made some significant lifestyle changes. He recently quit drinking and joined a twelve-step program, transferred from his stressful company, and was attending marital counseling.

Still, just looking at George's health picture and labs, even aside from the cancer, there were so many complicating factors. He had autoimmune thyroiditis. He was fully diabetic. He had gout. He had hyperlipidemia. Basically, he was a hot mess.

I kept it simple. First, I strongly encouraged his sobriety and therapy, then added some targeted supplements: fish oil, vitamin D3, an herbal anti-inflammatory blend, and modified citrus pectin. The biggest change was the process of cleaning up his diet. He absolutely had to do this. I prescribed a Mediterranean low-carbohydrate diet with no grains or legumes and predominantly fish as his protein source. We also initiated subcutaneous (SC) mistletoe therapy with Helixor A, three times per week.

George had been in serious trouble, and this therapeutic plan was focused simply on turning off the spigot of pro-inflammatory foods, providing targeted supplements according to his labs, and incorporating mistletoe therapy. That's it. The transformation this fostered was dramatic. Within two months, George lost 36 of the 80 pounds he needed to lose, he was no longer symptomatic with gout or his other aches and pains, and his outlook on life was more positive.

Within three months, his PSA went from 11.5 to 6.7, his HbA1C dropped from 6.7 to 5.6, and his insulin plummeted from 22 to 7. His PAP went from 4.5 to 2.3 (I like it below 2). His CRP went from 8.4 to 1.2! Essentially, his inflammation was drastically reduced and near normal levels. His wife noted a huge change in his personality, too. His usual rage patterns were now few and far between, and they were enjoying a rekindled connection with one another. We continued with three-month check-ins and labs for two years.

Across the board, George's health turned around. Eventually he lost the full 80 pounds that he wanted to lose, and he felt fantastic. His conventional practitioners wanted him to come in for follow-up exams, but in George's usual way, he refused. He was watching the labs that I had insisted on, and he was personally experiencing the vast improvements in his health. He felt that was good enough. But after two years of our ongoing health-oriented care, he did go in for a follow-up MRI, DRE, and blood tests. All these confirmed that his prostate cancer was in remission. He and his wife were trying to retire and move to another town, so I congratulated him, and we agreed to check in annually. But I didn't hear from George again for quite some time.

In December 2016, after three years of no communication, I received a phone call. George had been hospitalized with severe GI symptoms (serious pain and constipation), which led to a CT scan that noted a mass in his transverse colon. An emergency surgery to remove the mass and create an ostomy elucidated a malignant melanoma. Further imaging revealed metastasis to his lungs and lymph nodes in his right armpit—the same arm where he'd had melanoma before. Only now did George mention his history with this other cancer. He'd had melanoma, six years before he first consulted with me. It had been fully excised, and he thought it didn't matter, so he didn't mention it during our intake. Melanoma has a very high recurrence rate; his conventional team should have been monitoring him for this. I would have myself if I'd known about it! Now he had a Stage IV recurrence.

Though George had completely recovered from prostate cancer, he had slowly let his diet and lifestyle slide back to his pre-cancer ways, gaining back about half of the 80 pounds he had lost and taking on another major work project that was loaded with stress.

While recovering from his most recent GI surgery, he and his wife went to MD Anderson to discuss immune therapies. He was placed in a Phase I Clinical Trial, using a combination of a BRAF inhibitor (Tafinlar) and a MEK inhibitor (Mekinist), though no one ordered a molecular profile on his recently resected tissue to see if he even had the two targets addressed by those drugs.

Because he was hesitant to try anything else while on the clinical trial, he just wanted me to know his status and said that he'd "be in touch again, once the trial was over." Then we could "get back to the terrain work." I urged him to include an integrative approach while on the trial, as I had seen some poor outcomes with such therapies, but he was insistent about waiting. At our last 2013 check-in, his Core Terrain Labs (see chapter 5) were perfect. Now, following surgery and initiating the trial therapy, his labs were more concerning than ever. I had to just hold space for him and pray he found his way back to some supportive therapies before it was too late.

Within a few months, when most of the trial participants were already succumbing to their cancers or the subsequent side effects of this drug combination, George realized this trial was not the miracle he'd hoped for. His own labs and symptoms were worsening, and his scans showed minimal (if any) response. He finally had another consult with me. He admitted he was terrified to stop what they were doing at MDA, but he was the only one still alive in his trial arm! He knew he had to do something different. We evaluated his Single Nucleotide Polymorphisms (SNPs) and learned that his VDR, CYP2R1, and MAO SNPs made him prone to depression, fear, anxiety, and addiction. His SNPs also made him vulnerable to low circulating vitamin D levels—a vitamin crucial to keeping his immune system in balance and dopamine levels on track.

On his own, George sought the counsel of a local nutritionist who put him on a raw food vegan diet that was unfortunately sugar-laden (tons of grains, legumes, and fruits). This caused his tumors to explode and progress wildly. His D3 levels worsened down to a level of 17—another major driver of melanoma process. The nodes in his armpits were now visible as well as palpable and causing discomfort and loss of mobility. His breathing was getting worse, and his recent scan also noted some new activity around the colon surgical borders. Even more, a new biopsy showed he was both BRAF- and MEK-negative, meaning the MDA trial was *never* appropriate for him, and likely worsened his outcomes.

In March 2017, again without checking with me, George started a TIL (tumor infiltrating lymphocyte), an IL2 (think fever therapy), and a PD-1 inhibitor (checkpoint inhibitor, pembrolizumab). George did have PD-1 targets on his tissue assay, so that wasn't completely off base. He took all these along with Cytoxan and

Fludarabine to wipe out his stem cells, with the plan of re-infusing his own T cells. This all sounded wonderful, but the reality was a horrifying failure.

George described the first round as "intolerable." The medical community was just beginning to learn that people with non-functioning immune systems were not good candidates for immune therapies, particularly those with high platelets, poor NLR ratio, elevated LDH, or liver disease, as well as those over the age of 52. Patients with three or more of those factors should not pursue these therapies. George had all those rule-out factors. So, this therapy combination shot him into autoimmune gastritis, worsened his Hashimoto's autoimmune thyroiditis, and caused other joint issues that we suspected were autoimmune as well. At this point, George had pursued an assortment of mis-applied therapies for his recurrent melanoma for almost two years. Finally, he was ready to allow me to support him again.

His CRP was 14.7, ESR was 56, and LDH was 629. Believe it or not, George still had a chance to remedy some of the damages— both from his own lifestyle choices and from poorly applied SOC. But I wasn't sure that we could do more than stabilize him and improve his quality of life (QOL). He agreed to take a break from the MDA therapies and work on stabilizing all his systems. I immediately started him on LDN and provided an autoimmune flare protocol that included: high-dose vitamin D3, emulsified vitamin A, fish oil, probiotics, a five-day water fast, and then two weeks of an autoimmune paleo diet, along with intermittent fasting.

We managed to stabilize George with this autoimmune protocol. Then he resumed the supportive diet that we had established for him three years before. He was able to enter into therapeutic ketosis, and I started him on SC mistletoe (pini), three times per week.

After three months of this approach, George had not only stabilized, he felt good. His LDH was seriously improved (218), and other labs were responding too. After six more months, George got confirmation via tests and scans that he was in remission. This was completely unexpected!

In addition to celebrating his remission, we were all celebrating his change in outlook and attitude as well. This second experience with cancer had brought him through a much deeper spiritual shift. He had a clear resolve that he was never going back to the stressful, unhealthy lifestyle, and a poor diet that had set the stage for his cancers. He joined a faith community, and he and his wife were in a much better place relationally once again.

George has never resumed the MDA immunotherapy treatments, simply because he hasn't needed them. We've continued to regularly monitor his LDH as his main tumor marker. We run a twice-yearly CBC with full Trifecta Labs, and MDA continues to monitor him too. George continues his terrain-based dietary care (primarily a modified ketogenic diet) and SC mistletoe therapy. He has not taken any other treatments in the past three years. He still has some lung and lymph activity on his scans, though it is stable and not symptomatic. His labs have completely normalized, and his QOL is exceptional. He has connected deeply to his faith, and he is now finally retired and enjoying the fruits of his labor.

PART 4:

WEAVING IT ALL TOGETHER: SPECIAL APPLICATIONS IN CLINICAL PRACTICE

"Illnesses do not come upon us out of the blue. They are developed from small daily sins against nature. When enough sins have accumulated, illnesses will suddenly appear." —HIPPOCRATES

CHAPTER 10

UNIQUE SCENARIOS

Novel Mistletoe Administration Routes and Understanding Tissue-origins of Specific Cancer Types

Dr. Mark Hancock, MD and Dr. Marion Debus, MD

"Give me the power to produce a fever and I'll cure all disease."
—PARMENIDES

Throughout this book, we've primarily looked at subcutaneous and IV-administered mistletoe as therapies that awaken the immune system during cancer care. There are alternate administration routes for VAE therapy that trigger even stronger immune activity, either as a fever therapy or through intratumoral injection (high doses injected directly into the tumor itself) and other variations of these therapies provided in certain European clinics. We'll first look at these less common VAE administration methods. Then we'll look at several complex cancer types that require greater scrutiny in determining how mistletoe may best serve as an appropriate adjuvant (additional supportive therapy).

Most practitioners who provide mistletoe therapy in the U.S. focus primarily on standard (not fever-inducing) subcutaneous (SC) and supportive IV infusions. But as a curious practitioner or patient, it's good to at least know of other options. These high-intensity administration routes should be provided only by a physician who has completed additional training and mentoring in these methods.

Fever induction: A case for controlled and guided fever

In chapter 1, we considered a brief history of cancer research, including a look at the medical community's evolving understanding of immunotherapy. This included reports, particularly in the nineteenth century, noting spontaneous remission of cancer linked to resolution of an acute infection. More recent studies have found anywhere from 28 to 80 percent correlation between febrile illness and cancer remission.[1,2] In 2001, European researchers noted that patients who had never experienced a fever were at least 2.5 times more likely to develop cancer at some point in their lives than those who'd had fevers in the past.[3]

As uncomfortable as it can be, there's something immensely important about experiencing a fever. It has a crucial role in training and exercising the immune response.[4] In the early twentieth century, Rudolf Steiner and Dr. Ita Wegman had an understanding of this when they first used mistletoe in cancer treatment and referred to the importance of creating a "mantle of warmth" around the tumor.[5] Even conventional medicine is aware of the value of medical hyperthermia and its documented cytotoxic and immune-stimulating effects (see chapter 9).

That said, Mistletoe Fever Induction Therapy (MFIT) is far more intense than the effects experienced with SC injections at conventional dosages. Keep in mind, this does not necessarily mean that MFIT's oncological impacts are always better than those provided by SC therapy. As with all mistletoe therapies, it's far more important to evaluate the patient's constitution, condition, and goals. There are situations where lower-dose SC mistletoe is more effective than MFIT. The goal is to match the patient to the best therapy, in that moment in the patient's journey. MFIT is powerful, but it's not for everyone.

It takes effort to experience a fever! In fact, the energy required to raise the body temperature a single degree is equivalent to the energy required to complete a four- to five-kilometer walk (about two miles).[6]

There's a reason that MFIT has been referred to as *High-Challenge Induction Therapy.* When screening patients for fever therapy, we say "no" far more often than we say "yes." Fever induction therapy is not as hard on the body as most chemotherapies, but it is work and it is often uncomfortable. Patients need the vitality to endure a fever for up to three days. They need to have a strong desire and will to fight, and to clearly understand the value of therapeutic fever for its immunostimulatory effects.

MFIT is generally contraindicated for: glioblastoma prior to surgery; brain edema; most patients with less than a six-month life expectancy; those with heart conditions or severe co-morbidities; and patients currently undergoing chemotherapy, radiotherapy (in many cases), and other conventional immunotherapies. (Although it might well be that fever-inducing therapy would enhance the efficacy of checkpoint inhibitors and other immunotherapies; research in this field is urgently needed.) Also, patients with extensive liver metastases often lack the vitality needed for this kind of treatment. Fever therapy can alter PET scans and other conventional monitoring, so it is best to schedule MFIT with at least six weeks between the end of the fever therapy and diagnostic imaging.[7]

In addition to assessing the patient's overall vitality and screening for any serious contraindications, in the U.S. we also need to confirm there is a supportive home life for the patient. In Germany and Switzerland, MFIT patients can be admitted to an anthroposophic hospital and provided their treatment and follow-up monitoring there. In the U.S., we don't have that option. The MFIT injection is provided in clinic, but then patients go home with aftercare instructions. The fever often does not appear until the next day. It's crucial that they have at least one loved one who can care for them appropriately in that time and is willing to connect with the overseeing practitioner regarding any fever care questions that come up. It is the doctor's responsibility to ensure availability any time by phone in the days following the injection.

For the right patient, MFIT is intense but worthwhile. When Dr. Hancock speaks with patients and their loved ones, he describes the cancerous state as characterized by *chronic inflammation*. This chronic inflammation is like a truck spinning its wheels in the mud and getting nowhere. With fever therapy, we are causing a heightened and useful immune crisis, a healing crisis, with a high level of *acute inflammation*. This is active, organized inflammation that brings about substantial change. It's like putting that truck into four-wheel drive. It may make a big mess in the moment, but it gets you out of trouble quickly!

Mistletoe fever induction therapy (MFIT)

MFIT involves subcutaneous mistletoe doses high enough to induce fevers of 100.4 to 104.0 Fahrenheit (38.0 to 40.0 degrees Celsius). Fever induction works particularly well for patients who are "mistletoe naïve," meaning they have never been administered mistletoe before or have had only very low doses in the past. MFIT is usually provided using a high-lectin mistletoe,[8] although occasionally a lower-lectin mistletoe (such as Helixor A®) has, unintentionally, evoked fever in highly sensitive patients.[9] For the majority, we typically use the highest-lectin option, namely AbnobaViscum Fraxini®. If provided after chemotherapy, sufficient time should be allowed for recovery before administering the fever therapy. MFIT is more effective with an intact immune system. Fever therapy may be provided a couple of weeks *before* chemotherapy to enhance the effects of the conventional treatment. It is a powerful adjuvant in this regard.

When practitioners are trained in fever therapy, they're given guidelines and starting points for developing the treatment plan. But much like the SC injection "protocol," we hold two factors equally: the plan and the patient response. Typically, an initial injection of 10 mg AbnobaViscum Fraxini is sufficient to spark a fever. (In contrast, typical supportive SC injections usually start at 0.2 mg to 1 mg, depending on brand, to achieve the desired small local reaction.) A week later, we may increase to 20 mg to induce a second fever. Or we may keep it at 10 mg if the patient's initial response was dramatic. The patient's response always takes precedent over the initial dosage plan.

In lead up to the initial 10 mg fever-inducing injection, Dr. Hancock often provides 60 mg of IV mistletoe for three consecutive days. Because the mistletoe lectins have a half-life of 24 hours in the body, these IV infusions build up and prime the body for the 10 mg injection on the third day. Dr. Debus also encourages timing the MFIT injection based on biorhythm cycles, as first discovered and proposed by Dr. Reiner Penter. Ideally that injection is provided around 3:00 p.m. There are clear day and night warmth cycles in the body, and this afternoon injection time results in a fever peak at about noon the next day, which is an optimal time for that peak when working with the body's normal temperature cycles.[10]

Though adjustments will likely be made because of patient response, there needs to be some sort of rhythm to MFIT administration. It should not be chaotic. Patient and practitioners need a span of time to work with this and create that rhythm. For instance, fever therapy might be provided once a week for four weeks as an "induction phase," followed by "maintenance therapy" every three or four weeks until the fever reaction subsides. In between, we might provide supportive SC mistletoe, often from a different host tree and at a dose low enough that it does not trigger fever. We want to ensure a true rhythm and resolution in the fever cycle and avoid creating a rollercoaster of fever. As long as the dose is low enough, supportive SC VAE therapy between fevers can actually enhance the effects of the high-dose MFIT.

What happens in the body during MFIT

The fever will reach about 103.0 degrees Fahrenheit (39.5 Celsius). This is not as hot as medical hyperthermia (see chapter 9), and that's good from a safety standpoint. But it is hot enough to cause some tumor cell death—it just won't happen at the same fast rate as medical hyperthermia. Any increase in dead tumor cells means the immune system can come in, clean up the dead cells, and begin to recognize them as cancer. This cascade is characterized by *immunogenic cell death*. That means the cancer cells die in a process that activates the immune system. When that happens, the immune system learns to recognize the cancer cells as cancer and step into action. That is a powerful self-healing process, which we try to elicit as an immune-educating effect in all immunotherapies. If you can breach the immune-evading wall around the tumor, kill some of the cells, and allow the immune system to handle those dead cells, you give the body a chance to start eliminating the cancer cells on its own. During fever, heat shock proteins (HSPs) also form on the surface of stressed tumor cells. These HSPs act like a highlighter circling the troubled cells. These marked cells are not dead yet, but HSPs attract immune system cells to come over and eliminate them.

The fever, the dying tumor cells, and the HSPs all translate into a lot of heightened immune activity. In all honesty, that can feel awful. There may be some swelling of the tumor itself (see appendix A). Lymph nodes may swell too. These are normal signs that MFIT is working. The most common side effect is a raging headache, followed by nausea (sometimes vomiting), and significant soreness at the injection site. All of these are normal and not cause for concern. If the injection site becomes incredibly painful, it's fine to apply some *Aloe vera* or the AM topical preparation of Arnica Nettle Gel from Uriel Pharmacy.

It's important to let patients know that past, present, and future often unite within the increased warmth of fever therapy. Old or recent traumatic experiences can be stirred up during a fever and, ultimately, released.[11] This is good, but not always comfortable! On a more positive note, difficult decisions regarding the future can sometimes be facilitated through the fever experience. In our experience, patients sometimes come out of fever therapy with greater certainty about a major decision (such as whether to do chemotherapy or not) or newfound inspiration about their life purpose. Both fever and these inner experiences are hard work. If patients have jobs, we encourage them to take several days off to allow enough time for both the fever therapy and recovery time afterward.

On the whole, most patients tolerate MFIT well and describe it as more manageable than chemotherapy. In over twenty combined years of guiding MFIT, we've never seen a fever get out of hand or

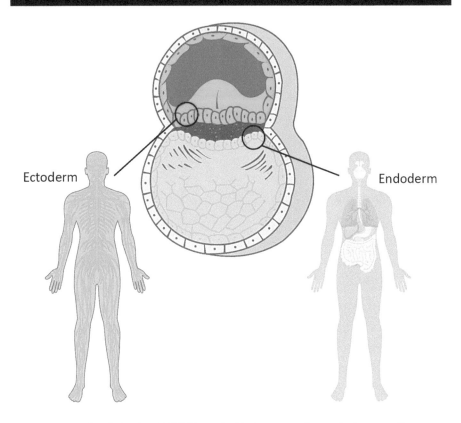

ECTODERM AND ENDODERM:
THE BOUNDARY/SHEATH AND METABOLIC ORGAN SYSTEMS

Ectoderm

Endoderm

turn non-physiologic. MFIT is safe. It does not degrade into malignant hyperthermia and does not cause organ toxicity. The body remains in control of the response. For patients who are ready for the exertion of dealing with a fever, it's very effective.

Mistletoe intratumoral injections

Intratumoral (or *intralesional*) injections are, as they sound, high-dose injections (usually starting at 10 to 20 mg) of VAE directly into or around the tumor area. Most often, these are injections to easily acces-sible sites (for example peripheral lymph nodes or breast lumps).[12] Like MFIT, this is a therapy that is provided only by practitioners who have received special instruction and mentoring. It is primarily provided in

European clinics, but also practiced worldwide by experienced doctors in their outpatient clinics.

Intratumoral (IT) injection is, of course, a powerful way to introduce viscotoxins (VTs) and lectins directly to the tumor itself. This can lead to immediate breaching of the tumor microenvironment, death of some of the cancer cells and, most importantly, education of immune cells in the region. IT injection is not for everyone. Like fever therapy, it can be quite uncomfortable. Patients need to know that. Though the injection site does not show the same reaction as an SC injection, there can be some tumor swelling due to the increased immune activity. Occasionally we have seen the tumor area get quite inflamed for days after the injection. This therapy is best for patients with a strong will and a desire to fight the cancer in their own way.

What happens in the body during intratumoral injection

With the tumor's defenses breached and many of the tumor cells experiencing stress, healthy immune cells can rush in and learn about the tumor. The mistletoe lectins act like a beacon, drawing more and more T cells and natural killer cells into the area. The immune system is finally able to educate itself about the tumor and take that information throughout the body. Potentially, it could use that information to address metastases.[13]

That latter step is known as something called the *abscopal effect.* This is an effect occasionally seen in radiation treatment: *Irradiate one tumor and the other metastases shrink or disappear.* It's not incredibly common, but it does happen.[14] We're not sure of the exact method of action, but it probably has to do with immune cell recognition and flagging. Irradiating the tumor results in some breaching of its immune-evading barriers. The immune cells come in, deal with the dying tumor cells, and learn about them in the process. They take that knowledge with them to other parts of the body where they're able to address metastases. Once again, this is a process defined by immunogenic cell death, which also can be evoked and enhanced by fever therapy, as we have seen above, or by hyperthermia.

Ultimately, the goal of any immunotherapy is to breach the walls of the tumor's microenvironment. It's not the tumor that paralyzes the immune system; it's actually the obscuring wall around it that causes the failure of the body's surveillance systems. In a sense, IT injection is an *in-situ* vaccination. It not only kills some of the cancer cells, but also educates the immune system by enhancing antigen presentation. As Dr. Debus puts it: *We have to make the cancer visible in some way, at the same time that we strengthen the body's metabolic warmth-producing forces and immunologic resources.*

Combining therapeutic synergies for best personalized care

It's often the combination of multiple forms of mistletoe application that mobilizes a whole-body response. Whichever administration routes are available in a patient's situation, it can be most effective to combine two or three and use more than one host tree. Always include SC injections in some way. As powerful and directed as these alternate approaches are, a profound *immunogenic* effect comes from simple SC injection.[15] After all, the skin is an extensive immune system organ. Even if a patient wishes to try IT injections, they should combine it with SC therapy as well. All the routes have a place and a purpose. IV therapy is highly supportive. MFIT awakens the whole system and heightens all immune activity. IT injection focuses and directs that immune activity. Each method allows the mistletoe to work at different points within the immune response.

Advanced uses of mistletoe in European clinics

In addition to MFIT and IT injections to easily accessible sites, there are a few other IT mistletoe administration routes that European practitioners are exploring right now (i.e., intrapancreatic injection).[16] Many of them are described in detail in the *Vademecum of Anthroposophic Medicines*.[17] These are not practiced in the U.S.; a patient interested in these therapies would need to travel to receive them. The following clinics in Germany regularly provide such therapies for international patients: Gemeinschaftskrankenhaus Havelhöhe (Berlin), Gemeinschaftskrankenhaus Herdecke (near Dortmund), Filderklinik (near Stuttgart), Paracelsus Krankenhaus (in Unterlengenhardt near Bad Liebenzell), Klinik Öschelbronn (near Pforzheim), as well as Klinik Arlesheim (near Basel, Switzerland).

Mitigating cancer-related fluid build-up

Malignant pleural effusion refers to a build-up of fluid in the space between the lungs and the chest cavity. It is a challenging problem in many advanced cancers. Fortunately, mistletoe has demonstrated significant success as an adjuvant therapy in this situation. In one comparison study, mistletoe extracts injected into the pleural cavity outperformed standard treatments by 15 percent and led to complete resolution in 79 percent of the treated patients.[18] Another study concurred that mistletoe was both better than talc and had fewer side effects, with a 96 percent success rate.[19]

Ascites refers to build-up of fluid in the abdominal cavity, often due to cancer that has spread to the abdominal lining. The use of mistletoe injected into the abdominal cavity to treat recurrent ascites is another advanced use.[20] There is one published case report of a woman with recurrent ascites from her cancer. She had the ascites resolve after instillation of mistletoe into her peritoneum.[21-23]

Novel bladder cancer adjuvant

VAE can be administered via bladder instillation, during which a high dose of mistletoe is periodically instilled through a catheter into the bladder and held there for several hours. This has been highly effective in caring for patients with bladder cancer. It appears to enhance immune stimulation directly at the tumor site. In a German study (see chapter 3 for study summary), a camera examination was performed and noted that marker tumors had disappeared in over half of the cases. In the remaining cases, surgical resection was performed. All the patients received additional bladder instillations and were followed carefully. In all the mistletoe-treated patients, the rate of recurrence was below the expected rate.[24] A Phase III study using this technique is currently underway.[25] The technical procedure is described in the *Vademecum of Anthroposophic Medicines.*[26]

Understanding organ system origins: Lymphoma, sarcoma, and glioma

Anthroposophic and integrative practitioners personalize the treatment plans for every cancer patient but also take into consideration the characteristics of the organ system from which the malignancy originates. Most cancers (solid tumors) originate from the epithelium of the glandular system, arising from the *endoderm*. However, lymphoma and sarcoma arise from the mesenchyme, which develops out of the *mesoderm,* and gliomas (brain/CNS cancers) originate in the glial cells arising from the *ectoderm*. Treatment decisions are better informed when we have a deep understanding of the organ systems from which each cancer arises. Let's learn more about those organ systems, how they form, and then discuss these cancer types as well.

Embryonic origins: Development of body systems, connections to cancer types

In embryonic development, when organs begin to form, there are two basic gestures in organ formation:

One is directed inwardly, originating from the endoderm, forming the organs of the gastrointestinal tract, from the mouth to the intestines, with all its associated glands, including the liver and pancreas. The lungs are included here too. These organs and body tissues, though diverse, hold in common the quality of taking in a substance from outside the body and metabolizing it in some way, whether food or water or air.

The other is directed outwardly, forming boundaries to the outside world and a protective sheath around the inner space of the body. The skin forms a palpable, physical barrier to the outside world, while the immune system, as it manifests itself in all our lymphatic tissues, represents an invisible, functional skin. Throughout life, this immune "skin" matures with each infection that it overcomes. The immune system represents a highly personalized sheath.[27]

These differences in the gesture of organ formation (inward vs. outward, metabolic vs. boundary-forming) are also reflected in the cancer risk factors for the associated body systems. The major risk factors for solid tumors, which predominantly affect organs associated with metabolism, tend to be lifestyle-oriented, such as: lack of exercise, metabolic syndrome associated with poor diet, and depression.[28,29] (The latter often appears long before cancer diagnosis has been made; the cancer-depression correlation is as high as 60 percent for hepatocellular carcinoma and 78 percent in pancreatic cancer.) It's more commonly known that Type 2 diabetes is a risk factor for pancreatic cancer,[30] and fatty liver is the most common cause of liver cancer.[31] These conditions are generally associated with metabolic syndrome and unhealthy Western dietary and lifestyle choices.

With all these factors, metabolic processes experience a certain stagnation. This lack of movement is physical, but also reflects in the soul life, which manifests as depressive tendencies. The soul does not connect properly to the body, causing a sense of stuck-ness, both physically and psychologically. One of Dr. Debus' patients described it as, "Standstill at high velocity." The dynamic and speed of modern city life not only prevent us from moving physically, but often also distract us from tackling biographic (life story) issues that are urgently calling for change. Instead of cultivated inner development, tumor development starts in the parts of the body that aren't really being organized by the body-oriented aspect of soul and spirit. We have mentioned earlier the resulting "cool-down" phenomena; our modern-day reduction in average body temperature and the rarity of febrile diseases. These patients greatly benefit when they cultivate more movement in their lives,[32] both in terms of physical exercise and inwardly by inciting enthusiasm for the truly important issues in life. Thus, soul warmth and physical

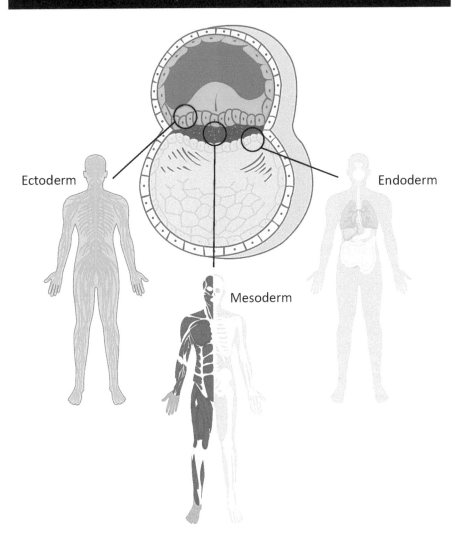

**THE THREE ORGAN SYSTEMS:
ECTODERM, MESODERM AND ENDODERM**

Ectoderm

Endoderm

Mesoderm

warmth will develop. Mistletoe treatment enhances and facilitates this warmth-generating process.

Both cancers of the skin (namely melanoma) and lymphoma originate in the different "sheaths" of the body. With these cancers, we see a unique gesture. Some of the known risk factors for these cancers include emotional shocks and traumas.[33] Somewhere in the person's story, there might be a major shock—a divorce, a physical injury, a death, a natural disaster, or an assault. Something broke through the patient's skin literally, figuratively, or both. Unlike the cancers associated with the metabolic organ systems, lack of movement or depression are not typically associated with lymphoma and, in clinical observation, are not characteristic for melanoma patients either.[34,35] Lüder Jachens, an anthroposophic dermatologist, describes the soul qualities of many melanoma patients as empathetically taking on a lot of social responsibility for others.[36] They may begin to transgress certain soul boundaries, in their frequent focus on being available to others. Eventually this allows outside forces to breach their soul boundaries. This might show in their warmth organism; melanoma patients tend to have exceptionally low body temperatures, often around 95.0 to 96.8 Fahrenheit (35.0 to 36.0 Celsius). One gets the impression that the warmth-generating, metabolic process is working, but energy (heat) is given away constantly to the outside world. Think of a house that is heated well, but all the windows are open. For both lymphoma and melanoma patients, there is a sense that the boundary system is broken.

From the perspective of the warmth organism, if we looked at the gesture of these two general types of cancer, we could say that solid tumors are more associated with *metabolic warmth production that has become stuck.* With cancers that involve the body's protective sheath, *warmth is lost because of injury to the sheath.*

Now breast cancer, which is the most common cancer in women,[37] can bear within itself both gestures. Being a gland, the breast has a strong relationship to the inner *metabolic system.* Yet it is a cutaneous gland and thus also belongs to the *skin* (sheath or boundary system). Patients with postmenopausal breast cancer tend toward more metabolic-type risk factors, whereas young, premenopausal women often have a constitution more associated with the boundary system type.

Lymphoma and other "body boundary" cancers

There are dozens of types of lymphoma and other blood cancers. They all stem from the progenitor *hematopoietic* stem cells in the bone marrow. About 178,000 people in the U.S. were diagnosed with leukemia, lymphoma, or myeloma in 2020, and these cancers were responsible for almost 10 percent of all cancer deaths in the same year.[38,39] Survival rates have definitely increased in the past 40 years, but treatment regimens are typically highly aggressive and hard on the patient. Blood cancers tend to affect people at the extremes of age—either the very young or the elderly. In both cases, there is a sense that the person's inner immune sheath is vulnerable, either from being newly incarnated or from the stress of the aging process. Integrative care can be especially nurturing for these patients.

Immune system development: It is helpful here to look at the immune system as an "interior skin" with which we meet the world. When we think of newborns, we see how they are entirely open to the world—both with their sense organs and more inwardly with their immune systems. At that age, the immune cells have yet to meet the world. As children grow, their immune cells encounter infections with viruses and bacteria, as well as pollen and food. This interior skin of the immune system becomes fuller and more multifaceted. The immune system includes all these "naive" B lymphocytes, which are not fully mature until they meet their antigen match. When a B lymphocyte meets an antigen match, it enters a process in the germinal center of the lymph nodes where the lymphocyte rearranges its genome to produce the best matching antibody for that antigen. These mature B cells propagate so that during an infection, millions of antibodies of the same type are produced to fit that precise antigen. After the infection resolves, these B lymphocyte cells then must die back and reduce in number. In the antigen-matching process, B lymphocytes open themselves up and physically cut their own DNA to produce a precise, high-affinity antibody. *This is a vulnerable process in which the cell opens itself to the outside world.* This could be one reason why we see so much greater vulnerability to B-cell lymphoma over T-cell lymphoma—95 percent of lymphomas originate from B lymphocytes.

Regardless of that risk, whenever infections resolve appropriately, each exposure to a childhood illness directs our forces inward, forming and maturing the differentiated "vital skin" of our immune system. The lymphatic tissue in children is very active and dynamic (hyperplastic) because it is dealing with infections all the time. Children are strikingly open toward the outer world—both in terms of their immune system development and in their impulse to imitate the adults around them. The more the lymphatic system matures toward puberty, the more an inner soul space develops (with all the unpredictable emotional states that go along with it). The hyperplastic lymphatic tissues recede, being shaped and formed by the soul and "I"-organization that have intensely worked through them during childhood infections.

The question may be asked, "Are there instances where this maturing process has not taken place properly during childhood?" There is some evidence pointing in this direction. For example, one study has noticed that self-reported history of measles or whooping cough during childhood seems to convey a 15-percent risk reduction for Non-Hodgkin-Lymphomas (NHL) later on in life.[40] In another recent study of 1,102 NHL cases and 1,708 population-based controls, researchers found that people who had rubella, whooping cough, and other childhood infectious diseases had lower incidence of B-cell NHL occurrence later on and, conversely, those who had not experienced such childhood illnesses, had a higher incidence of B-cell NHL later on (inverse association).[41]

That's a challenging way to acquire immune system strength, and there may be additional ways to nurture the immune sheath. Recent research has found that such protection may also be developed through artistic and educational means. A multicenter cross-sectional study of 84,000 students found a protective trend for a whole array of health issues in adult life for children who attended a Waldorf school. (Waldorf schools use a holistic pedagogy, based on Rudolf Steiner's work, providing academic, artistic, and physical activities in a balanced form.) Although continued studies are needed, the initial study saw a 20 percent protective effect against cancer later in life.[42] This study was not solely looking at lymphoma and boundary system cancers, but all cancers. Regardless, it would seem that there is some significant crosstalk between intensive soul-nurturing (strengthening the child's personal identity and boundaries) and healthy development of the immune system (a cellular sense of self and non-self).

Constitutional qualities: We cannot universally generalize the constitutional predisposition of a lymphoma patient. But some constitutional tendencies appear more pronounced in a number of the patients we encounter in our clinics. Again, the maturing of the immune system (during the course of various childhood infections) walks hand-in-hand with the maturing of soul life in later childhood and puberty. Thus, an inner space is created not only in terms of immune function, but also in terms of self-reflection and starting to live one's own individual biography (or life story).

In lymphoma patients, the lymphatic system seems to regress to the hyperplastic (immune naïve) state of childhood, quite often including enlarged cervical lymph nodes or mediastinal mass. Associated with this, we sometimes find a wonderful childlike openness, an outwardly directed, loving soul life that touches many people. These patients also like to explore all the varied, original, and adventurous possibilities that life can offer. Simultaneously, they might show a certain insecurity as to which passion they ought to pursue as "their own" within their distinctive biography. Their caring nature is beautiful. But taken to an extreme, it leaves them with a dysregulated balance between "becoming one with the world" and "being present with oneself." It can be especially nourishing for these patients to begin inner work using adjuvant anthroposophic soul care therapies. Biographical journaling can be overwhelming but also deeply healing for them.[43]

The most extreme and studied example of this constitutional quality is found among people with Down syndrome. In this condition there is a ten- to twentyfold greater risk of acute lymphoblastic leukemia and acute myeloid leukemia and a much lower risk of solid tumors.[44] In statistically supported medical literature, people with Down syndrome are typically described as "affectionate, sociable, and cheerful."[45] This is a strong, outwardly oriented soul tendency. This outward-focused self can find it challenging to form an "inner skin." Correspondingly we see a much higher risk of severe infections as well as blood cancers. However, this constitutional imbalance does not seem to be associated with a higher risk for solid tumors—the cancers that arise from being stuck both metabolically and biographically.

Lymphoma care strategies: The general therapeutic approach in lymphoma is to use remedies that help form boundaries and define an inner space.[46] This often translates into rhythmic administration of both mistletoe and *Helleborus niger.* Unfortunately, many integrative practitioners believe that mistletoe is contraindicated for lymphoma. The concern is that if mistletoe stimulates the immune cells, wouldn't it stimulate lymphoma growth? On the contrary, several retrospective analyses suggest a significant extension of survival time for lymphoma resulting from mistletoe therapy.[47] Furthermore, complete and incomplete remissions have been described when VAE therapy was used.[48,49] Mistletoe therapy can be safe and beneficial alone or alongside chemotherapy for lymphoma patients. It is, however, important to distinguish between high-grade and low-grade lymphomas when determining the best VAE administration route, dosage, and rhythm.

> *Low-grade non-Hodgkin lymphoma:* Includes chronic lymphatic leukemia (CLL), follicular lymphoma grade 1 and 2, Waldenstrom's Disease and marginal-zone lymphoma. These are slow-growing and either symptom-free or present few symptoms. Conventional oncology often adopts a "watch and wait" strategy here, since the natural course of the disease is, in many cases, only slowly progressive and is not likely to lead to any severe impairments in the long term. In this situation, chemotherapy is usually unnecessary and is used only at a later stage, as the patient gains no prognostic advantage from it. In this waiting time, the scope opens up for mistletoe therapy's immune-stimulating function to delay progress or even to achieve remission
>
> *High-grade lymphoma:* This refers to highly malignant, aggressive, non-Hodgkin lymphomas (i.e., diffuse large-cell B-cell lymphoma). Chemotherapy is the primary recommendation,

and in most patients, this leads to remission and healing. Here mistletoe therapy has a predominantly supportive character, as adjuvant treatment alongside chemotherapy and as follow-up treatment to maintain remission and to improve fatigue and susceptibility to infection.[50]

Regardless of low- or high-grade status, the most appropriate host trees are pine (pini) and fir (abietis).[51,52] These coniferous trees give structuring and focusing forces that are needed in lymphoma. Iscador® P (pini) is the most well-reported for lymphoma care in Europe. But Helixor A (abietis) or P (pini) are also useful for either high- or low-grade lymphoma. Helixor products are often more readily available in the U.S. With slow-growing tumors, we tend to provide supportive intravenous Helixor A or P or Iscador P.

In low-grade lymphomas such as CLL, where there is no excess proliferation, we may use MFIT with due caution. In these cases, the fever can improve fatigue and lead to stabilization or even remission of the disease.[53] IT therapy combined with MFIT has also been applied successfully in primary cutaneous B-cell lymphoma.[54] When providing normal, low-dose, SC mistletoe, significant fatigue sometimes responds better to deciduous, higher-lectin host trees, such as AbnobaViscum Fraxini or Helixor Mali. These more nuanced treatment choices typically are not provided for fragile patients or in aggressive cancers.

When lymphoma patients begin to understand the need for boundary-building as part of their entire treatment plan, they become curious about other adjuvants. *Helleborus niger* is especially helpful. If a patient is anxious or otherwise seems poorly grounded, *Helleborus niger* helps them feel more comfortable within themselves. It also fosters rhythm and a harmonious distribution of warmth within the warmth organism. Mistletoe helps to *generate* needed warmth, while *Helleborus niger* helps to structure and *retain* that warmth (see chapter 8). In addition to VAE and *Helleborus niger*, we encourage lymphoma patients to explore adjuvants that are more focused on soul development. Anthroposophic art therapy and biographical journaling are especially useful.

Leukemia care strategies: Many practitioners who provide VAE therapy for other cancers (including lymphoma) may not provide it for *acute leukemia* (AML and ALL). Practitioners who do provide VAE tend to direct the mistletoe in a more constitutional way, as a low-dose remedy. Iscucin® A through D are helpful here. A large skin reaction is not always necessary or desired. However, there is precedent for use of more substantial dosing of mistletoe in leukemia. One preclinical study found a therapeutic synergy in dosing mistletoe alongside doxorubicin in chronic myeloid leukemia (CML) cells. Six times more cancer cells were killed when mistletoe was added to doxorubicin than when doxorubicin was used alone.[55] A similar synergy was found between mistletoe extracts with high triterpene levels and cytarabine in acute myeloid leukemia cells.[56] In clinical practice, with CML (which is usually well-controlled with tyrosine kinase inhibitors), higher doses of lectin-rich mistletoe preparations, from deciduous trees like AbnobaViscum Fraxini or Helixor M (mali), can be very helpful and strengthening.

Clearly, we are still learning how VAE interacts with leukemia. Conservative practitioners will likely look for other adjuvant options that have more research and case reports associated with them. Integrative and anthroposophic practitioners frequently recommend *Helleborus niger* alongside conventional treatment for leukemia. This is a safe and gentle starting point that can be helpful in addressing anxiety and conventional treatment side effects. It also cares for that deeper need for boundary-creation seen in most patients with blood cancer.

Melanoma care strategies: Melanoma is obviously not a lymphoma. But as mentioned earlier, it does display some constitutional similarities with lymphoma. Both of these cancer categories involve a boundary, either the body's inner or outer sheath. Our colleague Dr. Nasha Winters once said, "A lot of people get confused about melanoma, and it overwhelms them. I don't consider melanoma a skin cancer; I consider it a *systemic cancer* very much like blood cancers. When I approach it that way, I have much more positive outcomes."

There are notable intersections between melanoma and lymphoma. Certain lymphomas can appear as dermal nodules, lesions, or rashes, and melanoma patients often have the same constitutional character-istics as lymphoma patients. In our clinics, we've seen melanoma and blood cancers respond exceptionally well to the boundary-forming effect of *Helleborus niger*. The patients who try *Helleborus niger* often report inner experiences of greater wellbeing and feeling more centered. We've also found mistletoe therapy to be essential in melanoma, par-ticularly the supportive administration of SC VAE from birch (betulae), almond (amygdali), and pine (pini) host trees. Melanoma is well-known as responsive to immune-enhancing treatments, such as PD1 inhibitors, which take the brakes off the cancer-killing T cells.[57]

Sarcoma: The cancer "in between" the inner and outer body

Earlier we looked briefly at embryonic development and how that development differentiates between inner and outer body systems. In biology, we actually refer to three layers of cells in that differentiation stage. The *endoderm* gives rise to those inner organ systems, and the *ectoderm* develops into the skin and nervous system. A third cellular category resides between those two layers: the *mesoderm*. This middle layer develops primarily into the muscles, connective tissue, bones, and the reproductive and urinary tracts. Sarcomas develop within these tis-sues of the mesoderm.

Generally, sarcomas are divided into tumors arising from bone or from soft tissue. They make up less than one percent of all adult cancers, but up to 15 percent of pediatric cancers.[58] Sarcoma is lightly related to leukemia and lymphoma, which arise from myeloid progenitor cells. These ultimately originate from the mesoderm. This relationship can be seen in the fact that there can be transformation between lymphoma, leukemia, and sarcoma. Sarcoma's statistical tendency toward pediatric patients indicates that this cancer tends to be a cancer of youth. From an anthroposophic perspective, we notice what we call "unrestrained youth forces"—growth and vitality that lacks balance and boundaries.[59]

Constitutional qualities: For patients with sarcoma, there is often a history of one distinct instigating trauma, while in carcino-mas (solid tumors), there is more often a history of repetitive "mini

THE IMMUNE EFFECTS OF INTRATUMORAL INJECTION WITH VISCUM ALBUM EXTRACT (VAE)

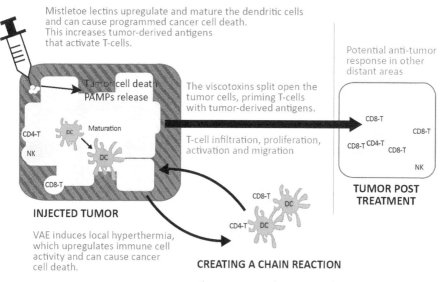

Mistletoe lectins upregulate and mature the dendritic cells and can cause programmed cancer cell death. This increases tumor-derived antigens that activate T-cells.

Potential anti-tumor response in other distant areas

Tumor cell death
PAMPs release

The viscotoxins split open the tumor cells, priming T-cells with tumor-derived antigens.

Maturation

T-cell infiltration, proliferation, activation and migration

INJECTED TUMOR

TUMOR POST TREATMENT

VAE induces local hyperthermia, which upregulates immune cell activity and can cause cancer cell death.

CREATING A CHAIN REACTION

The tumor is used against itself. The IT cascade activates T-cells, increases recognition of tumor antigens, mediates tumor cell death, and releases a new array of tumor-derived antigens.

traumas."[60] The latter might be felt as the monotonous daily grind of everyday life, out of alignment with the soul and spiritual direction of the individual. Sarcoma is a cancer of incarnating (feeling one is not "in life" enough) while the solid tumors are cancers of excarnating (feeling too "stuck" in life).

The mesoderm, or *mesenchyme* (from which sarcomas arise), is the "glue" that holds the bodily organism together, structurally and functionally. It includes connective tissue, as well as interstitial fluid. It is responsible for providing structure, as well as all the processes that are necessary for information exchange between organs. In its intense fluid exchange, the etheric forces (life forces) prevail, whereas all the messenger substances that circulate in this fluid, regulating cell growth and differentiation, as well as metabolic processes, are part of the forming principle of the astral body (soul).

From an anthroposophic perspective, we look for how we may support connections within the fourfold human. One other anthroposophic remedy provided for patients who have sarcoma is *Cetraria islandica* (Icelandic moss—a lichen, which is composed of a symbiosis of fungus and algae). This remedy is provided to help regulate the connection between the astral and etheric body—which strengthens the mesenchymal tissues.[61]

Warmth is also crucial for patients with sarcoma. When the "I"-organism has a healthy connection to the bodily processes, this manifests as warmth. Through this insight, we can also understand why enkindling warmth is such a key to successful therapy for sarcoma. There is much evidence for this in conventional therapy, and mistletoe can also help enkindle such warmth.

Sarcoma care strategies: Sarcomas, depending on the type, are often resistant to chemotherapy and other standard of care (SOC) modalities. They are stubborn cancers! However, even conventional medicine acknowledges that therapeutic medical hyperthermia (see chapter 9) has been found to improve survival.[62] With this finding in mind, it is not so surprising to note that Coley's successes with early forms of "fever therapy" involved patients with sarcoma. Warmth enhancement is indeed a powerful component in sarcoma care. So, yes, there is a definite role for VAE therapy, especially fever therapies and IT injection.

A compelling European case series described remissions and robust tumor responses in six sarcoma patients with varied mistletoe extracts.[63] In this case series, there was a patient on a high-lectin mistletoe who declined chemotherapy. With the high-lectin mistletoe, the patient experienced reduction in tumor size. The practitioner changed host trees, and the regressed tumor began to grow again. The doctor changed back to the high-lectin mistletoe and this patient achieved a complete and durable remission of over 16 years.

Another illustrative case from Tbilisi, Georgia involved a 58-year-old patient with an inoperable sarcoma after multiple failed conventional treatments. AbnobaViscum Fraxini, initially in a low dose of 0.2 mg, was injected into the tumor (IT therapy), followed a few days later by a 2 mg injection. Initially the tumor was expectedly inflamed, and later it became markedly smaller. The dose was gradually increased and the injections continued until the twelfth dose, after which the patient experienced a remission. An ultrasound found an area of necrotic tissue where her tumor had been. The tissue was biopsied and found to be composed of fibrotic tissue, white cells, and no tumor cells.[64]

In a small, randomized study looking at osteosarcoma (see chapter 3 for summary), patients who were given mistletoe therapy as a sole maintenance therapy after surgery for second relapse, showed a considerably longer post-relapse, disease-free survival (PRDFS) compared to those who received oral etoposide only, as seen 12 years after the start of the trial. A trend for an advantage in overall survival (OS) was also evident. The mistletoe therapy group also had notably improved immune parameters.[65] It is worth noting that this study used the lectin-free Iscador P, whereas in clinical practice and published case stories a high-lectin mistletoe is typically used, such as AbnobaViscum Fraxini or Quercus, or Helixor P (pini).[66]

Sarcoma presents a compelling case for the use of IT therapy and MFIT in carefully selected patients. Sarcomas have a clear relationship to the immune system. There are several documented sarcoma cases showing an abscopal response to conventional radiation therapy, in which only one tumor was treated but the entire tumor load regressed.[67,68] These responses show the importance of the immune system in sarcoma elimination. Even the conventional cancer research community has documented the value of medical hyperthermia for sarcoma.[69] Local hyperthermia also significantly prolongs survival in this tumor type.[70]

Warmth is powerful. Both IT mistletoe and MFIT can increase warmth. That's an obvious assertion regarding fever therapy, but IT therapy produces warmth, too. It causes an acute inflammatory response inside the tumor, which is a kind of local hyperthermia. At the same time, the high viscotoxin content of the mistletoe will cause cancer cell necrosis. This involves release of many inflammatory compounds as the cell splits apart and breaks down. As mentioned earlier, this is when immune system education can finally occur as specific cancer cell markers become visible.

Glioblastoma and other cancers of the CNS

Only about 24,000 adults in the U.S. are diagnosed with a primary central nervous system (CNS) tumor each year, which is less than one percent of annual cancer diagnoses.[71] For glioma (brain tumor) and glioblastoma (Stage IV glioma) the annual incidence is six in 100,000.[72] Gliomas make up 81 percent of all malignant brain tumors. Unfortunately, SOC treatment for these tumors has advanced little in recent decades. In glioblastoma, average survival with treatment is about 14 months.[73] There is clearly a lot to be gained from integrative therapies that do more than just focus on the tumor. We need to expand our focus to include addressing underlying causative factors in these cancers.

Constitutional qualities: From an anthroposophic threefold perspective, it is understandable that tumors in the restful, quiet area of the CNS are very rare. The nerve cells themselves have little to no metabolic activity in an anthroposophic sense. A nerve cell works hard—that is for sure—but its main function of polarizing and depolarizing is itself like a mini death process.[74] One way to determine if a cell is alive or dead is to find the difference between inside and outside concentration charge. Nerve cells depolarize as part of their activity—so by this definition they are undergoing tiny death-like states on a continuous basis. Nerve cells do not move and have little regenerative capacity, and so, they almost never become cancerous.

Though other brain tumors can arise from other tissue types, gliomas arise from the more metabolic *glial cells* in the brain, which arise out of the *ectoderm*.[75,76] Glial cells are not nerve cells. Glial cells exist solely as metabolic helpers to the nerve cells.[77] It is fascinating that primary brain tumors are far more common in pediatric populations—where the etheric life forces are still stronger. It is usually embryologic cells, or cells lining or supporting the nerves, that are affected.[78]

Glioma care strategies: Due to glioma's location in the center of the nerve–sense system, we tend to select mistletoe from tree types that are more *structuring* and less *metabolic*. Usually these are the coniferous trees—pine and fir. Fir (abietis) mistletoe is more supportive and indicated when undergoing brain irradiation. It is also used for support during chemotherapy, though pine mistletoe can often be transitioned to during this time. Generally, in the U.S., only low-dose, low-lectin mistletoe therapy is provided when caring for CNS tumors.

A significant reason for using these lower-lectin, more structuring host trees is that the brain is an enclosed space. Swelling is a crucial concern. With any space-occupying lesion, mistletoe therapy should be utilized only under the direction of a clinician whose training and mentorship has focused on this skill. One clinician in Prague uses fever induction with high-dose mistletoe and has several case reports of long-term survival.[79] But this approach is not available in the U.S. In Europe, this therapy is provided only within a participating hospital center with supportive care that can quickly address any transient tumor swelling. In the adjuvant situation, when the actual tumor has been removed, lectin-rich mistletoe preparations may be considered if scans confirm there is no longer any brain edema (swelling), and the location of the tumor is not critical (i.e., brainstem).

In case of edema, boswellia—also known as frankincense (*Boswellia serrata*)—can be helpful as it possesses strong anti-inflammatory properties. It may be used in high doses (several grams per day) to more quickly wean off of the steroids that are often needed for swelling related to surgery and radiation.[80] Steroids can have marked side effects if used over a longer period of time (diabetes, immune suppression, sleeping disorders, etc.) Ironically, this only promotes cancer growth further and diminishes treatment efficacy. Ultimately steroids are known to reduce survival in glioma and glioblastoma.[81] There is a need for strategic balance here, as steroids are often necessary, but it is best to aggressively wean off them. It's good to know that boswellia can help make that possible.

In addition to boswellia, *Helleborus niger* (see chapter 8) is another effective adjuvant. It is used when we see brain edema. It's also extremely useful for mitigating cognitive issues associated with the tumor or resulting from chemotherapy or radiation. It seems to take the edge off memory, concentration, and cognition challenges. Indeed, one of the more common uses of *Helleborus niger* is for the "brain fog" associated with chemotherapy in any cancer, not solely brain cancers. It also seems to help some patients with cancer-related fatigue, whether stemming from the disease or its treatment.

In addition to these adjuvant therapies, a therapeutic ketogenic diet is emphasized as essential in GBM care by many practitioners in the U.S., including Dr. Hancock and Dr. Winters. Dr. Hancock understands the ketogenic diet as regulating or even "pruning" the etheric body. As discussed in greater depth in chapter 9, ketosis induces several effects simultaneously on immune, metabolic, and genetic aspects of the cancer process. A therapeutic ketogenic diet is particularly beneficial as a foundational therapy for brain cancer because of its ability to reduce inflammation, enhance anti-tumor immune system activity, and make tumor cells more vulnerable to many other SOC and adjuvant therapies.[82]

Researchers have found that a therapeutic ketogenic diet creates metabolic conditions that restrict the growth of tumor cells, while supporting immune function in the brain.[83] Though large clinical trials finding significantly improved survival are currently limited to animal trials,[84] human studies are accumulating, including a small trial with several long term (three to four-year) survivors,[85] and a long-term survivor with GBM recurrence treated with ketogenic diet as a standalone therapy.[86] Dr. Winters has over 50 long term survivors with GBM largely due to the ketogenic diet working in conjunction with addressing the terrain of each patient. Dr. Hancock has an esteemed conventional neuro-oncologist colleague who refers patients to him specifically for the integrative approaches he is able to employ, including the ketogenic diet. Ketogenic diets have long been used as a natural method to prevent seizures, which are common with brain tumors.[87] This is a fascinating "side benefit" of implementing a ketogenic diet during brain cancer care.

Concluding thoughts

In this chapter we've shown that it is possible to use mistletoe to vigorously upregulate the immune system, prompt a transformative fever, and even direct the body's anticancer forces with IT injections of mistletoe. This is the strongest, most dramatic mistletoe administration route and is only for carefully selected patients. Most patients will find that supportive SC or IV mistletoe therapy provide transformative benefits on their own, but it's still empowering to know about less common VAE therapy methods. We also looked at novel uses of mistletoe in problematic situations such as pleural effusion and ascites. By varying the host tree type and manufacturer, mistletoe therapy can be used in practically every therapeutic situation in integrative oncology.

We've expanded our understanding of different cancer types, recognizing the constitutional tendency of patients with lymphoma, leukemia, and sarcoma to be "too open" and "not grounded enough." This differs from patients with solid tumors where the opposite tendencies are present. We also looked at the constitutional aspects of glioma and glioblastoma. For all these unique cancers, we explored how integrative care fits into the therapeutic picture, including: mistletoe, *Helleborus niger*, boswellia, and therapeutic dietary change. When SOC has a poor prognosis, it is heartening to know there are other options that can provide the unexpected positive results we all hope for. May some of these new options bring healing!

CASE STORY ONE: ROBIN

Fever Therapy as Primary Treatment Strategy				
Physician: Dr. Mark Hancock	Patient: Robin	First seen: (May 2018)	Age: 45 (at first visit)	Sex: Female
Cancer Type & Stage:	Left breast cancer (ER-, PR-, HER2-negative). One involved left-side axillary node, and involvement of left anterior mediastinal nodes; Stage 3c at time of recurrence in 2018.			
Risk Factors:	High stress work environment; high anxiety. Severe childhood trauma.			

When Robin came to my clinic, Humanizing Medicine, in May of 2018, she was already well into a journey of battling breast cancer. In 2016, she'd been diagnosed with Stage II left sided triple negative (ER- PR-, HER2-negative) breast cancer. This is a very aggressive cancer. She opted for a lumpectomy and, due to her personal beliefs, she declined radiation and chemotherapy. She did go to

Mexico for four rounds of dendritic cell therapy followed by two months of intravenous vitamin C (IVC, see chapter 9).

Robin worked on an inner spiritual practice and focused on healthy eating and managing her stress response in a healthier way. Prior to her diagnosis, she was employed in a high-stress position as an insurance executive, so these soul- and spirit-care practices were likely very needed. Robin was disease-free from this aggressive cancer for several months. She tried to put it all behind her; she did not do any follow-up imaging but focused on a healthy lifestyle.

Her efforts had been helpful, but only to a point. Unfortunately, Robin had a recurrence in the same breast in July of 2017. Because of her beliefs and previous difficult encounters with medical doctors, she attempted to manage her cancer on her own focusing on her diet and self-treating with dozens of supplements. Still her tumor continued to grow. By the time she met with me in May 2018, she had a fist-sized tumor in her left breast. Despite this situation, Robin remained insistent that she would not under any circumstance do chemotherapy or radiation. As she put it, "I would rather die than do those treatments." This is a deeply personal choice, and we respect and support patients, whatever course they choose.

A PET CT showed a centrally necrotic 4.2 x 6.7 cm tumor in the left breast, with one involved left-sided axillary node and involvement of the left anterior mediastinal nodes. There was no evidence of bone or organ metastasis. A Biocept cancer biomarker test showed: 0 cytokeratin + circulating tumor cells and 19 cytokeratin positive cells in her blood. This meant that Robin was Stage 3c (T3N3bMo(i+)) with the most aggressive form of breast cancer. I explained this clearly: "With the best of all conventional care, long-term survival is estimated to be less than 50 percent."

After careful discussion with Robin, she opted for fever therapy with IV AbnobaViscum Fraxini via IT injection. She initially declined not only chemotherapy and radiation, but also surgery. She demonstrated a good understanding of the risks that she was taking on. So, we proceeded.

In the first week, I provided three days (spaced three to four days apart) of IV and IT therapy, building from 10 mg to 40 mg IT. For the next three weeks, Robin came in once a week for similar IV and IT therapy, working up to 110 mg IT injection. After the second injection, she reported that her breast was sore and inflamed. The IT injections successfully provoked fever, initially 100.9 degrees Fahrenheit (38.3 Celsius) and then reaching up to 104.3 Fahrenheit (40.2 Celsius). During her first fever, Robin reported a lucid dream where she began turning into a mistletoe plant. She also said that she worked through some severe childhood trauma during this fever.

After the first four weeks, Robin had a two-week break from this therapy course. Then we began another three-week, once-per-week therapy course, again with IV and IT together. By day 63, we had worked up to 200 mg for the IT injection. During this series, her fevers held at about 102.3 to 102.6 F (39.1 to 39.2 C). From day 3 to 63, Robin's tumor was notably enlarged and inflamed, up to 9 cm on exam. I explained that this is a normal response and a sign of enhanced immune activity. But we also decided to pause therapy for a few weeks to let the immune response resolve.

At this point, we once again discussed the possibility of surgery. The tumor was obviously stressed by the treatment, and this could be a highly effective moment to remove it. We managed to persuade Robin to pursue lumpectomy with a surgeon. A week later, just prior to surgery, Robin was excited to report that her tumor was much smaller, 6 x 6 cm by palpation. Ultrasound confirmed a 4.3 x 4.8 cm mass with prominent nodes.

The lumpectomy was completed on day 98, a little over three months after starting VAE fever therapies. The pathology report described a *"well circumscribed cavity with necrotic center 2.8 x 2.2 cm.... Breast tissue with abscess cavity, abundant necrosis, numerous histiocytes, dense fibrosis and fibroblast proliferation admixed with recent and old blood. Remaining breast tissue shows fibrocystic changes."* In other words, no evidence of malignancy! Robin was understandably elated. We discussed and decided on a post-surgery clean-up therapy strategy. For the next four weeks, she came in for IV mistletoe (working down from 200 mg to 100 mg) plus IVC (working up from 30 g to 90 g). The first two weeks, she experienced fevers of 102.0 and 99.7 F. respectively. The final two weeks, the therapy did not provoke any fever. This is expected as we increased the dosage of the IVC—the cooling therapy in this warm-cool therapy combination.

In the long-term, Robin continues SC mistletoe three times per week at home and comes into the clinic every six to eight weeks for IV mistletoe. In her third year of remission, we added breaks between her SC mistletoe injections. She obtains yearly ultrasounds which show resolution of her previously enlarged lymph nodes. Robin is still cancer-free and living an active life.

CASE STORY TWO: MAX

Fever Therapy for Stage IV Hodgkin's Lymphoma				
Physician: Dr. Mark Hancock	**Patient**: Max	**First seen**: March 2020	**Age:** 29 (first visit)	**Sex:** Male
Cancer Type & Stage:	Refractory Stage IV Hodgkin's Lymphoma (with lung metastases), at time of diagnosis in 2017.			
Risk Factors:	Alcohol and tobacco exposure, stress, diet high in processed foods and sugar.			

When Max first came to my clinic, he had been living with his lymphoma diagnosis for two years. Originally, he was diagnosed upon experiencing an inexplicable 30-pound weight loss and night sweats. After his diagnosis of Stage IV Hodgkin's Lymphoma (with lung metastases), Max initially declined chemotherapy and started a therapeutic ketogenic diet and took several supplements instead. He did find that his B symptoms diminished with those self-treating choices. But this self-care was not enough. A year later, a CT scan showed progression, and Max opted to start the chemotherapy combination ABVD (Adriamycin, Bleomycin, Vinblastine, Dacarbazine). That did not provide a complete response, and he started on brentuximab vedotin. He also had radiation on one remaining area in his mediastinum. This is when Max met with me.

Max was only 29. As I got to know him during patient intake interviews, he shared that he was a musician. Before cancer, he was in a band and he taught; he was just starting his career. He wanted to do everything he could to maximize his chances of success.

We discussed some integrative and anthroposophic options he hadn't tried. We began with high-dose melatonin at 300 mg per day, to synergize with his radiation. Max also started mistletoe therapy: Helixor Pini IV, to which he responded with fever to 101 F. He transitioned to SC Helixor Abietis (5 mg, two times per week) and *Helleborus niger* 4x (three times per week). Max also took stibium powder three times per day.

Within six weeks of beginning these therapies, Max reported that his neuropathy was 95 percent better. His energy had improved. He felt "more secure in life." Soon Max was able to work again, as well as play in his band. After six months, Max had a follow-up scan and a biopsy of a small area that was found to be benign. After a secondary follow-up scan, he was declared to be in full remission by his oncologist. Max continues using both the *Helleborus niger* as well as the Helixor Abietis, with a one-week break between series.

CASE STORY THREE: LUCY

SC Mistletoe & Ketogenic Diet for GBM				
Physician: Dr. Mark Hancock	**Patient:** Lucy	**First seen:** October 2019	**Age:** 65 (at first visit)	**Sex:** Female
Cancer Type & Stage:	Glioblastoma Multiforme of the right temporal lobe. Wild type IDH1 unmethylated tumor at time of diagnosis in 2019.			
Risk Factors:	High carbohydrate diet, alcohol use, stress, pesticide exposure, turbulent divorce.			

When Lucy came to me in 2019, her life had been completely upended by a sudden and highly aggressive cancer diagnosis. Three months earlier, she had gone to the ER with a severe headache. A scan was ordered, and it showed a brain hemorrhage with a tumor being the cause. She underwent an emergency craniotomy with resection of her tumor. Lucy was diagnosed with glioblastoma multiforme of the right temporal lobe. Pathology revealed a wild type, IDH1, unmethylated tumor. Tumors with this genetic profile tend to be the least responsive to conventional treatment.

Lucy was 65. In a matter of 24 hours, she'd gone from being a small business owner of a trucking company, who loved caring for her three dogs, to having a cancer diagnosis that left her fighting for her life. In the days that followed, Lucy began subsequent radiation therapy for six weeks, two months of Temodar, and dexamethasone to control inflammation. She decided to stop the Temodar due to her unfavorable tumor genetics and the side effects. She established care with us three months out from her diagnosis.

At least Lucy had supportive family members. Her two sisters were caring for her extensively, but it was clear that all three women felt lost and overwhelmed. Lucy had already started a whole-food plant-based diet, and she had successfully weaned off the dexamethasone. I saw room for improvement in her diet, and she was willing to try other therapeutic approaches. At my suggestion, she began a therapeutic ketogenic diet, restricting carbohydrates to 20 grams per day and protein to 1 gram per kilogram per day and increasing her fat intake to meet her core caloric needs with healthy fats. She tracked her macronutrient intake on an online app, and her sisters regularly reported her numbers to me.

Lucy's two sisters became integral to her recuperation. She still had severe fatigue and needed full assistance to move about her house. Lucy suffered from debilitating nausea and severe brain fog after her radiation treatments and chemotherapy. Fortunately, she showed no neurological deficits.

I recommended *Helleborus niger* injections twice per week for the brain fog and brain edema. Lucy also started on SC Helixor Abietis three times per week, for the sheltering and supportive effects of this host tree. She was very sensitive to this mistletoe and had robust skin reactions. She also started taking boswellia in high doses and several repurposed off label meds: mebendazole, metformin, atorvastatin, and niclosamide. These were used to block key metabolic pathways of cancer cells and ideally trigger apoptosis (healthy cell death).

Over the first six weeks, Lucy's nausea abated, and her brain fog lifted. Over the next few months, her strength returned to the point where she became independent again. She could walk easily, dress on her own, and make her own meals. She was able to start IVC infusions. Lucy also strategically used her diet and a ketone supplement prior to several weeks of hyperbaric oxygen therapy (HBOT), to address any residual microscopic disease.

After 20 months of these therapies, her inflammatory markers showed a marked reduction in C-reactive protein (CRP), from 7 down to 0.4. A recent MRI (at 18 months out) showed no recurrence of her glioblastoma. Lucy is once again leading an active life—something she thought would never be possible. She continues with the SC Helixor Abietis. Lucy's story is a striking turnaround that demonstrates the power of implementing the best combination of therapies in an appropriate order and rhythm. In her case, some conventional therapies (such as chemotherapy) played little role, due to the genetics of her tumor. Finding a synergy with natural and conventional therapies was key to her success. Above all, her two loving sisters stayed by her side through thick and thin. They were the support circle that held her when she could not care for herself.

Chapter 11

Using Mistletoe Therapy in Advanced Disease and End-of-Life Care

Dr. Steven Johnson, DO

"Go into yourself and see how deep the place is from which your life flows." —Rainer Maria Rilke

In North America, most people who seek out mistletoe therapy do so late in their cancer-fighting journey. When other treatments have failed, they hope that mistletoe might improve their quality of life (QOL), prolong their lives, and perhaps facilitate remission. As you will learn in this chapter, we can make a good case for why trying mistletoe therapy during the latter stages of cancer often proves to be a beneficial decision. However, anthroposophic doctors and integrative clinicians would always hope to have the opportunity to help their patients as early as possible.

For some patients with advanced cancer, mistletoe therapy can be used in palliative care and even hospice care. In my practice and among my colleagues, there are many reports of mistletoe helping to improve appetite and sleep; reduce nausea, emesis, fatigue, and depression; and decrease the necessary dosage of pain and anxiety medications. For patients who want to be more alert and awake during the dying process, in order to interact with loved ones, mistletoe therapy can play a helpful role. It can foster a deeper sense of dignity and humanity during the dying process and improve QOL.[1,2] While mistletoe therapy is more widely encouraged at earlier stages of cancer, it does provide many unique properties that can help in late-stage and palliative phases.

In reality, using mistletoe for these benefits is difficult in our current hospice and healthcare system. In a hospital environment, most providers will not see the value in using an injectable integrative therapy in this manner. Though I know of patients who used mistletoe during their dying process, typically they died at home and had already incorporated mistletoe into their integrative care plan long before. Integrative and anthroposophic physicians rarely use mistletoe exclusively for palliative care unless the patient or family specifically requests it. (This can be quite different in some European hospitals, where mistletoe is more commonly used in the hospital and larger clinic settings.) For the purposes of this chapter, we will not focus on palliative hospice care scenarios. Rather, we'll look at situations where mistletoe helped extend life and improve QOL for patients who were still ambulatory and fairly independent but had been told they had no further realistic conventional treatment options. Still, I think it is good to know that a doctor or nurse trained in mistletoe therapy and anthroposophic or holistic nursing can offer a great deal to a patient and family during end of life hospice care.

No matter the prognosis, I am always hopeful when a new patient comes to me asking about mistletoe therapy. So often patients enter my clinic with an advanced disease and a poor prognosis. Either they have been told they have a short time to live, or they will have to endure many potential side effects that will drastically compromise their enjoyment of life. While mistletoe is not a miracle medicine, the integrative community has seen some remarkable outcomes.

For instance, patients with advanced stage breast cancer who are undergoing chemotherapy experience far less intense side effects when also provided adjuvant mistletoe therapy.[3] Other studies have found that patients with breast and colorectal cancer experience greater physiological and mental resilience when they are provided mistletoe therapy alongside chemotherapy. This effect has been seen repeatedly, and it hints at how mistletoe seems to improve regulation of the autonomic nervous system (ANS). It's the ANS which, in turn, regulates most of our bodily processes.[4,5] Another randomized study looked at 123 patients with breast cancer (Stage I-IIIA) who received chemotherapy alone or along with adjuvant Iscador® M or Helixor® A. Researchers found that several QOL measures improved for those who were provided mistletoe therapy. The QOL measures included: pain, nausea, vomiting, poor appetite, diarrhea, and insomnia—all familiar chemotherapy side effects. In addition to side effect mitigation, the patients who received mistletoe therapy also experienced improved mood and ability to engage socially. These benefits have been seen in multiple studies.[6,7]

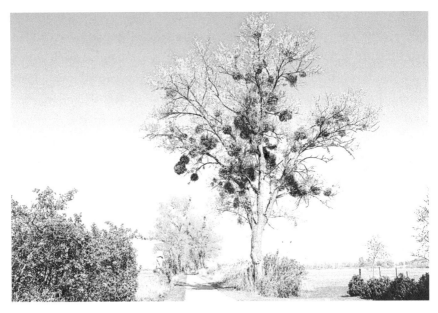

Pancreatic cancer (see case story below) is incredibly difficult to treat effectively and is often diagnosed late in its progression. In a Phase III randomized, controlled study, researchers examined QOL measures for 220 patients who had Stage III or IV pancreatic cancer. Due to poor prognoses, these patients were receiving the "best possible supportive care" (no longer in active treatment). The study participants either received that supportive care only, or supportive care plus mistletoe therapy. In the mistletoe therapy group, 13 of 15 QOL scores improved notably, including: appetite, fatigue, insomnia, pain, and nausea[8] In another study looking at 396 patients with pancreatic cancer, those who received adjuvant mistletoe therapy as part of a larger cancer treatment program experienced fewer chemotherapy side effects. They also experienced fewer life-limiting symptoms of the cancer itself, compared to patients who didn't receive mistletoe therapy.[9] There are plenty of examples and studies like these for most solid tumors. The studies show consistent benefits of mistletoe therapy in improving both QOL and extension of life. The result is frequently not a full remission, but rather a state in which the patient is living in a vital and coherent state with their cancer.

We can see there is strong scientific support for providing mistletoe when prognosis is poor. But when I was asked to provide instruction on this topic, I was drawn far more to share case stories than to share a long list of scientific study results. There is nothing more delicate, personal, and deeply spiritual than facing death and discussing a plan for one's own care during the dying process. Some concepts are explained better through real-life narratives instead of abstract study results. The anthroposophic application of mistletoe therapy in the face of a dire prognosis is one of those concepts.

For the remainder of this chapter, I want to share two case stories with far greater depth and personal detail than we've used in any of the other case summaries in this book. You'll see readily that these two patients are very dear to me. They both inspired me in different ways by their resilience, courage, and unique attitudes toward both life and death. Living well with cancer for an unexpected and prolonged period can be a special and unexpected gift. Both of these case studies illustrate that possibility.

CASE STORY ONE: LINDA

"One more Christmas dinner with the family"

When she first came to my clinic, Linda was 62, and it had been one year since she had chemotherapy and surgery (Whipple procedure) for pancreatic cancer. Just three months earlier, her scans showed that the cancer had metastasized to her liver. She was struggling with nausea, abdominal pain, poor appetite, and a 20-pound weight loss over the previous two months. She was just starting her second round of palliative chemotherapy when she came to my office to inquire about mistletoe. A close friend had a positive experience with mistletoe therapy when she had breast cancer and encouraged Linda to explore the possibility.

Linda was not usually open to holistic or alternative medicine, so this was a big step for her. She researched mistletoe therapy and anthroposophic medicine a little on her own. While she was impressed to see hospitals and clinics using this therapy in Germany and Switzerland, she also found plenty of online criticism of anthroposophic medicine and mistletoe. She was clearly tentative at her first visit. She wasn't sure how much time she had left to live and did not want to waste any of it.

Linda was six treatments into her second round of chemotherapy, and she definitely felt worse than during the earlier rounds she had received. She was losing weight, was nauseated, and food was rarely a pleasure. She often said to me, "Thank God for mashed potatoes!" Linda was sick to her stomach day after day and struggling just to get out of bed, with no desire to embrace the morning sunshine or spend time with her horses and farm—which had always been her passion. Instead, her life was defined by steadily increasing dosages of pain and anti-nausea medications. This wasn't the life she wanted, and yet she truly wanted to live. Linda's oncologist told her that a cure was unlikely, and she probably had six to twelve months to live. I remember she said, "I still have a lot of love to give. I love my horses and riding around my land, taking in the views." She wanted to be able to do just that once again.

Because mistletoe therapy was being studied at the Sidney Kimmel Comprehensive Cancer Center at Johns Hopkins,[10] Linda found the confidence to give it a try. Her friend told her that mistletoe helped her feel more hopeful, and it was an integral part of her cancer remission. Linda still had some doubts but decided she would try this new treatment for a set amount of time. It was early October when we conversed. She very much wanted to enjoy Christmas dinner with her family—and feel good eating it! We decided together that this was a good three-month goal.

After Linda and I spoke, she decided to stop chemotherapy for those three months, as she had received a substantial dose already, and she was tolerating it so poorly. Her CEA (tumor marker) had come down slightly, though not dramatically. We repeated a CT scan, and it showed a small reduction of some liver metastases, but several new liver lesions had also appeared. We discussed how mistletoe might help regulate her immune response and hopefully change her internal balance. We hoped it would up-regulate her immune surveillance and possibly slow the tumor growth. Having had so much chemotherapy, and after losing so much weight, I wasn't sure her body could mount a good immune response against the tumor. I had to be honest and tell her I wasn't sure how much she would benefit at her current stage of illness.

We ran lab tests looking for signs of inflammation and other biological clues to guide the choice of her supplemental treatments. Linda started on an intermittent fasting protocol, three days a week. This may sound counter-intuitive, but we certainly weren't doing this with a goal of further weight loss. Rather this was to help her gain weight during her eating days. Gaining weight is often a good sign in this type of cancer. She also started on subcutaneous (SC) Helixor P (pine) mistletoe alternating with AbnobaViscum® Fraxini (ash). She began biography counseling and therapeutic eurythmy, which is a special anthroposophic movement therapy based on the gestures of sounds, the spoken word, and musical tones (see chapter 8). Linda had heard of movement therapies like qigong and decided to give therapeutic eurythmy a try. We also agreed that, from this point onward, we would work from a position of hope and not fear. A new journey would begin.

Eventually Linda transitioned from SC to IV mistletoe therapy, still alternating different types of Helixor and AbnobaViscum mistletoe. We regularly alternated several anthroposophic homeopathic medicines and adjusted other supplements based on common tumor markers for pancreatic cancer. Linda's general condition did improve during that three-month period, and she did get to eat and enjoy that Christmas dinner with her family. Her journey didn't end there either.

I have been working with Linda for over three years now. She still has pancreatic cancer at the time of writing this account. Her liver still shows metastatic lesions, though they are smaller than before. Her CEA is less than half of its original number. Her liver and metabolic markers such as liver function studies and LDH (lactic dehydrogenase, see chapter 9) are normalized now. Linda occasionally takes anti-nausea medicine and prescription pain medications for abdominal pain. But these are her only prescription medications now. Her weight has improved, and she enjoys many foods—not just mashed potatoes! Though she's quick to note that she's limited herself to a much healthier diet. Linda works on her land once again and rides her horses often. Most days she would characterize as "good and fulfilling." She also sleeps through the night and wakes with hope and vitality to enjoy each day. Of course, she has to take it easy, but she does not spend her days stuck inside her house or unable to get out of bed. She is no longer depressed. She has had several Thanksgiving and Christmas dinners with her family now and was able to enjoy eating some of her favorite foods.

Linda did not get the full remission she wanted, but she is very grateful to be where she is in this moment. Three years ago, she and her oncologist didn't think she would be well enough to spend Christmas with her family. At 66, she now embraces her life journey living with cancer. Linda appreciates that she still has the option to use conventional therapies if needed, as she is more resilient now and has returned to a healthier weight. Most importantly, she is hopeful about living longer than expected. As she said, "I am so much stronger now." She appreciates and enjoys every moment she has with her horses, friends, and family.

Thinking About Linda: Remissions are not likely in scenarios like these. However, I have seen some remissions of pancreatic cancer, when integrating conventional care, anthroposophic mistletoe therapy, and holistic support. Linda's story is not so atypical. It is possible for patients with advanced cancers to outlive life expectancies with decent QOL. They can even experience a high QOL, despite being told they will need strong palliative care to be comfortable. Instead, they live in a state of proactively managing their cancers.

Mistletoe therapy within a larger integrated oncology care plan can initiate a remarkable turn of events, even when a patient presents in such an advanced state that short-term palliative care seems the only option. In Linda's case, as well as the next, there was an unexpected *extension* of life with an exceptional *quality* of life, while using minimal pain and other medications. Unexpected improvements in QOL and survival are indeed seen in multiple meta-analysis studies that examined the effects of mistletoe therapy.[11,12] Certainly, my colleagues and I have witnessed this often with our own patients.

CASE STORY TWO: ARTHUR

"I can accept my fate, but before I go…"

There are certain patients who make an impression on you that never fades. Arthur demonstrated a level of dignity, faith, love, and hope which is forever imprinted in my memory and soul. I remember when he first came to my clinic with his wife. Arthur was 71 years old, with an infectious sense of humor and a glint in his steely eyes. He had been in an ongoing battle with an unusually aggressive adenocarcinoma of the prostate. He had received radiation and hormone therapy over the past three years, but now presented in Stage IV, with metastases to his lungs, liver, pelvic lymph nodes, and bones. He had lost almost 25 pounds. He was given a poor prognosis of less than six months to live. His oncologist offered chemotherapy but told him he couldn't promise that the treatment wouldn't be worse than the disease. He advised Arthur to enter the local hospice program to receive palliative care. Arthur opted against chemotherapy. He had heard of European mistletoe, and his curiosity brought him to my clinic.

One of the first things Arthur said to me was: "Doc, I know I am going to die. I am a devout Catholic and retired army man, so I can accept my fate. But before I go, I want to travel to Europe and visit the churches dedicated to my dearest Virgin Mary. Can you help me do that?"

Arthur was quite serious. I told him the best we could do was try. Needless to say, I was concerned about getting his hopes up. But we agreed to embark on this journey together nonetheless.

That day, Arthur gave me a bar of fine European dark chocolate. This chocolate would come to symbolize our relationship. Every time we saw Arthur, he gave our staff and me a wonderful bar of Belgian or Italian chocolate. His wonderful attitude and appreciation for everyone was infectious, and our entire team always looked forward to his appointments.

Over that spring, Arthur started on an alternating course of IV vitamin C therapy (see chapter 9) and IV AbnobaViscum Fraxini (ash) mistletoe (sometimes enhanced with SC Iscador Quercus (oak) on the same day, to simulate a mild fever response; see chapter 10). We supported this intermittently with glutathione and chelating agents, as Arthur's bloodwork had shown very high levels of lead. He opted for a mostly vegetarian and alkaline diet, and we worked with many nutritional supplements to bring his high CRP (inflammatory marker) down to a normal level. We were able to adjust all his supplements in light of his tumor markers. Arthur took several anthroposophic remedies including formica 6X, astragalus 3X, and vitis stibium to help stabilize the accelerating metastasis. He also worked with art therapy, specifically focusing on contrasts of darkness and light. The art therapist encouraged him to think about strengthening his own forces of inner light as a counter image to the tumor. This idea rang true for Arthur, and he embraced this spiritual and creative practice.

The first six months resulted in a stabilization of Arthur's tumor metastases. His PSA dropped slightly, and the lymph node and liver lesions decreased in size. He felt more energetic and gained about ten pounds. Most importantly, he did indeed travel to Europe that summer. He was there for three weeks and visited several churches in Italy and France. On his return, he was ecstatic—and I promptly began gaining several pounds from all the chocolate he brought me!

After about six months of a fairly stable course, we decided to change the mistletoe regimen and began a higher IV dose of high-lectin AbnobaViscum Fraxini. We continued to intermittently add SC mistletoe at the same time as the IVs to induce fever responses. This was successful in that Arthur's PSA dropped even further, and his liver, lung, and lymph nodes showed significant improvement. However, there was not much change in the bone lesions—at least that meant "no progression." Arthur felt good, with a fair amount of energy and sense of wellbeing.

We completed several rotations of this therapy combination over the course of the next nine months, while continuing to rotate detoxification support and other treatments to build him up and strengthen his vitality. In addition to art therapy, we also added warming essential oil baths. Over time, all these efforts paid off. The following summer, Arthur traveled to many religious sites around the Baltics and other places in Europe associated with appearances and revelations of the Virgin Mary. He was elated, and for many months he was visibly beaming with joy. Around that time, in addition to more chocolate, he also gave me a medallion of the Virgin Mary.

During the second year of treatment, some of the bone metastases started to progress again and became painful. We decided it was worth it to try some palliative radiation. This was successful in reducing the painful lesions. Arthur was still able to avoid any conventional pain medications, relying on the mistletoe therapy and anthroposophic medicines instead. We rotated different forms of mistletoe that year, both subcutaneously and intravenously. Arthur had some ups and downs with fatigue and bone pain, but overall, it was a good year. He was grateful for all our successes so far.

Arthur remained dedicated to his treatment, and he actually took a third trip to Europe during his third year since we began working together. Heading into the fourth year of care, Arthur developed a bone metastasis to the skull, and it eventually grew dangerously close to his brain. After a lot of back and forth, we decided to risk radiation. Unfortunately, this procedure proved tragic. Shortly after the radiation treatment, Arthur developed sepsis and pneumonia, dying later that year. He was 75 and had outlived his predicted life expectancy by almost four years.

Arthur was thankful right up to the moment of his passing. But I will always wonder if I made the wrong decision in encouraging him to pursue that final radiation treatment. In truth, when I met him, I never thought he would live so long. Yet now I still wonder if he could have lived even a bit longer.

The end to this story is still deeply meaningful to me. Arthur died on a Sunday evening. I was at home, cooking dinner for my family. I remember reaching into the oven and badly burning my hand. The oven had a clock, so I happened to notice the time. When Arthur's family called me from the hospital to let me know that he had passed, I realized it was only minutes away from the time that I had burned my hand. There seemed to be a special connection between us that has remained lasting.

I was honored to attend Arthur's funeral, and now, almost ten years later, I still think of him often. The medallion of the Virgin Mary that he gave me is a little tarnished. But every now and then, I still hold it in my hand and remember Arthur's incredible dignity and kindness. I hope to be as full of hope and joy as him someday. That way of being never left him, even at the end of his life.

Thinking About Arthur: It is fairly common for patients to look for mistletoe or other integrative therapies when they have advanced disease and a poor prognosis. Though I often wish we could treat patients earlier in the course of their disease, I am often amazed how much mistletoe therapy can improve QOL and extend life too. I see this happen even in late-stage disease when we might otherwise stop all treatments and transition the patient to hospice care. Often, even in late-stage cancer, mistletoe seems to strengthen the spirit of many individuals in such a way that they are able to overcome a very poor prognosis. Arthur's story is an extraordinary one. As I often say to my patients, while late-stage cancer is a serious matter, it doesn't stamp an expiration date on our journey through life.

A *few closing thoughts*

There is an interesting common thread that runs throughout mistletoe survival studies and clinical observations. Often, when QOL improves, so does the tumor response to mistletoe. This again points to the self-regulating and self-empowering aspects of mistletoe therapy. Unlike so many conventional cancer treatments, mistletoe improves cancer outcomes, while also improving quality of life, which is so important to most people. This includes physical and emotional wellness and the intangible aspects of the human spirit that define our sense of wellbeing.

There is a strong principle of healing taught in anthroposophic medicine. My interpretation goes like this: *Health is not simply the absence of disease. It is a state of inner and outer coherence with ourselves and the world in which we live.* Mistletoe therapy embodies this principle. It is a symbol of what medicine could be in the future: Multiple harmonious practices that treat the disease while also improving the frequently overlooked intangibles of wellness that help us to look forward to life.

CHAPTER 12

WHAT THE HORIZON HOLDS
FOR MISTLETOE THERAPY . . .
and for an Expanding Integrative
Approach to Cancer Care

Dr. Nasha Winters, ND, FABNO

Special thanks to Dr. Steven Johnson
for his contributions to this chapter

"[One] who has health, has hope; and [one] who
*has hope has everything." —*THOMAS CARLYLE

What a journey! We have explored a brief history of oncology and immunotherapy, discussed humankind's evolving relationship with mistletoe, and learned about some of the interactions and synergies between VAE and other therapeutic interventions. With over a century of use as an adjuvant (additional and supportive) cancer therapy, mistletoe therapy has been established as safe, affordable, and clearly effective for enhancing quality of life (QOL). I hope the immunological understanding, research findings, and patient case stories have heightened your curiosity about this special plant.

The most important question you can ask and answer for yourself right now is: *How and where can I connect with mistletoe as a patient, practitioner, or supporter of integrative cancer care?* In these next few pages, I hope to provide some practical stepping stones. Initially, I'll speak solely to patients and loved ones who are in the midst of a cancer care journey right now. Later, I'll share opportunities for practitioners and integrative health philanthropists, too.

The challenges of accessing mistletoe

Today, many patients with cancer in Germany and Switzerland utilize mistletoe therapy at some point in their care. Mistletoe is offered as an accepted adjuvant therapy in some other European countries as well.[1] We hope to see mistletoe become a similar standard of care (SOC) therapy here in the United States. There are genuine challenges with accessing mistletoe in the U.S. right now, with ease of access varying from state to state. That's our reality. VAE is not yet covered by insurance—though its out-of-pocket cost pales in comparison to the conventional cancer care costs that often exceed insurance limits and are passed along to patients. Yes, there are challenges, and we need to take some time to state and face them head on. There are also clear solutions, both regarding physical access and financial support. Let's look at these challenges and their solutions, along with a vision for a better future for all of integrative oncology.

Financial Access: In terms of ballpark cost, mistletoe remains a relatively low-cost therapy at about $150 to $300 (U.S.) per month for SC injections and about $5,000 to $10,000 for aggressive IV or IT interventions (this varies broadly, depending on dosage and frequency of infusions). My colleagues and I urge any patient who struggles with covering this cost to connect with Believe Big (www.BelieveBig.org), a nonprofit organization focused specifically on providing wellness grants to cover mistletoe therapy. This organization has also funded a clinical research trial at Johns Hopkins Hospital[2] with hopes of bringing this therapy into the SOC realm.

When discussing the issue of cost with new mistletoe patients, the question that inevitably comes up is, "If this therapy is so effective, why isn't it covered by insurance?" In short, our current conventional healthcare and insurance systems are incapable of covering personalized medical therapies like mistletoe.

Our U.S. insurance system, down to the DNA of how it codes office visits and drug-based treatments, has no room for a therapy that is successfully administered through hours-long conversations with the patient; deep knowledge of their physical, emotional, and spiritual goals; and significant real-time, response-based adjustments to dosage and even product brand. Both the current insurance system and FDA drug-approval process are set up to approve and apply patentable pharmaceutical drugs. They have *no categorical framework* to acknowledge the existence of highly effective non-drug therapies. Mistletoe has no insurance code, therefore it can't be covered. This lack of insurance coverage has nothing to do with whether VAE therapy is effective; rather it's due to a structural flaw in our healthcare and insurance system.[3,4] Because of this flaw—prioritizing business efficiencies over humanized patient care—we now have a drug development system that fast-tracks the approval of new cancer drugs that have little evidence of life extension, while ignoring non-pharmaceutical treatments that have well-documented benefits for QOL and overall survival.[5]

Insurance-based healthcare does not incentivize holding the patient at the center of care decisions. Rather short-term financial streamlining takes precedent even though, over the long-term, patient-oriented care likely costs us all less. Mistletoe as an inherently personalized therapy, puts the patient back in the center of the equation. It walks upstream against the flow of the conventional insurance-based system in the U.S.—though mistletoe therapy does have some insurance-coverage in several European countries.

So yes, for now, patients in the U.S. must cover the cost of VAE therapy. Yet, it is a comparatively low-cost cancer care therapy. If cost is an issue, please connect with Believe Big. Also connect with anthroposophic, naturopathic, or integrative oncologists in your region. Ask if there are regional community funds that support cancer patients who want to access holistic care. On a longer timeline, consider sharing your story with your senator and representatives. Insurance law and FDA regulations will not change without a groundswell of public concern.

Geographic Access: Your first step in connecting with mistletoe is, of course, finding a provider who offers it. My coauthors and I have created a multi-year educational initiative to increase awareness, access, and training regarding mistletoe therapy in the U.S. It will take time to see the fruit of these efforts. But it is possible for you to access this course-altering therapy from where you are right now. Realize it may take a little creativity and some initial travel.

Begin with reaching out to the Physicians' Association for Anthroposophic Medicine (PAAM) at www.AnthroposophicMedicine.org. There are currently AM physicians in 25 states and many other mistletoe therapy providers trained by PAAM. Email this organization to find out who offers VAE therapy in your state or nearby region. If there are no VAE therapy providers in your state, consider telemedicine options with an out-of-state provider. You will need to travel for your initial patient exam and to learn how to self-administer the subcutaneous (SC) injections. But, at that point, most patients can complete their own care at home, and follow-up questions and check-ups are addressed via telemedicine. Mistletoe providers are also happy to work with your local integrative practitioner to help with coordinating your care.

If you already have an integrative or holistic practitioner working with you, and they don't know about mistletoe, please share this book with them! Let them know that PAAM offers VAE therapy trainings to anthroposophic physicians, as well as MD, DO, ND, NP, and PA practitioners. This book is based on several core classes we offer during our VAE Therapy Practitioner Trainings. In recent years, a growing number of practitioners at these trainings are attending because their patients have asked them to learn about mistletoe. Right now, patient requests are driving the expansion of the list of U.S. mistletoe therapy practitioners.

Practitioner Awareness: There are challenges with awareness and, sometimes outright opposition stemming from misinformation about efficacy and research. Even though a majority of the 45 NCI-designated cancer care centers in the U.S. claim to have an Integrative Medicine Department, those departments are rarely aware of well-vetted efficacious therapies that provide researched anti-cancer benefits. Instead, they tend to focus on spirit- and soul-care therapies only.[6,7] These offerings are powerful—practices like yoga, meditation, and acupuncture—but they are only one component of integrative oncology.

There are so many more therapeutic offerings that provide well-studied and proven effects for the patient's physiology, biochemistry, immune system, and metabolic system. These Integrative Medicine Departments should not feel threatened by well-vetted therapies like mistletoe and others described in this book and in the books listed in our Resources section. As we've stated repeatedly, in clinical practice within true integrative oncology, we tend to combine mistletoe with conventional care to enhance SOC effects.

Every therapeutic option works better, and patient outcomes improve, when we're all working together and aware of each other's treatment strategies. Maintaining a wall between conventional and integrative therapies achieves only one outcome: patients feel caught in the middle. Indeed, in the U.S., about 80 percent of all patients with cancer seek some form of alternative care, and 30 to 40 percent report this choice to their conventional oncologists.[8]

Too often, patients feel they must pick one or the other. They choose herbal medicine instead of chemotherapy, or they pursue chemotherapy and radiation and do nothing on the nutritional and integrative side. People shouldn't have to make these either-or decisions. Those choices only hurt patients. As practitioners, we take our patients farther and achieve better results when we work together. When it comes to finding the best solution for their cancer care journey, patients need to be at the center. Patients need to feel comfortable assembling all their practitioners, their lab results, their unique risk factors, and their deeply personal goals, and then collaborating to create the treatment strategy that works best for them.

In addition to introducing you to one specific integrative therapy, my coauthors and I hope that this book has served as a broader invitation to more bridge-building dialogue. We hope the rich research and findings shared in these pages earn even more trust with conventional oncology teams and mainstream integrative departments. As the U.S. research base continues to grow for mistletoe and many other integrative oncological therapies, we hope that trust grows exponentially.

We are especially grateful for the growing, bridge-building organizations such as the Society for Integrative Oncology (SIO), which support stronger research and review of integrative care models in academic and mainstream medicine. Because of organizations like SIO, many conventional oncologists are awakening to the value of mistletoe and all of integrative oncology. SIO is shedding light on the strongest research findings and helping innovative practitioners find and connect with each other.

Mistletoe research horizons

At the time of publication, the Sidney Kimmel Comprehensive Cancer Center at Johns Hopkins concluded its first-ever Phase I clinical trial of IV application of mistletoe therapy for Stage IV solid tumor patients. We are awaiting the results now. We hope publication of this trial will further establish the conventional-integrative bridge.[9]

We have also learned of other trials soon to matriculate in academic institutions around the U.S. This includes a SC VAE QOL breast cancer trial, a SC VAE glioblastoma trial, and another trial examining the effects of mistletoe injected into the portal vein for hepatocellular carcinoma (HCC – liver cancer). We hope these will be underway soon. Our book's website (www.TheMistletoeBook.com) maintains a list of published clinical studies where we post new results as soon as they are published. A European mistletoe educational website (www.mistletoe-therapy.org) also maintains a similar study summary list.

Over 150 studies have examined the effects of VAE therapy.[10] It is one of the most researched integrative oncology treatments in the world. In contrast, a 2021 study reviewed 100 cancer pharmaceutical drugs that have entered the market in the past 17 years. Less than 44 percent were properly evaluated to meet FDA standards. Yet all were fast-tracked into the patient population. The overall survival extension for these drugs was a mere 2.4 months.[11]

Meanwhile, mistletoe has decades of contemporary research showing its benefits for QOL and life extension. Yet it remains remarkably unknown in conventional circles. We practitioners can and must do better in our awareness-building efforts. We owe it to our patients!

Calls for future lines of inquiry

As practitioners and authors, my colleagues and I hope to see more research on several major mistletoe frontiers. We hope to build more conventional oncology confidence through U.S.-based studies, particularly looking at these topics:

- *Host Tree Specific Effects:* In chapter 4, Dr. Hinderberger mentioned studies that looked at the benefits of certain VAE host trees for specific cancers. We do need more research looking at host tree specific effects in various cancer types.

- *Conventional Immunotherapies and VAE-Immunotherapy Combinations:* Up to 80 percent of patients do not respond well to cancer immunotherapies.[12] More research is needed to look at how VAE might enhance or interact with the new conventional immunotherapies.

- *Mistletoe Use in High-risk Cancer Environments:* As patients become more aware of BRCA, ATM, Lynch, CHEK2, GATA3, and other genetic predispositions, future studies could explore whether VAE therapy can be used in "previvor" scenarios, as a prophylactic therapy.

We would like to see more U.S.-led research focused on lesser-known mistletoe administration routes. This includes varied intratumoral (IT) applications (see chapter 10). We also know of one colleague, outside our coauthor group, who has developed an oral mistletoe capsule. All current research and findings regarding mistletoe benefits have been focused on SC, IV, intravesical (injection into the bladder), and IT administration. To the best of our knowledge, most of the bio-actives in VAE (particularly the lectins) would break down in the digestive tract and would not enter the body via oral consumption. However, we don't know that for sure. Perhaps future studies will find otherwise, and we would be provided another valid administration route.

Yet another mistletoe research frontier involves its use for pets who have cancer. The Florida-based veterinarian, Dr. Loren Nations, is especially known for his successful use of mistletoe along with metabolic therapies (dietary change) for dogs and cats with cancer. As people explore more humanized and integrative care options for themselves, it was a matter of time before we wondered if these options could foster better outcomes for our four-legged companions. For now, Dr. Nations has numerous positive veterinary case stories. We hope to see funding materialize to support companion animal studies that might validate these methods.

A future vision for integrative oncology: Increasing access through a nonprofit integrative research hospital model

When conventional practitioners first learn about mistletoe, it is often a first introduction to truly personalized medicine. Throughout this book we've described the need to evaluate the person's constitution, their life history, and their current spiritual challenges, in addition to their tumor type and lab results. The whole person needs to be taken into consideration before even selecting the right mistletoe host tree. Then administration and dosage itself is personalized, based on the body's response. This is what it means to let the patient lead the care. It is not easy to shed the old insurance-code model and embrace such a responsive and deeply spiritual care philosophy. But it is invigorating and hopeful!

Right now, I am working with a diverse group of co-founders to develop the plans for an integrative residential hospital and research institute. This research and wellness model would provide a safe space where patients and practitioners can embrace this emerging paradigm shift. Such wellness-care hospital models do not exist yet in the U.S., but they are not unheard of elsewhere. Our European coauthor, Dr. Marion Debus, practices at the Klinik Arlesheim in Switzerland. This is a hospital offering both in- and outpatient care, with chemotherapy alongside VAE, IV vitamin C, medical hyperthermia, and hyperbaric oxygen, among many other holistic patient care offerings. We know of similar examples in other European countries, Southeast Asia, South America, and Mexico. (In addition, PAAM is currently conducting a feasibility study for developing an innovative anthroposophic clinic in the U.S. modeled after those in Europe such as Klinik Arlesheim.)

In the U.S., we'd like to take that integrative hospital model one step further. Our nonprofit wellness-model hospital, the Metabolic Terrain Institute of Health, would include a research arm with in-house data analysis capabilities. Through high-tech big data analysis, we now have the capability to analyze multiple variables and multiple outcomes at once. We really aren't limited to the reductionist single-input single-outcome study model that makes it so challenging to research and establish efficacy for whole-plant extracts like mistletoe—or multiple-variable care strategies of any kind. We need solid research to examine the real-world effects of integrative care. We can do that now with large patient pools and big data analysis. I've already begun gathering data for a global project involving several thousand integrative cancer care patients, and the research hospital will exponentially expand our ability to draw solid statistical conclusions.

As a philanthropic nonprofit, we would also make integrative oncology available to all patients—much like the St. Jude's model of charitable care. Integrative access would expand broadly through philanthropic donations, research grants, wellness grants and, hopefully in the future, insurance coverage. We hope that someday this integrative research institute will replicate itself, that we would eventually have several such academic nonprofit hospitals worldwide, offering mistletoe along with a complete metabolic and integrative approach.

We need to pair this patient-centric paradigm shift with gold-standard clinical trials and real-world observational data analysis. Solid research can establish that this approach to medicine provides quantifiable positive outcomes. This is how we embody what my anthroposophic colleagues call "spiritual science." This is how we build a better bridge.

Fully integrative: Translational medicine and multiple practices, all working together

I envision a hospital setting where genuinely integrated, patient-centered, and precision-driven approaches to changing cancer outcomes coexist under one roof. In such a space, before an individual undergoes a single treatment, whether for a first diagnosis or recurrence, they will have a complete biomedical work up, including fresh tissue or liquid blood biopsy, and comprehensive laboratory testing to qualify what is driving their process including metabolic, inflammatory, and toxic exposure risk factors. Each patient will have their epigenetics evaluated along with testing based on personal and family history. We'll do a deep dive into their emotional, spiritual, stress, and lifestyle histories—uncovering everything that might have contributed to the diagnosis and prognosis. All these inquiries will be provided in addition to more conventional imaging and cancer marker testing.

This residential hospital and research institute will be housed on a nature-dense campus that aims to restore health in a wellness-based, deeply nourishing, and spiritually supportive environment. This will be accomplished in a systems-based approach, where research and translational medicine move elegantly from laboratory bench, to bed, to greater community, and beyond.

Today, the World Health Organization forecasts a doubling of cancer diagnosis rates by 2030.[13] Meanwhile, a majority of those living through cancer now, will experience a recurrence at some point in their lives.[14] At a global scale, we have not approached this problem appropriately or successfully. I believe our greatest flaw is our *focus on the disease* instead of focusing on building *the patient's foundational health.* We want to create a reproducible hospital model that provides actual healthcare—not solely disease management. We want to provide the empowerment for lifestyle change and the therapies that help patients become well again.

Taking the next step: Solutions Summary

We have some big hopes and goals for improving mistletoe access and access to integrative oncology in general. Maybe you're in a space where you can join us in embracing those visions. Maybe you're a patient focused solely on your own health right now. You can't think of major paradigm change in the medical world when you're simply trying to survive. I understand that. Really. As a 30-year thriver of Stage IV ovarian cancer, I know. Sometimes you need tiny steps broken down. Here are a few basics for each of our readers, wherever you're at.

Financial access

> *Connect with Believe Big:* Visit www.BelieveBig.org and learn about their patient resources. Apply for a wellness grant.

> *Reach out locally:* Ask your anthroposophic or holistic care provider about regional grants and local support for integrative oncology patients in need.

Geographic access

> *Consider telemedicine:* If there are no VAE therapy providers in your state, research the possibility of telemedicine options with an out-of-state provider. Uriel Pharmacy (see Resources) keeps a list of mistletoe therapy practitioners. You may also reach out to PAAM (www.AnthroposophicMedicine.org) to find the mistletoe therapy practitioner nearest you. Take the first step and make a call.

> *Persuade your own physician:* If you already have an integrative physician, functional medicine doctor, naturopathic doctor, or other provider who simply doesn't know about mistletoe, offer this book to them. Encourage them to contact

PAAM about our Mistletoe Therapy Trainings. These patient requests are driving a major wave of practitioner training right now!

Practitioner training

Contact PAAM: Ask to be notified about upcoming mistletoe therapy trainings (see Resources). Attend an in-person training and then join a mentoring cohort. Much of mistletoe administration nuances are learned in close contact with a mentor, while caring for the patients in your clinic right now.

Connect with SIO: The Society for Integrative Oncology (www.IntegrativeOnc.org) provides conferences, shares integrative oncology advances, and helps integrative practitioners connect with each other.

Survivor and thriver stories

Share your story: Practitioners and patients who have intriguing mistletoe therapy experiences are invited to share their stories. Visit this book's website at (www.TheMistletoeBook.com), where you may add your story to our collection. We hope these testimonials will encourage further research and collaboration.

Visionary supporters

Fund a trial: Support clinical trials and the research institute! We do not expect research dollars to funnel in from NIH or NCI. We welcome visionary supporters, angel investors, major donors, and other passionate individuals who are interested in supporting research. If you are interested, please contact the Metabolic Terrain Institute of Health at: info@MTIofHealth.org.

Political Action

Speak out: Contact your state representatives and senators to let them know your story. Insurance law and FDA regulations will not change without a groundswell of public concern.

Visit www.TheMistletoeBook.com for guidance on how to speak with your representatives—in a way that increases awareness but doesn't put your own rights at risk.

Understand your "right to try": Patients, loved ones, practitioners, and integrative oncology supporters all benefit from educating themselves on the Right to Try Act. As FDA describes, "This law is another way for patients who have been diagnosed with life-threatening diseases or conditions who have tried all approved treatment options and who are unable to participate in a clinical trial to access certain unapproved treatments."[15] In my own practice, this law protects the choices of more than half of my patients.

The proceeds from this book go directly toward education and research. Funds will be split between PAAM's educational initiatives for practitioners and the Believe Big fundraising initiatives to support wellness grants for patients and the Phase II and III Johns Hopkins Clinical Trial. See the Resources section for more information about these organizations and the research institute.

There is a whole community of like-minded, health-oriented patients and practitioners, and we welcome you into this space. We would love to hear your own ideas about how you might like to get involved. It is our hope and our expectation to be the thought-leaders and vision-builders of the oncology world. We are building a world where cancer doesn't have to be a death sentence, where we can enhance outcomes, and where prevention is the best cure. Join us as we make this vision a reality.

Afterword

Holly Lucille, ND, RN

Growing up the daughter of two pharmacists, I was well versed in the "here, take this" approach to medicine. An ailment, a diagnosis, then a drug. Funny, it never really resonated with me. That's why, later in my life, I found myself searching beyond my conventional nursing training for something more. This search ended with a postgrad immersion into the science and credentials of holistic nursing, which eventually led to my degree as a Naturopathic Doctor.

It just made sense: being able to look at an individual comprehensively, caring for the whole human, understanding the unique contributing factors behind a clinical presentation, identifying and treating the root cause, respecting the innate healing abilities of the body. This was how I could and would practice medicine. No more reducing anyone to his or her signs, symptoms, diagnoses, or lab tests. No more protocols. Instead, I saw "wake-up calls" in each and every person I cared for throughout over twenty years of practice.

This made the practice of medicine meaningful for me. I respected the rigor of science, the time-tested history of natural medicine, and the essence of caring for and truly seeing someone who came to me for help and assistance.

Then the tables turned. While I was lying in my infrared sauna—walking my talk—with a bentonite clay mask on my face and chest, rubbing the sweat around, I bumped into something. Something peculiar.

Something not right. A *lump*. A lump the size of a nickel around five o'clock on my left breast.

The first MD dismissed it as "nothing; perhaps trauma from an ill-fitting bra." I got a second opinion. My breast surgeon called me the day after I had a biopsy and said, "You have inner and outer ductal breast cancer."

After a subsequent MRI, I chose to have a double mastectomy. The surgery went well, and I healed wonderfully. My surgeon referred me to a western, allopathic (conventional) oncologist. She was the head of the department and had a stellar reputation. Even with my background and beliefs, after the shocking diagnosis of breast cancer at age 55, it was the one appointment that I felt too scared *not* to make. I first saw her nurse, then her PA, and then finally her.

She came into the exam room with my pathology report in hand. She reviewed the prognostics and offered her treatment. Yes, a drug. That was it. No questions about me, my diet, or my lifestyle. No blood-work or further tests. Just a drug. Oh, and the mention that if I had too many uncomfortable side effects from this particular drug, we could try some others. Then a quick note that she would like to see me in six months.

I am not exactly sure why I was surprised, but I left that appointment shocked and more scared than before. My body had just demonstrated that it was vulnerable to influences that stimulate abnormal cell division. I knew from my studies, having recently given a presentation on cancer stem cell research, that most people diagnosed with cancer don't perish from the original tumor. They die from metastasis occurring before conventional treatment has begun, from cancer recurrence after conventional treatment, or from immunosuppression and other toxicities resulting from both chemotherapy and radiation.

Enter integrative oncology and anthroposophic medicine.

I was lucky enough, because of who I am and who I knew, to have an amazing contact willing to care for me post-mastectomy. Unlike the Western oncologist that I was too scared not to see, my anthroposophic doctor asked me questions. *Many, many questions.* Questions about my history, my environmental exposures, the kind of water I drank, my diet, my lifestyle, my exercise habits, my parents, my marriage, my work. She asked me questions about my body, my soul, and my spirit. Then she drew from all these biographical details and my prognostics, ordering precise individualized testing to uncover root causes in my terrain. After all, if I simply pointed my finger at the cancer, as so many do, I still had three fingers pointing back at me. Yes, my surgeon removed the tumor. Now we, as a team, needed to tend to my terrain.

This wasn't a scary process. In fact, despite the recent cancer diagnosis and major surgery, this new process was a warming one. I still felt the loss of innocence and the fear of future metastasis or complications. But this new path helped me feel contained, comforted, and relieved that I was being monitored, measured, and treated. That treatment included evidenced-based natural interventions and therapies like mistletoe. I also incorporated specific dietary and lifestyle recommendations, and we monitored my labs monthly. Changes in my lab results informed tweaks to my initial treatment choices. This was a true partnership with someone who practices root-cause, whole-person, evidence-based, anthroposophic medicine. With each passing month, I started to feel more and more confident in my body, my health, and my future.

Yes, I went from being a practitioner to being a patient. At first, I was seduced by the "here, take this" approach out of fear and anxiety about the "C" word. I forgive myself. I was gently reminded how powerful nature is, how amazing our bodies are, and how holistic principles, with their roots spanning thousands of years, are still relevant and deeply needed today. One year after my initial diagnosis, I am here and strong and dedicated to this path.

I am so grateful to see this collaborative book out in the world, connecting with both practitioners and patients. We all need the message in these pages—both the education regarding mistletoe therapy and the greater call to see and care for the whole person.

APPENDIX A

BASICS OF MISTLETOE ADMINISTRATION

*Special thanks to Dr. Nasha Winters, Dr. Peter Hinderberger,
and Dr. Steven Johnson for contributions to this section*

As we often say in our trainings, "Mistletoe is not a protocol therapy." There is no height and weight chart or tumor type chart that
immediately tells the practitioner what dosage to recommend for each
patient. Optimal dosage is determined by starting low, titrating up,
and observing patient response. That optimal dose will change over
time. The guidelines that follow in this appendix are solely starting
points, and this is not intended as a comprehensive treatment manual.
This material is intended as a general introduction so that practitioners
and patients alike may familiarize themselves with the basic principles
of VAE therapy administration. This is a brief overview of a well-vetted, research-supported off-label drug use (OLDU) of *Viscum album*
extract (VAE). Like any other botanical therapy, this is not an FDA-
approved cancer treatment.

VAE therapy is incredibly nuanced and requires specialized training.
Practitioners should administer VAE only upon completion of accred-
ited training and ongoing mentorship by an experienced VAE therapy
practitioner. Patients should seek out practitioners who have completed
such training. Uriel Pharmacy, Believe Big, and PAAM maintain lists
of such practitioners (see Resources). These physicians follow the VAE
best practices established at European clinics and approved by the
anthroposophic hospitals in Switzerland.

Before subcutaneous (SC) injections or IV administration even
begins, VAE therapy starts with appropriate host tree selection (see

chapter 4 and appendix E). Once host tree(s) is/are decided upon, SC injection is administered—typically in the abdomen (preferred), thigh, or upper arm, avoiding all radiation fields, recent surgical sites, or infected areas. It is crucial that the injection be administered with a half-inch needle at a 45-degree angle to the skin to ensure the extract reaches the immune-cell rich region just below the skin surface. Patients need to be taught how to use one hand to spread the skin of the injection site, while holding the syringe with their other hand at the appropriate angle and injecting at the correct depth. When patients say they have never experienced a desired VAE reaction, it is almost always because of poor injection technique. Practitioners who complete PAAM-accredited training programs are provided the instruction necessary to teach correct technique to their patients. The first SC injection should always be completed in-office to monitor tolerance and to ensure correct injection angle. Patients may self-administer at home thereafter.

Most SC schedules begin with injections three times per week. Dosage begins low and slowly titrates upward to find the dose at which the patient experiences a desired injection site reaction (see Image 1 "VAE Therapy Dose Escalation Decision Tree"). When a desired reaction occurs, the primary immediate effect is a reddening and swelling of the injection site, no larger than a silver dollar and, for some, a low-grade fever (one to two degrees above normal). Lymph nodes near the injection site may swell slightly. This reaction lasts for 24 to 72 hours. These are not adverse reactions; they are desired responses that indicate immune system activation.

Wait until this reaction has subsided before providing the next SC injection. For some patients, this may necessitate adjusting the dosage schedule (i.e., injections two days/week instead of three days/week). Reaction (redness, swelling) larger than the size of a silver dollar or a fever over 100.4 F may indicate a need to temporarily cease injections and begin again at a lower dose. Conversely, a reaction that is the size of dime or smaller (or no reaction at all) indicates that the patient should graduate to the next dosage level at their next injection. Always

Image 1: VAE Therapy Dose Escalation Decision Tree

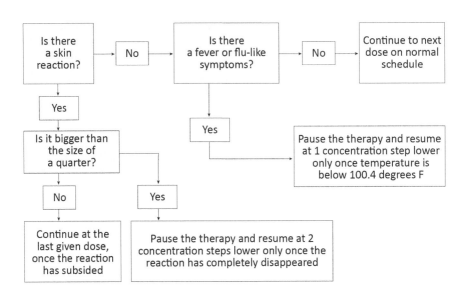

be ready to adjust the dose to the patient in order to maintain an optimal injection site reaction.

When the patient achieves their optimal reaction, they should remain at that dosage level. If they reach a point where that dosage no longer incurs a reaction, increase to the next dosage level. As we have mentioned frequently throughout this work, patient response leads the treatment progression.

Each VAE manufacturer provides their own dosage guidelines for how to begin SC mistletoe therapy. Helixor®, the manufacturer that we often recommend for practitioners who are new to VAE therapy, provides some simple dosing guidelines.

Start with Series 1 (1 to 10 mg) three days/week (i.e., on Monday, Wednesday, and Friday).

If Series 1 is tolerated well, increase to Series 2 (10 to 20 mg), again three days/week.

If needed, progress to Series 3 and then Series 4 (20 to 50 mg).

Image 2: VAE Therapy Sample Schedule

TIME	MONDAY	WEDNESDAY	FRIDAY	PACK
Week 1	1 mg	1 mg	1 mg	SE I
Week 2	5 mg	5 mg	5 mg	
Week 3	10 mg	10 mg	10 mg	SE II
Week 4	20 mg	20 mg	30 mg	
Week 5	30 mg	30 mg	20 mg	SE IV
Week 6	20 mg	30 mg	30 mg	
Week 7	50 mg	50 mg	50 mg	
Week 8	70 mg (20+50)	70 mg (20+50)	80 mg (30+50)	SE IV + 50 mg OP
Week 9	80 mg (30+50)	100 mg (50+50)	100 mg (50+50)	
Week 10	100 mg (50+50)	150 mg	200 mg	100 mg GP + 50 mg OP
Week 11 and on	100 mg	150 mg	200 mg	100 mg GP + 50 mg OP

Image 2: "VAE Therapy Sample Schedule" shows how this could play out for a specific patient. Remember, the dose escalation schedule will vary from patient to patient. Depending on the stage of the cancer, aggressiveness, and risk of recurrence, Helixor recommends that patients continue administering their "optimal-reaction dose" three days per week for two to five years. An alternative to that would be to cycle through the above protocol (from Series 1 to 4) repeatedly with breaks in between. After the initial treatment years, depending on the patient's lifestyle and recurrence risk, they may transition to a maintenance pattern of cycling through Series 1 and 2 just twice per year.

What if the visible SC response subsides?

Patients often ask what to do if they get to a point in the maintenance pattern where they no longer experience a reaction at the injection site. A lack of reaction does not necessarily mean the VAE is no
longer working. Dr. Hinderberger recommends a technique called the
"thigh test" to determine whether the current dosage is still effective. At
the next scheduled SC injection, instead of administering in the abdomen, inject it in the outer surface of the thigh, about two inches below
the hip bone. There's a little fat there. If there is a reaction in that location, the dosage is still adequate. If there's no reaction, we would then
discuss how we might increase to a higher maintenance dose or change
host trees.

Ultimately, the local inflammatory reaction is one sign that mistletoe is working. But there are many other indicators too. Practitioners
should check in regularly with patients, asking about their whole picture of health. Is there improvement in mood, vitality, sleep, appetite,
strength, and uprightness in posture? Have they experienced increases
in temperature? Even a half-degree shift is meaningful if it occurs pre-
dictably in relation to the VAE therapy. Improvements in heart rate and
pulse quality are significant and so are shifts in warmth distribution.
Did they have cold hands at the first patient visit, and do they have
warm hands now? All of these are measures of self-regulation. If these
shifts occur and persist, it is a good sign that VAE is still conveying
beneficial effects.

*This section was intended solely as a basic introduction to SC
VAE therapy. Practitioners who want to learn more about SC
mistletoe, as well as IV administration and intratumoral applications, should connect with the Physicians' Association for Anthroposophic Medicine (PAAM, see Resources) and attend a PAAM-
sponsored mistletoe therapy training.*

Dramatic Responses to VAE Therapy

Understanding Tumor Lysis, Pseudo Progression, and Allergy Potential

Tumor Lysis and Pseudo Progression

Tumor lysis syndrome and *pseudo progression* are two dramatic treatment responses that can occur in the presence of VAE therapy. *Tumor lysis syndrome* has been referred to as a state in which

> tumor cells release their contents into the bloodstream, either spontaneously or in response to therapy, leading to the characteristic findings of hyperuricemia, hyperkalemia, hyperphosphatemia, and hypocalcemia. These electrolyte and metabolic disturbances can progress to clinical toxic effects.[1]

Tumor lysis syndrome indicates that the tumors have been severely stressed by the therapy and subsequent immune system activities. However, we do need to stabilize and slow the tumor destruction in that situation, because of the potential for severe toxicity. The tumor destruction is good, we just don't want too much too fast. We need to harness and manage this response. If signs of tumor lysis syndrome occur, we pause VAE therapy and restart at a lower dose.

Pseudo progression refers to an increase in the size of the primary tumor or the appearance of a new lesion, as seen on scans, ultimately followed by tumor regression. It is a common response to immunotherapies, including VAE therapy. Pseudo progression is actually good; it is a sign that the immune system is highly active at the tumor site.

This is a normal therapeutic response, not an undesired reaction or side effect. However, it can be disturbing for the patient and conventional oncology team if they see such a response on scans. For this reason, it is best to avoid scans for six to eight weeks after the start of VAE therapy. After that time period, the typical regression phase begins.

Allergies and Other Precautions

As noted in chapter 2, latex, banana, avocado, kiwi, and chestnuts have lectin structures similar to those found in mistletoe extract. However, cross-reactive allergy is extremely rare. Both the Anamnestic Form and MD Anderson Prognostic Scoring System (see appendices C and D) screen for allergy concerns. Additionally, all VAE therapy practitioners should provide a skin prick and intradermal test at initiation of treatment.

VAE therapy is highly nuanced and must be personalized. Trained mistletoe practitioners understand how to address allergy potential, manage cytokine release syndrome, and provide appropriate therapeutic alternatives when mistletoe is contraindicated. Practitioners who wish to learn more about these topics should connect with the Physicians' Association for Anthroposophic Medicine (PAAM, see Resources) and attend a PAAM-sponsored mistletoe therapy training.

Appendix C

Anamnestic Form

Helixor® and other manufacturers provide an Anamnestic Form for practitioners to use when screening patients for mistletoe therapy. The word *anamnestic* refers to a heightened immune response in the presence of an antigen that is similar to previously encountered antigens. The Anamnestic Form seeks to identify people who might experience a hypersensitivity or true allergy or might simply need to begin with a low-lectin VAE (i.e., *Viscum album abietis*) and very low dose. Most anamnestic screening forms ask the following:

- Patient's age, gender and general state of health
- Tumor type and stage
- Previous treatment history and current treatment: What treatments have already been utilized (chemotherapy, radiation, surgery, targeted therapy, hormone blockade, checkpoint inhibitor)? What was the response? Any side effects? What current conventional treatments are being pursued?
- Any history of allergies, asthma, or eczema?
- Any history of autoimmune disease?
- Any current issues with autoimmune disease?
- Any concurrent disease processes?
- Any previous treatment with VAE? What type and dose? What was the response?

Detailed answers are crucial. The patient's answers will not necessarily "rule them out" for mistletoe therapy. Autoimmunity or allergies do not immediately contraindicate mistletoe. Rather, these details help the skillful practitioner select the appropriate host tree and dosage as a starting point. This is vital to ensure a positive treatment response.

When we hear of patients experiencing a hypersensitivity reaction to their initial mistletoe injection, it is often due to poor (or no) anamnestic screening or host tree selection that did not take anamnestic factors into consideration.

M.D. Anderson
Prognostic Scoring System

In addition to the anthroposophic Anamnestic Form (see appendix C), U.S. mistletoe practitioners also may utilize the M.D. Anderson (MDA) Prognostic Scoring System[1] to evaluate potential mistletoe therapy patients. The two tools are similar in that they seek to flag individuals who may have a complex or negative response to any immunotherapies, including mistletoe therapy. The MDA Prognostic Scoring System asks if patients:

- are over age 52
- have elevated LDH
- have elevated neutrophil count
- have diminished lymphocyte count
- are experiencing liver issues (metastases, fatty liver, or liver disease)
- have elevated platelets
- have a poor ECOG score (a basic measure of quality of life and ability to care for oneself)

According to MDA, patients who demonstrate three or more of these risk factors are at a greater risk of side effects and lack of treatment response to *any immunotherapy*. Similar to evaluating anamnestic factors, the patient's answers may not result in immediate contraindication. Some of these factors (elevated LDH, concerning immune cell counts, etc.) may be addressed through lifestyle and dietary choices and other therapies. However, it is imperative to address such factors before beginning VAE therapy in order to ensure an optimal response and positive patient experience.

Dr. Winters follows the same scoring system noted above but includes more functional ranges on the lab results (see appendix F). She includes *low* platelet counts (as this can be a sign of autoimmune platelet issues like ITP) and any flaring autoimmune issues in general (such as Hashimoto's or rheumatoid arthritis). She also screens for tissue involvement beyond the liver such as lung, kidney, thyroid, and GI tract. All of these are sites where immune therapies can wreak havoc when applied at the wrong time and dose.

Host Trees and Cancer Types: Basic Matching Guidelines

Compiled by Steven Johnson, MD, Peter Hinderberger, MD, and Nasha Winters, ND, FABNO. Based on manufacturer materials, clinical experience, and the handbook Mistletoe Therapy for Cancer *by Johannes Wilkens (2010)*

The following are intended as initial guidelines only. Trained mistletoe therapy practitioners learn to match host tree products to each patient based on several factors, including the individual patient's constitution, energy levels, vitality, and personal health goals.

Other general considerations regarding host tree matching

Beyond looking at tumor type, there are several other constitutional considerations that we look at when selecting the most appropriate host tree. In general:

- Consider quercus or pini for men (both generally and more specifically for male organ cancers).
- Consider mali for women (both generally and more specifically for female organ cancers).
- Also consider mali for patients who have more weight below the waist.
- Consider abietis for patients who are more nervous-sensitive type (slim, low fat storage, nervous).
- Consider pini for patients who are more athletic type.

When looking more generally at the body (not necessarily organ systems), certain host trees seem to serve certain body regions more optimally. For cancers located in the:

- Head and neck region: consider abietis and pini
- Chest (lungs, esophagus, mediastinum): consider abietis and pini
- Periphery (brain, sense organs, skin): consider abietis and pini
- Soft tissues: consider abietis, pini, and fraxini
- Retroperitoneal region: consider mali and pini

Additionally, fraxini and pini seem the most beneficial in pancreatic cancer. Sensitive or weak patients (universal responders) tolerate low-lectin mistletoe (abietis) better than high-lectin mistletoe (fraxini). These are primarily clinical observations that have been noticed and documented by practitioners over several decades.

Cancer – Location/Origin	Brand & Host Tree – Preferred	Brand & Host Tree – Alternates (if applicable)
CNS (Central Nervous System)	Helixor Abietis	Abnoba Abietis, Abnoba Betulae, Iscador Pini, Iscucin Pini
ENT	Helixor Abietis, Iscador Pini	Abnoba Abietis, Abnoba Amygdali
Endocrine	Abnoba Abietis, Abnoba Amygdali, Helixor Pini, Iscador Pini, Iscucin Pini	
GI Tract	Helixor Mali, Iscador Quercus, Iscador Mali	Abnoba Quercus, Abnoba Pini, Iscucin Abietis
Gynecological or Breast	Abnoba Mali, Helixor Mali, Iscador Mali, Iscucin Mali	
Leukemia, Lymphoma	Abnoba Fraxini, Helixor Pini	Abnoba Abietis, Iscador Pini, Iscucin Mali, Iscucin Quercus
Male Cancers	Abnoba Quercus, Helixor Abietis, Helixor Pini, Iscador Quercus, Iscucin Pini, Iscucin Populi	
Pediatric	Abnoba Abietis, Abnoba Fraxini, Helixor Abietis	
Respiratory Tract	Helixor Abietis	Abnoba Abietis, Iscador Pini, Iscador Quercus, Iscucin Tiliae
Sarcoma (connective tissue)	Abnoba Fraxini, Iscador Pini	Abnoba Abietis, Iscucin Mali, Iscucin Quercus
Skin	Helixor Pini	Abnoba Abietis, Abnoba Betulae, Iscador Pini, Iscucin Pini
Urogenital Tract	Helixor Abietis, Helixor Pini	Abnoba Mali, Abnoba Pini, Abnoba Crataegus, Abnoba Quercus, Iscador Mali, Iscador Pini, Iscador Quercus, Iscucin Tiliae, Iscucin Salicis

Host trees and cancer types

Terrain-centric Core Lab Tests and True Healthy Ranges

*© 2021 DrNasha, Inc. and the
Metabolic Terrain Institute of Health*

These tables provide the core labs that anthroposophic, naturopathic, and integrative doctors often monitor. Some are familiar, commonly ordered during any patient's annual physical. Some are not so well-known. Almost all of the listings provide optimal ranges that differ significantly from what is listed as "healthy" on a standard lab report. The ranges below are based on what is associated with optimal health, rather than the "normal averages" of a generally unhealthy population group (see chapter 5 and its references).

For best treatment outcomes, it's crucial to test, assess, address, and not guess. Practitioners who want to learn more about all the testing available to the oncology patient and how to interpret and apply results in an effective holistic fashion, should connect with the Physicians' Association for Anthroposophic Medicine (PAAM) or take the *Metabolic Approach to Cancer, Mastermind Course* through DrNasha, Inc. (see "Resources").

Trifecta Labs (see Chapter 5)	
CRP (C-reactive protein)	Less than 1 (or < 0.1, depending on lab)
ESR	Less than 10
LDH	Less than 175 (or <450, depending on lab)

Complete Blood Count (CBC)		
Test	Units	Range
WBC (White blood cells)	x10E3/uL	5 to 7
RBC (Red blood cells)	x10E6/uL	4 to 5
Hemoglobin	g/dL	13 to 15
Hematocrit	Percentage (%)	40 to 45
MCV	fL	~ 90
MCH	pg	~ 30
MCHC	g/dL	~ 32
RDW	Percentage (%)	12.3-14.5
Platelets	x10E3/uL	175 to 250
Neutrophils	Percentage (%)	N:L Ratio = 2:1
Lymphocytes	Percentage (%)	N:L Ratio = 2:1
Monocytes	Percentage (%)	7
EOS (Eosinophils)	Percentage (%)	Less than 2
Basophils	Percentage (%)	0

Complete Metabolic Panel (CMP)		
Test	Units	Range
Glucose, serum	mg/dL	55 to 85
BUN	mg/dL	Less than 20
Creatinine, serum	mg/dL	Less than 1
eGFR	mL/min	Less than 59
BUN:Creatinine ratio		~ 20
Sodium, serum	mmol/L	Greater than 140
Potassium, serum	mmol/L	Greater than 4.0
Chloride, serum	mmol/L	In standard range
Anion gap		Less than 15
Carbon dioxide	mmol/L	Less than 25
Calcium, serum	mg/dL	8.8 to 9.5
Protein, total	g/dL	Greater than 7
Albumin, serum	g/dL	Greater than 4
Globulin, total	g/dL	In standard range
A:G ratio		In standard range
Bilirubin, total	mg/dL	In standard range
ALP, serum	IU/L	Less than 90
AST (SGOT)	IU/L	~ 20
ALT (SGPT)	IU/L	~ 20
GGT	IU/L	Less than 15

Additional Labs	
Homocysteine	About 7
Ferritin	35 to 75
Fibrinogen	Less than 300
Insulin	~3
IGF-1	~100
HbA1C (HgA1C, Hemoglobin A1C)	Less than 5
VEGF, serum	Less than 350
VEGF, plasma	Less than 50
Galectin-3	Less than 10
GGT	Less than 15
Triglycerides	Less than 90
HDL	Greater than 70
LDL	50 to 200
VLDL	5 to 40
Total Cholesterol	160 to 300
Vitamin D3 1,25 OH	Less than 70
Vitamin D, 25-OH	80 to 120
TSH	About 0.8 to 2.0
Total T4	7 to 9
Free T4	Greater than 1
Free T3	Greater than 3
T3	100 to 159
T3 uptake	30
Reverse T3	Less than 17
Anti-thyroglobulin antibody	Less than 5
TPO antibodies	Less than 5
Ceruloplasmin	Less than 20
Copper, RBC	Less than 120
Zinc, RBC	Greater than 13
G6PD w/RBC	In standard range
AM cortisol	15 to 17
Uric acid, serum	Less than 4
Iron, serum	35 to 155
Total iron binding capacity	250 to 450
Percent (%) iron saturated	25 to 55
UIBC	150 to 375
D-dimer	Less than 0.5 (or <300, depending on lab)
PAI-1	In standard range
LDH Isoenzymes	
LD isoenzyme 1 - heart and RBC	Less than 24
LD isoenzyme 2 - reticuloendothelial (immune)	Less than 33
LD isoenzyme 3 - lungs	Less than 21
LD isoenzyme 4 - kidneys, placenta, pancreas	Less than 7
LD isoenzyme 5 - liver and striated muscle	Less than 14

DIY *tracking and home monitoring*

Integrative practitioners often recommend several at-home monitoring smart phone apps and devices. These are a few of our favorites:

Blood glucose and ketone monitoring: Keto-Mojo™ Meter or
Abbot's Precision Xtra®
Nutrition and macronutrient tracking: Cronometer or
MyFitnessPal™
Heart rate variability (HRV) trackers: Oura Ring, Fitbit®, or
Biostrap™
Vitamin D reminder: Dminder, an app that flags optimal sun
exposure times in your region

Resources

A more comprehensive and regularly updated list of Patient and Physician Resources is maintained at www.TheMistletoeBook.com.

Books

Büssing, Arndt. *Mistletoe: The Genus Viscum* (CRC Press, 2004).

GAAD and the Medical Section of the School of Spiritual Science. *Vademecum of Anthroposophic Medicines: Best Practices for Mistletoe Use in Cancer Care*, 2019).

LeShan, Lawrence. *Cancer as a Turning Point: A Handbook for People with Cancer, Their Families, and Health Professionals* (Plume, 1994).

McKinney, Dr. Neil. *Naturopathic Oncology: An Encyclopedic Guide for Patients and Physicians* (Liaison Press, 2020).

Murphy, Christine. *Iscador: Mistletoe and Cancer Therapy* (Lantern Books, 2001).

Parmar, Dr. Gurdev (Dr. Tina Kaczor, ed.). *Textbook of Naturopathic Oncology: A Desktop Guide of Integrative Cancer Care* (Medicatrix Holdings, 2020).

Stengler, Dr. Mark, and Dr. Paul Anderson. *Outside the Box Cancer Therapies* (Hay House, 2019).

Turner, Kelly A. *Radical Remission: Surviving Cancer against All Odds* (HarperOne, 2015).

Ward, William. *Traveling Light: Walking the Cancer Path* (Lindisfarne Books, 2008).

Weirauch, Wolfgang. *Ita Wegman and Anthroposophy: A Conversation with Emanuel Zeylmans* (SteinerBooks, 2012).

Wilkens, Johannes, and Gert Böhm. *Mistletoe Therapy for Cancer* (Floris Books, 2010).

Winters, Dr. Nasha, and Jess Higgins Kelley. *Metabolic Approach to Cancer: Integrating Deep Nutrition, the Ketogenic Diet, and Nontoxic, Bio-individualized Therapies* (Chelsea Green, 2017).

PATIENT RESOURCES

Believe Big

Nonprofit patient support organization focused on improving access to mistletoe therapy in cancer care. Financial assistance through Wellness Grants program available.

Website: www.BelieveBig.org

See Supporting Organizations listing for full contact info.

Oncology Nutrition Institute

Provides a 90-minute webinar on deep interpretation of basic CBC as a cancer patient (or anyone striving for truly optimal health).

Website: www.OncologyNutritionInstitute.com

Click on "Trainings and Classes" and select "Nutrition and CBC Blood Testing."

Physicians' Association for Anthroposophic Medicine (PAAM)

Provides a patient resource page and provider directory. See expanded listing under Supporting Organizations.

Website: www.AnthroposophicMedicine.org

Terrain Advocacy Program (TAP)

Teaches patients and caregivers how to apply tools, techniques, support, and inspiration for themselves and others on the cancer journey. Fosters partnership with terrain-based practitioners to help patients improve clinical and quality of life outcomes.

Website: www.DrNasha.com/terrain-advocate-program/

Practitioner Training and Mentoring

Physicians' Association for Anthroposophic Medicine (PAAM)

Mistletoe therapy training, anthroposophic oncology education, one-to-one mentoring, and free training materials for practitioners. Visit the main website and click on "Training and Continuing Education."
Website: www.AnthroposophicMedicine.org
Mistletoe Page: www.AnthroposophicMedicine.org/Mistletoe/
PAAM Education Calendar: www.AnthroposophicMedicine.org/Subscribe-to-the-Education-Calendar
Email: paam@anthroposophy.org
Mailing Address: PO Box 4039 / Grand Junction, CO 81502

Metabolic Approach to Cancer, Mastermind Course

Physician training and certification program focused on highly personalized integrative patient care, via extensive inquiry into the patient's biography, tissue and blood biopsies, imaging and labs.
Website: www.DrNasha.com/mastermind-matc/
Email: info@DrNasha.com

Anthroposophia Foundation

Recorded and live Webinars, resources and mentoring opportunities for mistletoe and anthroposophic medicine
Website: www.AnthroFoundation.org
Email: hello@AnthroFoundation.org
Mailing Address: 317 Church Street / Phoenixville, PA 19460

The International Federation of Anthroposophic Medical Associations (IVAA)

See their English-language website for current information, research links, and downloadable brochures about Anthroposophic Medicine.
Website: www.ivaa.info

SUPPORTING ORGANIZATIONS

Anthroposophic Health Association (AHA)

Formerly AAMTA, AHA is an umbrella association, made up of professional associations for Anthroposophic Medicine, Anthroposophic Naturopathy, Anthroposophic Nursing, Anthroposophic Psychology, Eurythmy Movement Therapy, Rhythmical Massage, Art Therapy, Music Therapy and Singing Therapy.

Website: www.AnthroposophicHealth.org

Believe Big

A nonprofit patient support organization focused on improving access to mistletoe therapy in cancer care. Financial assistance through the Wellness Grant program. Provides information on current mistletoe clinical trials in which patients may be able to enroll.

Website: www.BelieveBig.org

U.S. Phone: 1.888.317.5850

Mailing Address: 4821 Butler Road, Suite 1D, Glyndon, MD 21136

Metabolic Terrain Institute of Health

Virtual organization; forthcoming research hospital campus in Arizona and patient funding resources.

Website: www.MTIofHealth.org

Email: info@MTIofHealth.org

Oncology Association of Naturopathic Physicians (OncANP)

Licensed Naturopathic Doctors (NDs), naturopathic medical students, and allied providers from across North America. Focused on enhancing survival and quality of life through the integration of naturopathic medicine with conventional cancer care.

Website: www.OncANP.org

Email: info@ OncANP.org

U.S. Phone: 1.800.908.5175

Physicians' Association for Anthroposophic Medicine (PAAM)

Practitioners, please see additional links in "Professional Training" section above.

General Information: www.AnthroposophicMedicine.org

Anthroposophic Medicine Provider Directory: www.Anthroposophicmedicine.org/Provider-Directory

Society for Integrative Oncology (SIO)

Professional organization for integrative oncology. Facilitates communication, education, and research by bringing together practitioners from multiple disciplines, focused on the care of people with cancer and survivors.

Website: www.IntegrativeOnc.org

Email: info@IntegrativeOnc.org

U.S. Phone: 1.202.964.0824

Mailing Address: 4301 – 50th Street, NW / Suite 300 PMB 1032 / Washington, DC 20016

Uriel Pharmacy

Provides Helixor-type mistletoe and Iscucin-type products for U.S. clinics. Also maintains a VAE therapy provider directory; call to inquire. More information in the "Ordering Information" section below.

Website: www.ShopUriel.com

Email: orders@UrielPharmacy.com

U.S. Phone: 866-642-2858

LAB COMPANIES

Labcorp: Website: www.LabCorp.com

Quest Diagnostics: Website: www.QuestDiagnostics.com/

Nutrition Genome: DNA testing focused on genetic insights to inform a personalized diet and lifestyle choices.

Website: www.NutritionGenome.com

CLINICAL TRIALS AND RESEARCH UPDATES

Anthromed Library

List of recent articles on anthroposophic medicine and mistletoe research.
www.AnthroMed.org/mistletoe

Believe Big

See previous listing under Supporting Organizations for complete contact information. Believe Big also helps connect patients to current open clinical trials.
www.BelieveBig.org

www.ClinicalTrials.gov

Search a database of over 300,000 clinical trials in the U.S. and internationally. To find global clinical trials on mistletoe therapy in cancer care, fill out the search fields with:
Condition or Disease: cancer
Other Terms: mistletoe
Country: (leave blank)
Find detailed information about the Johns Hopkins trial by conducting the same search, but selecting "United States" from the "Country" list.

www.TheMistletoeBook.org

Maintains a regularly updated list of leading mistletoe studies and case stories.

www.mistletoe-therapy.org/scientific-literature

European resource. Maintains a comprehensive, regularly updated list of published laboratory findings and human clinical studies focused on mistletoe therapy.

Mistletoe Ordering Information

Current as of autumn 2021; for practitioners only.

Practitioners: Ordering protocols vary. Attend a PAAM training or connect with your mentor to learn of current mistletoe ordering opportunities.

Uriel Pharmacy

Provides Helixor-type mistletoe and Iscucin-type products for
U.S. clinics.
Website: www.ShopUriel.com
Email: orders@UrielPharmacy.com
U.S. Phone: 866-642-2858

AbnobaViscum

Provides abnobaVISCUM mistletoe.
Website: www.abnoba.de

Weleda

Provides Iscador mistletoe products.
Website: www.FeelGoodNatural.com/brand/weleda-iscador/

TEAM ACKNOWLEDGEMENTS

There are people behind the scenes of every project, without whom the endeavor could not come to fruition. First, our deepest gratitude goes out to the mistletoe practitioners and researchers who explored this therapy long before us. The deep spiritual collaboration between Dr. Rudolf Steiner and Ita Wegman, MD in the early 1900s gave birth to the anthroposophic approach to medicine and to *Viscum album* (European mistletoe) therapy. Their vision to bridge science and the deeper mysteries of healing has inspired thousands of doctors and therapists all over the world. We also remember Rita Leroi MD, one of the founders and the Chief Physician of the former Lucas Klinik (now Klinik Arlesheim). Dr. Leroi was a great teacher to a generation of doctors to follow.

Our coauthor team will be forever grateful to the past President and CEO of SteinerBooks, Gene Gollogly (1950–2021), whose encouragement, enthusiasm, and support for this project pushed us all forward to finish the book. We are equally grateful to Maurice Orange, MD (1953–2021). Dr. Orange was a modern pioneer of mistletoe therapy and a great mentor of many doctors around the world including the coauthors Steven Johnson, DO and Mark Hancock, MD. Marion Debus, MD was also a close colleague of Dr. Orange, and both of them inspired Dr. Johnson to organize the mistletoe and integrative oncology training course that led to the development of this book.

We also want to thank the nonprofit organization Believe Big and its founder Ivelisse Paige for working so hard to fund the recent mistletoe research trial at the Sidney Kimmel Comprehensive Cancer Center at Johns Hopkins. Believe Big educates the public about mistletoe therapy and helps make mistletoe available to patients who are held back by cost. It is also important to acknowledge the lead investigators of the Johns Hopkins mistletoe trials: Luiz Diaz, MD and Channing Paller, MD. We are grateful to have such scientific leaders turn their curiosity toward the potential benefits of mistletoe therapy. A special thank you goes to coauthors Nasha Winters, ND, FABNO and Peter Hinderberger, MD, who supported Believe Big's efforts and helped develop the first Johns Hopkins mistletoe trial. This Johns Hopkins trial has gleaned significant public attention. But this is not the first time U.S. researchers have investigated mistletoe. That ground-breaking honor belongs to Patrick Mansky, MD, one of the first mistletoe researchers in the U.S. Dr. Mansky's research led to further academic investigations as well as clinical interest in mistletoe. We thank Phillip Incao, MD and Paul Scharff, MD. Their pioneering work as well as so many others in the U.S. and around the world deserves to be mentioned. They laid the foundations for mistletoe therapy to gain the recognition it has today.

We want to acknowledge the Physicians' Association for Anthroposophic Medicine (PAAM), which donated many resources to the training and mentoring courses for doctors across the country. Thank you to PAAM's coordinator Amanda Jacobs who was often behind the scenes, organizing these initiatives. We acknowledge the hard work and constant encouragement of Kirin Buckley (a mistletoe therapy patient and cancer survivor herself), who kept pushing us forward and coordinated so many of the book's puzzle pieces: seven authors, an editor, multiple donors, and the publisher.

We offer a special thank you to Anika Hanisch who provided invaluable guidance and crucial insights into the organization, flow, and writing of the manuscript. We thank Kristen Dorn for her expertise with graphic design and Pamela Askins for organizing our final steps as we polished the manuscript for the publisher and for providing draft feedback. Several other friends and colleagues read drafts and provided needed feedback during the editing process, including: Donna DeRosa, Sandragail Dunn, RN, Eileen R. Hosking, Cindy

Kennedy, Ursula Morell, Amy L. Pass, Sergio Rico, Christian Swen-ingsen, and Linda Winters.

Finally, John Scott Legg at SteinerBooks has been instrumental in bringing this book into the world. We are grateful to the entire Steiner-Books publishing team, who saw our manuscript's promise and the great need for its insights.

Just like the training course that provided the foundation for this book, this was a team project with a community of dedicated individuals behind it. Each unique contribution to the manuscript has proved invaluable. It has been a monumental project. As we pass the book along to you, our readers, we also want to acknowledge all our patients and all the researchers and clinicians who are part of this journey with us. Thank you!

Individual Contributor Acknowledgements

Steven Johnson, DO

Thank you to all my colleagues and staff who give such wonderful care to our patients. Thank you to all of our patients who have touched our hearts with their courage to heal and their dignity in the face of hardship. A special thank you to Liz, my wife, who has been on this journey with me for over 21 years, managing the office and caring for our patients, always with an open heart.

Nasha Winters, ND, FABNO
Fellow of the American Board of Naturopathic Oncology

So many people and places have influenced my passion for integra-tive oncology and mistletoe in particular. My gratitude goes out to the many patients who continue to guide and teach me. If it weren't for you, this book wouldn't have been written. To my colleagues who inspire me with their curiosity and desire to change the cancer conversation—I celebrate you. And, to my family and friends, who continue to believe in me and my vision for the future: Thank you, and I love you.

Adam Blanning, MD

Deep thanks to Philip Incao, MD and Alicia Landman-Reiner, MD, for their mentorship, encouragement, and friendship in exploring anthroposophic medicine. Many loving thanks to my wife Lauren for her support.

Marion Debus, MD

I would like to thank Matthias Girke, who has been my clinical teacher for years of close collaboration in Havelhöhe. Working together with the wonderful members of the Vademecum Editorial Board has been inspiring and deeply influenced my clinical work. Maurice Orange was my most important teacher in oncology. Many anthroposophic doctors around the globe work with mistletoe therapy for the sake of their cancer patients and, in a self-sacrificing way, set up training courses to spread knowledge of the possibilities of anthroposophic oncology, namely: Maike and Yvan Villegas in Peru; Harihara Murthy, Srinivasa Rao, and Ravi Doctor in India; and Iramaia Chaguri, Sheila Grande, and Bernardo Kaliks in Brazil. Thank you all.

Paul Faust, ND, FABNO
Fellow of the American Board of Naturopathic Oncology

I want to thank my awesome wife, Ellen, who encouraged my pursuit of Naturopathic Medicine and who has been my bedrock of steadfast support. You have slogged through the trenches with me hand-in-hand over the past 25 years, and I could not have done any of it without you. Thank you so much, dear! And to my daughter, Isabel, who has kept my life in balance with her humor and *joie de vie*. Never stop dancing, Baby Honey Badger! You've both been the rays of sunshine in my life to light my path and provide inspiration during the stormy times.

Mark Hancock, MD

I would like to thank my patients who, when faced with a terrifying diagnosis, decided to place their trust in a higher purpose and have faith in enkindling the innate forces of healing. You have chosen me to care for you, but you have been my most personal and profound teachers during your healing journeys. I would like to thank my wife Enid, who brings her heart into all the clinical activities.

Peter Hinderberger, MD

I would not have chosen this comprehensive medical path were it not for a group of friends and fellow medical students (class of 1977), disillusioned by the analytical approach of medicine, who persuaded me to attend a presentation by Rita Leroi, MD. Dr. Leroi was head of oncology at the Lucas Klinik (now Klinik Arlesheim) in 1976. She has passed away, but was a wonderful human being, clinician, and teacher.

About the Contributors

Steven Johnson, DO, served as Co-chief Resident of Internal Medicine at the University of Massachusetts affiliated hospitals in Worcester (1996). He directed one of the first inpatient integrative medicine clinics in the U.S. and now directs the first European Mistletoe/Integrative Medicine Training Program in North America. Dr. Johnson has written numerous articles and lectured internationally. He is currently the president of the Physicians' Association for Anthroposophic Medicine (PAAM) and founder of the Foundation for Health Creation. Currently Dr. Johnson works part time in private practice at Collaborative Medical Arts (CollaborativeMedicalArts.net) in upstate New York and practices with adults with special needs at Camphill Village in Copake, New York. Dr. Johnson is an avid student of medicinal botany, and serves as a consultant for integrative and anthroposophic pharmacy.

Nasha Winters, ND, FABNO (Fellow of the American Board of Naturopathic Oncology), is a global healthcare authority and best-selling author in integrative cancer care and research (DrNasha.com). Consulting with physicians around the world, she has educated hundreds of professionals in the clinical use of mistletoe. She has created robust educational programs for both healthcare institutions and the public to incorporate well-vetted integrative therapies into cancer care to enhance outcomes. Dr. Winters is currently focused on opening a comprehensive metabolic oncology hospital and research institute (Metabolic Terrain Institute of Health) in the U.S., which will provide the best that standard of care has to offer alongside the most advanced integrative therapies. This facility will be in a residential setting on a gorgeous campus, against a backdrop of regenerative farming, EMF mitigation, and wellness-oriented retreat space.

Adam Blanning, MD, practices anthroposophic family medicine at the Denver Center for Anthroposophic Therapies (DenverTherapies.com) in Denver, Colorado. He is president of the Anthroposophic Health Association (AHA), an umbrella organization for groups working to bring anthroposophic insights into the realms of medicine, nursing, naturopathy, body therapies, artistic therapies, movement therapies, and counseling. Dr. Blanning lectures and teaches nationally and internationally on topics related to holistic medicine and the dynamics of human development. He is the author of *Understanding Deeper Developmental Needs: Holistic Approaches for Challenging Behaviors in Children.*

Marion Debus, MD, received her medical training at Ruhr-University Bochum (1989–1995). Her professional training in internal medicine includes her years at Klinik Öschelbronn Germany, Princess of Wales Hospital Bridgend GB, and Gemeinschaftskrankenhaus Havelhöhe in Berlin, Germany. Between 2002 and 2005, Marion further specialized in hematology and oncology at Robert-Bosch-Krankenhaus in Stuttgart, Germany. From 2005 to 2017, she was senior physician at the anthroposophic community hospital Havelhöhe Berlin with a large oncological outpatient clinic. She is currently Head of the Department of Oncology, Hematology, and Internal Medicine at Klinik Arlesheim (Klinik-Arlesheim.ch) near Basel, Switzerland.

Paul Faust, ND, FABNO (Fellow of the American Board of Naturopathic Oncology), is the Founder and Naturopathic Medical Director of the Chesapeake Natural Health Center (ChesapeakeNaturalHealth.com), established in 2001. He became the first Naturopathic Doctor licensed by Maryland's Board of Physicians in 2016 and has been retained by them as an Expert Witness for cases involving Naturopathic Medicine within the state. He also serves on the board of the Naturopathic Formulary Council. In 2020, he was selected to receive Maryland's first Naturopathic Doctor of the Year Award. Previously he has served on the editorial review board for the *Alternative Medicine Review,* a leading publication for complementary and alternative medicine.

Mark Hancock, MD, MPH, founded Humanizing Medicine in Atlanta, Georgia, together with his wife Enid, in 2015. The clinic is strongly rooted in the couple's belief that everyone should have quality integrative healthcare options. For his entire professional career, Dr. Hancock has worked with Anthroposophic Medicine, which originally introduced mistletoe as a cancer care therapy over one hundred years ago. Dr Hancock graduated *summa cum laude* from Saint George's Medical School in 2008 and was elected Chief Resident during his training at University of New Mexico Hospital. He was introduced to the advanced use of mistletoe by Dr. Maurice Orange, greatly influencing his life course. Dr. Hancock's journey through life has been full and varied and has taken him through art, philosophy, science, and even some farm work, before ultimately landing in medicine. Read about his journey and medical philosophy at HumanizingMedicine.com.

Peter Hinderberger, MD, was born and raised in Switzerland, where he also attended medical school. In 1978, he completed part of his internship at the Lukas Klinik in Arlesheim, Switzerland (now the oncology department of the Klinik Arlesheim), an integrative oncology clinic. In 1982, he spent another six months at that clinic to deepen his knowledge and practical experience in the use of subcutaneous and intravenous mistletoe. In the spring of 1984, Dr. Hinderberger opened his general practice at the Ruscombe Mansion Community Health Center in Baltimore. He now practices at the Raphael Clinic of Maryland (RaphaelClinicMD.com) in Towson, Maryland. Integrative oncology has always been a focus of his research and practice.

REFERENCES AND AUTHOR NOTES

INTRODUCTION

1. R. Steiner. *How to Know Higher Worlds: A Modern Path of Initiation* (CW 10). Hudson, NY: Anthroposophic Press, 1994.
2. H. J. Hamre, et al. "Use and safety of anthroposophic medicinal products: an analysis of 44,662 patients from the EvaMed Pharmacovigilance Network. *Drugs: Real World Outcomes* 4, 199–213 (2017). https://doi .org/10.1007/s40801-017-0118-5.
3. Qi Zhang, et al. "The path toward integration of traditional and complementary medicine into health systems globally: The World Health Organization report on the implementation of the 2014–2023 strategy," PMID: 31525106 DOI: 10.1089/acm.2019.29077.jjw.
4. A. Chaudhary and N. Singh. "Contribution of World Health Organization in the global acceptance of ayurveda," *Journal of Ayurveda and Integrative Medicine,* 2011(2):179–186.
5. M. A. Horneber, et al. "Mistletoe therapy in oncology," Cochrane Database Syst Rev, 2008:CD003297. DOI: 10.1002/14651858.CD003297 .pub2.
6. M. Kröz, et al. "Validation of the German version of the cancer fatigue scale (CFS-D)," *Eur. J. Cancer Care,* 2008;17:33-41. DOI: 10.1111 /j.1365-2354.2007.00799.x.
7. Per data published by Mistletoe-Therapy.org. "Currently 154 studies have been conducted on the anthroposophical mistletoe preparations abnobaVISCUM, Helixor, Iscador and Iscucin (status May 2020)," accessed Apr. 26, 2021.

CHAPTER 1

1. J. Wilkens and G. Böhm. *Mistletoe Therapy for Cancer: Prevention, Treatment, and Healing* (Edinburgh: Floris Books, 2010), p. 23.
2. Ibid.
3. M. Wood. *The Earthwise Herbal, vol. 1: A Complete Guide to Old World Medicinal Plants.* Berkeley, CA: North Atlantic Books, 2008.
4. Imhotep case 45: Breasted, *Edwin Smith Papyrus.*
5. H. E. Sigerist. "The historical development of the pathology and therapy of cancer," *Bulletin of the New York Academy of Medicine* 8, no. 11 (1932): 642–53.
6. C. Galen. *Methodus Medendi, with Brief Declaration of the Worthie Art of Medicine, the Office of a Chirgion, and an Epitome of the Third*

Booke of Galen, of Naturall Faculties. London: Thomas East, 1586, pp. 180–182.

7. S. Mukherjee. *The Emperor of all Maladies: A Biography of Cancer* (New York: Simon and Schuster, 2011), pp. 47–49.

8. B. Krone, et al. "The biography of the immune system and the control of cancer: from St Peregrine to contemporary vaccination strategies," *BMC Cancer,* 14, Article number: 595 (Aug. 14, 2014).

9. G. L. Rohdenburg, "Fluctuations in the Growth Energy of Malignant Tumors in Man, with Especial Reference to Spontaneous Recession," *The Journal of Cancer Research,* Apr. 1, 1918; 3(2):193–225. doi: 10.1158/jcr .1918.193.

10. B. Wiemann and C. O. Starnes. "Coley's toxins, tumor necrosis factor and cancer research: A historical perspective," *Pharmacology and Therapeutics,* vol. 64, no. 3, 1994, pp. 529–564, ISSN 0163-7258, https://doi .org/10.1016/0163-7258(94)90023-X.

11. A. Szurpnicka, et al. "Biological activity of mistletoe: in vitro and in vivo studies and mechanisms of action," *Arch. Pharm. Res.* (2020) 43:593–629 Online ISSN 1976-3786 https://doi.org/10.1007/s12272-020-01247-w.

12. B. Barlow. "Mistletoe in folk legend and medicine," *Australian National Herbarium,* Aug. 7, 2008; posted https://www.anbg.gov.au/mistletoe/folk -legend.html. Retrieved Apr. 30, 2021.

13. M. Grieve. *A Modern Herbal: vol. 2, I–Z and Indexes,* New York: Dover, 1971. Digital version of entry "Mistletoe," at https://www.botanical.com /botanical/mgmh/m/mistle40.html. Retrieved Apr. 29, 2021.

14. U. Pfüller. "Chemical constituents of European mistletoe (Viscum album L.), in A. Büssing (ed.), *Mistletoe: The Genus Viscum* (Amsterdam: Harwood Academic, 2000), pp. 101–122.

15. G. S. Kienle and H. Kiene. *Mistletoe in Oncology: Facts and Basic Concepts,* New York: Schatauer, 2003.

16. M. Giudici, et al. "Interaction of viscotoxins A3 and B with membrane model systems: Implications to their mechanism of action," *Biophys. J.,* 2003 Aug;85(2):971-81. doi: 10.1016/S0006-3495(03)74536-6. PMID: 12885644; PMCID: PMC1303218.

17. M. Yang and W. J. Brackenbury. "Membrane potential and cancer progression," *Front Physiol.,* 2013 Jul 17;4:185. doi: 10.3389/fphys.2013 .00185. PMID: 23882223; PMCID: PMC3713347.

18. M. Hashemzaei, et al. "Anticancer and apoptosis-inducing effects of quercetin in vitro and in vivo," *Oncol. Rep.,* 2017 Aug;38(2):819-828. doi: 10.3892/or.2017.5766. Epub 2017 Jun 28. PMID: 28677813; PMCID: PMC5561933.

19. H. Becker and J. M. Scher. "Short survey of the main components of European mistletoe (*Viscum album* L.)," in R. Scheer. et al (eds.), *Fortschritte in Der Misteltherapie,* Essen: KVC Verlag, 2005.

20. A. Szurpnicka, et al. "Biological activity of mistletoe: in vitro and in vivo studies and mechanisms of action," *Arch. Pharm. Res.* (2020) 43:593–629 Online ISSN 1976-3786 https://doi.org/10.1007/s12272-020-01247-w.

21. S. K. Ghosh. "Giovanni Battista Morgagni (1682–1771): Father of pathologic anatomy and pioneer of modern medicine," *Anatomical Science International*, vol. 92,3 (2017): 305–312. doi:10.1007/s12565-016-0373-7.

22. Y. Kaya and A. Sindel. "John Hunter (1728–1793) and his legacy to science," *Childs Nerv. Syst.*, 32, 1015–1017 (2016). https://doi.org/10.1007/s00381-015-2852-x.

23. L. Tonetti. "The discovery of the lymphatic system as a turning point iin medical knowledge: Aselli, Pecquet, and the end of hepatocentrism," *Journal of Theoretical and Applied Vascular Research* (2017);2(2):67–76.

24. P. Pott and J. Earles. *The Chirurgical Works of Percivall Pott, F.R.S. Surgeon to St. Bartholomew's Hospital, A New Edition*, London: Wood and Innes, 1808, 3:177.

25. R. D. Passey. "Experimental soot cancer," *The British Medical Journal*, 1922, 2 (3232): 1112–1113.

26. A. Dronsfield. "Percivall Pott, chimney sweeps and cancer," *Education in Chemistry*, vol. 43 no. 2. Royal Society of Chemistry, 2006. pp. 40–42, 48.

27. J. H. Wiener. *Great Britain: The Lion at Home: A Documentary History of Domestic Policy, 1689–1973*, New York: Chelsea House, 1974.

28. "Johannes Müller (1801-1858), anatomist, physiologist, pathologist," *JAMA*, vol. 214,11 (1970): 2049-51.

29. M. Schultz. "Rudolf Virchow," *Emerging Infectious Diseases*, vol. 14,9 (2008): 1480–1481. doi:10.3201/eid1409.086672.

30. R. R. Langley and I. J. Fidler. "The seed and soil hypothesis revisited: The role of tumor-stroma interactions in metastasis to different organs," *International Journal of Cancer*, vol. 128,11 (2011): 2527-35. doi:10.1002/ijc.26031.

31. Ibid.

32. Ibid.

33. P. Ehrlich. "Ueber den jetzigen Stand der Karzinomforschung," *Ned. Tijdschr. Geneeskd.*, 5 (1909), pp. 273-290.

34. G. P. Dunn, et al. "The immunobiology of cancer immunosurveillance and immunoediting," *Immunity*, vol. 21, no. 2, 2004, pp. 137–148.

35. Quangdon Tran, et al. "Revisiting the Warburg effect: Diet-based strategies for cancer prevention." *BioMed Research International*, vol. 2020 8105735. 4 Aug. 2020, doi:10.1155/2020/8105735.

36. T. Boveri. *Concerning the Origin of Malignant Tumors*, New York: Cold Spring Harbor, 2006.

37. V. Wunderlich. "Early references to the mutational origin of cancer," *International Journal of Epidemiology*, vol. 36, no. 1, Feb. 2007, pp. 246–247, https://doi.org/10.1093/ije/dyl272.

38. "Cancer mutations occur decades before diagnosis," European Molecular Biology Laboratory, Feb. 4, 2020; online at https://www.ebi.ac.uk/about/news/announcements/cancer-mutations-decades-before-diagnosis. Retrieved Apr. 29, 2021.

39. W. C Röntgen. "On a new kind of rays," *Nature*, 53, no. 1369 (1896): 274–76.

40. E. H. Grubbe. "Priority in therapeutic use of X-rays," *Radiology,* 21 (1933): 156–62.

41. W. S. Halsted. "The results of radical operations for the cure of cancer of the breast," *Transactions of the American Surgical Association* 25: 66.

42. L. F. Vernon. "William Bradley Coley, MD, and the phenomenon of spontaneous regression," *Immunotargets Ther.,* 2018;7:29–34. https://doi.org /10.2147/ITT.S163924.

43. E. F. McCarthy. "The toxins of William B. Coley and the treatment of bone and soft-tissue sarcomas," *The Iowa Orthopaedic Journal,* vol. 26 (2006): 154–8.

44. S. A. Hoption Cann, et al. "Dr William Coley and tumour regression: A place in history or in the future," *Postgraduate Medical Journal,* 2003;79:672-680.

45. R. Steiner. *Introducing Anthroposophical Medicine* (CW 312). Great Barrington, MA: SteinerBooks; 2010.

46. C. Murphy. *Iscador: Mistletoe and Cancer Therapy.* New York: Lantern Books, 2001. (AUTHOR NOTE: Ita Wegman was instrumental in developing the first recognized mistletoe extract product, Iscador®. Her story is covered in greater depth at https://www.mistletoe-therapy.org /information-for-patients/preparations/iscador.)

47. G. S. Kienle, et al. "Individualized integrative cancer care in anthroposophic medicine: A qualitative study of the concepts and procedures of expert doctors," *Integrative Cancer Therapies,* May 4, 2016, 15(4);478-494. DOI: 10.1177/1534735416640091 PMID: 27151589 PMCID: PMC5739166.

48. R. Steiner. lecture of Oct. 27, 1922 p.m., in *Physiology and Healing: Treatment, Therapy, and Hygiene* (CW 314). Forest Row, UK: Rudolf Steiner Press, 2014.

49. R. A. Weinburg. *The Biology of Cancer,* 2nd ed. (New York: Garland Science, 2014), 15(13).

50. R. R. Bartelme. "Anthroposophic Medicine: A Short Monograph and Narrative Review: Foundations, Essential Characteristics, Scientific Basis, Safety, Effectiveness and Misconceptions." *Global Advances in Health and Medicine.* vol. 9 2164956120973634. 29 Dec. 2020, doi:10.1177/2164956120973634.

51. J. Conant. *The Great Secret: The Classified World War II Disaster that Launched the War on Cancer.* New York: Norton, 2020.

52. S. Farber. "Temporary remissions in acute leukemia in children produced by folic acid antagonist, 4-aminopteroyl-glutamic acid (aminopterin)," *New England Journal of Medicine,* 238 (1948): 787-93.

53. D. R. Miller. "A Tribute to Sidney Farber—the Father of Modern Chemotherapy," *British Journal of Haematology,* 134 (2006): 20-26.

54. F. M. Burnet. "The concept of immunological surveillance," *Prog. Exp. Tumor Res.* 1970;13:1–27.

55. M. Burnet. "Immunological factors in the process of carcinogenesis." *Br. Med. Bull.* 1964;20:154–158.

56.   M. Smyth, et al. "A fresh look at tumor immunosurveillance and immunotherapy," *Nat. Immunol.*, 2, 293–299 (2001). https://doi.org/10.1038/86297.

57.   B. M. J.issell, et al. "How does the extracellular matrix direct gene expression?" *J. Theor. Biol.* 99, 31–68 (1982).

58.   M. J. Bissell and M. A. Labarge. "Context, tissue plasticity, and cancer: are tumor stem cells also regulated by the microenvironment?" *Cancer Cell,* vol. 7,1 (2005): 17-23. doi:10.1016/j.ccr.2004.12.013.

59.   A. L. Correia and M. J. Bissell. "The tumor microenvironment is a dominant force in multidrug resistance," *Drug Resistance Updates: Reviews and Commentaries in Antimicrobial and Anticancer Chemotherapy,* vol. 15,1–2 (2012): 39-49. doi:10.1016/j.drup.2012.01.006.

60.   M. J. Bissell and W. C. Hines. "Why don't we get more cancer? A proposed role of the microenvironment in restraining cancer progression," *Nature medicine,* vol. 17,3 (2011): 320-9. doi:10.1038/nm.2328.

61.   E. Schickler. "Ein neues Mittel gegen Carcinom," [A new remedy against cancer]; Case report series (German), 1924.
      62. R. A. Weinburg. *The Biology of Cancer,* 2nd ed. New York: Garland Science, 2014.

63.   E. Schickler. "Ein neues Mittel gegen Carcinom" [A new remedy against cancer], Case report series (in German), 1924.

64.   G. Salzer and L. Havelec. "Rezidivprophylaxe bei operierten Bronchuskarzinompatienten mit dem Mistelpräparat Iscador Ergebnisse eines klinischen Versuchs aus den Jahren 1969–1971" [Prevention of recurrence of bronchial carcinomas after surgery by means of the mistletoe extract Iscador. Results of a clinical study from 1969–1971]. *Onkologie,* vol. 1,6 (1978): 264-7. doi:10.1159/000213966.

65.   G. Kelter and H. H. Fiebig. "Absence of tumor growth stimulation in a panel of 26 human tumor cell lines by mistletoe (*Viscum album L.*) extracts Iscador in vitro," *Arzneimittelforschung 56* (6A): 435-40, 2006.

66.   A. Szurpnicka, et al. "Biological activity of mistletoe: in vitro and in vivo studies and mechanisms of action," *Arch. Pharm. Res.* (2020) 43:593–629; online https://doi.org/10.1007/s12272-020-01247-w.

67.   J. M. Braun, et al. "Standardized mistletoe extract augments immune response and down-regulates local and metastatic tumor growth in murine models," *Anticancer Res,* 22 (6C): 4187–90, Nov.–Dec. 2002.

68.   A. Pulliero, et al. "Genetic and Epigenetic Effects of Environmental Mutagens and Carcinogens," *BioMed Research International,* vol. 2015 (2015): 608054. doi:10.1155/2015/608054.

69.   "NIH complementary and integrative health agency gets new name," NCCIH Press Office, Dec. 17, 2014; online at https://www.nih.gov/news-events/news-releases/nih-complementary-integrative-health-agency-gets-new-name. Accessed Apr. 26, 2021.

70.   P. Barnes, et al. "CDC advance data report #343. Complementary and alternative medicine use among adults: United States, 2002." U.S. Department of Health and Human Services, Centers for Disease Control and Prevention, National Center for Health Statistics; May 27, 2004.

71. N. N. Sanford, et al. "Prevalence and nondisclosure of complementary and alternative medicine use in patients with cancer and cancer survivors in the United States." *JAMA Oncology*, vol. 5,5 (2019): 735-737. doi:10.1001/jamaoncol.2019.0349.

72. C. A. Buckner, et al. "Complementary and alternative medicine use in patients before and after a cancer diagnosis." *Current Oncology* (Toronto), vol. 25,4 (2018): e275-e281. doi:10.3747/co.25.3884.

73. C. M. Witt, et al. "A Comprehensive Definition for Integrative Oncology," *JNCI Monographs*, vol. 2017, no. 52, Nov. 2017, lgx012, https://doi.org /10.1093/jncimonographs/lgx012.

74. Per Society for Integrative Oncology website, www.integrativeonc.org. Accessed Apr. 26, 2021.

75. T. N. Seyfried and L. M. Shelton. "Cancer as a metabolic disease," *Nutrition and Metabolism* (London) 2010, 7:7. http://www .nutritionandmetabolism.com/content/7/1/7.

76. L. G. Boros, et al. "Submolecular regulation of cell transformation by deuterium depleting water exchange reactions in the tricarboxylic acid substrate cycle." *Medical Hypotheses*, vol. 87 (2016): 69-74. doi:10.1016 /j.mehy.2015.11.016.

77. A. M. Soto and C. Sonnenschein. "The tissue organization field theory of cancer: A testable replacement for the somatic mutation theory," *BioEssays: News and Reviews in Molecular, Cellular and Developmental Biology*, vol. 33,5 (2011): 332-40. doi:10.1002/bies.201100025.

78. T. N. Seyfried. "Cancer as a mitochondrial metabolic disease," *Frontiers in Cell and Developmental Biology*, vol. 3 43. July 7, 2015, doi:10.3389 /fcell.2015.00043.

79. Registered at https://clinicaltrials.gov/ct2/show/NCT03051477. Accessed Apr. 26, 2021.

80. A. Brodsky, "Cancer immunotherapy in 2020 and beyond," Cancer Research Institute, at https://www.cancerresearch.org/blog/january-2020 /cancer-immunotherapy-in-2020-and-beyond. Retrieved Apr. 29, 2021.

81. S. Kruger, et al. "Advances in cancer immunotherapy 2019: Latest trends," *J. Exp. Clin. Cancer Res.*, 38, 268 (2019). https://doi.org/10.1186/s13046 -019-1266-0.

82. AUTHOR NOTE: The data collection project is already underway for this project. Covered in greater detail in chap. 12.

83. Per data published by Mistletoe-Therapy.org, "Currently 154 studies have been conducted on the anthroposophical mistletoe preparations abno-baVISCUM, Helixor, Iscador and Iscucin (status May 2020)." Accessed Apr. 26, 2021.

84. C. Murphy, *Iscador: Mistletoe and Cancer Therapy*. New York: Lantern Books, 2001, p. 15.

85. "European Mistletoe," National Institute of Health (NIH) National Center for Complementary and Integrative Health (NCCIH)," digital fact sheet, Aug. 2020. At https://www.nccih.nih.gov/health/european -mistletoe. Retrieved Apr. 29, 2021.

86. *Vademecum of Anthroposophic Medicines*, Association of Anthroposophic Medicine in Germany (GAAD); 2017, 82-89.

87. P. J. Mansky, et al. "NCCAM/NCI phase 1 study of mistletoe extract and gemcitabine in patients with advanced solid tumors." *Evidence-based Complementary and Alternative Medicine: eCAM*, vol. 2013 (2013): 964592. doi:10.1155/2013/964592.

88. R. Madeleyn, et al. "Hirntumore bei Kindern: Therapieverläufe (Teil I)" [Brain tumors in children: therapy courses (Part 1)] *Der Merkurstab. Beiträge zur einer Erweiterung der Heilkunst.* 2001;54(6):397–407.

89. Ibid. (Teil II)." [Brain tumors in children: therapy courses (Part 2)] *Der Merkurstab. Beiträge zur einer Erweiterung der Heilkunst.* 2002;55(1):36–47.

90. A. J. Husemann and A. Orale. "Misteltherapie bei Riesenzellastrozytom" [Mistletoe therapy for giant cell astrocytoma"], *Der Merkurstab. Beiträge zur einer Erweiterung der Heilkunst* 2000;53(3):183.

91. *Vademecum of Anthroposophic Medicines*. Published by Association of Anthroposophic Medicine in Germany (GAAD); 2017, 82-89.

92. K. Hostanska, et al. "Recombinant mistletoe lectin induces p53-independent apoptosis in tumour cells and cooperates with ionising radiation," *Br. J. Cancer.* 2003 Jun 2;88(11):1785-92. doi: 10.1038/sj.bjc .6600982. PMID: 12771996; PMCID: PMC2377150.

93. J. E. Felenda, et al. "Antiproliferative potential from aqueous Viscum album L. preparations and their main constituents in comparison with ricin and purothionin on human cancer cells," *Journal of Ethnopharmacology*, vol. 236, 2019, pp. 100–107; https://doi.org/10.1016/j.jep.2019 .02.047.

94. G. S. Kienle and H. Kiene. "Review article: Influence of *Viscum album L* (European mistletoe) extracts on quality of life in cancer patients: a systematic review of controlled clinical studies," *Integr Cancer Ther*, 2010;9:142-157. doi: 10.1177/1534735410369673.

95. B. K. Piao, et al. "Impact of complementary mistletoe extract treatment on quality of life in breast, ovarian and non-small cell lung cancer patients: A prospective randomized controlled clinical trial," *Anticancer Research*, 2004;24:303-310.

96. Quangdon Tran, et al. "Revisiting the Warburg Effect: Diet-Based Strategies for Cancer Prevention." *BioMed Research International,* vol. 2020 8105735. 4 Aug. 2020. doi:10.1155/2020/8105735.

97. T. Seyfried, *Cancer as a Metabolic Disease: On the Origin, Management, and Prevention of Cancer*, Hoboken, NJ: Wiley, 2012.

98. N. K. LoConte, et al. "Lifestyle modifications and policy implications for primary and secondary cancer prevention: Diet, exercise, sun safety, and alcohol reduction," *American Society of Clinical Oncology Educational Book. American Society of Clinical Oncology. Annual Meeting*, vol. 38 (2018): 88-100. doi:10.1200/EDBK_200093.

99. J. R. Infante, et al. "Levels of immune cells in transcendental meditation practitioners," *International Journal of Yoga*, vol. 7,2 (2014): 147–51. doi:10.4103/0973-6131.133899.

100. Jiang Shui, et al. "Epigenetic modifications in stress response genes associated with childhood trauma," *Frontiers in Psychiatry*, vol. 10 808, Nov. 8, 2019. doi:10.3389/fpsyt.2019.00808.

101. J. J. Medina, "The Epigenetics of Stress," *Psychiatric Times,* Apr. 7, 2010; vol. 27, no. 4. https://www.psychiatrictimes.com/view/epigenetics -stress. Retrieved Apr. 29.2021.

102. S. P. Megdal, et al. "Night work and breast cancer risk: A systematic review and meta-analysis," *European Journal of Cancer* (Oxford, UK: 1990), vol. 41,13 (2005): 2023-32. doi:10.1016/j.ejca.2005.05.010.

103. E. McNeely, et al. "The self-reported health of U.S. flight attendants compared to the general population," *Environmental Health,* 13, 13 (2014); https://doi.org/10.1186/1476-069X-13-13.

104. D. Buettner and S. Skemp. "Blue Zones: Lessons from the world's longest lived." *American Journal of Lifestyle Medicine,* vol. 10,5 318-321, Jul. 7, 2016. doi:10.1177/1559827616637066.

CHAPTER 2

1. N. Sipeki, et al. "Immune dysfunction in cirrhosis," *World J. Gastroenterol,* 2014;20(10):2564-2577. doi:10.3748/wjg.v20.i10.2564.

2. Wu SY, et al. "Natural killer cells in cancer biology and therapy," *Mol Cancer,* 2020;19(1):120, Aug 6, 2020. doi:10.1186/s12943-020-01238-x.

3. D. Ostroumov, et al. "CD4 and CD8 T lymphocyte interplay in controlling tumor growth." *Cell Mol. Life Sci.,* 2018; 75(4):689-713. doi:10.1007 /s00018-017-2686-7.

4. M. Hoffman, et al. "Human acute and chronic viruses: Host-pathogen interactions and therapeutics," *Advanced Concepts in Human Immunology: Prospects for Disease Control,* 2020;1-120, Aug 12, 2020. doi:10.1007/978-3-030-33946-3_1.

5. A. Thakur, et al. "Intracellular pathogens: Host immunity and microbial persistence strategies." *J. Immunol. Res.* 2019;2019:1356540, Apr 14, 2019. doi:10.1155/2019/1356540.

6. A. M. van der Leun, et al. "CD8⁺ T cell states in human cancer: insights from single-cell analysis," *Nat. Rev. Cancer.* 2020;20(4):218–232. doi:10.1038/s41568-019-0235-4.

7. Ibid.

8. R. T. Lee, et al. "The sugar-combining area of the galactose-specific toxic lectin of mistletoe extends beyond the terminal sugar residue: Comparison with a homologous toxic lectin, ricin," *Carbohydr. Res.* 254, 269–276 (1994).

9. U. Pfüller. "Chemical constituents of European mistletoe (Viscum album L.)," in A. Büssing (ed.). *Mistletoe: The Genus Viscum.* Amsterdam: Harwood Academic, 2000, pp. 101–122.

10. W. Kreis. "Advances in structure elucidation of mistletoe constituents," in R. Scheer, et al. (ed.), *Die Mistel in der Tumortherapie 2.* Essen: KVC Verlag, 2009, pp, 17–29.

11. G. S. Kienle and H. Kiene. *Mistletoe in Oncology. Facts and Basic Concepts.* New York: Schatauer, 2003.

12. H. Li, et al. "The structural basis of T cell activation by superantigens," *Annu. Rev. Immunol.,* 1999; 17:435–466. doi: 10.1146/annurev.immunol .17.1.435.

13. A. Galelli, et al. "Selective expansion followed by profound deletion of mature V beta 8.3+ T cells in vivo after exposure to the superantigenic lectin Urtica dioica agglutinin," *J. Immunol.*, Mar 15, 1995; 154(6):2600–11. PMID: 7876535.

14. A. Galelli and P. Truffa-Bachi. "Urtica dioica agglutinin. A superantigenic lectin from stinging nettle rhizome," *J. Immunol.*, Aug 15, 1993; 151(4):1821-31. PMID: 8345184.

15. U. Pfüller. "Chemical constituents of European mistletoe (Viscum album L.)," in A. Büssing (ed.). *Mistletoe: The Genus Viscum*, Amsterdam: Harwood Academic, 2000, pp. 101–122.

16. M. Franz. *Struktur und biologische Aktivitäten der chitinbindenden Mistellektine* (dissertation), Tübingen, 2003.

17. W. Kreis. "Advances in structure elucidation of mistletoe constituents," in R. Scheer, et al. (ed.). *Die Mistel in der Tumortherapie 2*, Essen: KVC Verlag, 2009, pp. 17–29.

18. M. Giudici, et al. "Interaction of viscotoxins A3 and B with membrane model systems: Implications to their mechanism of action," *Biophys J.* Aug. 2003;85(2):971-81. doi: 10.1016/S0006-3495(03)74536-6. PMID: 12885644; PMCID: PMC1303218.

19. M. Yang and W. J. Brackenbury. "Membrane potential and cancer progression." *Front. Physiol.* Jul. 17, 2013; 4:185. doi: 10.3389/fphys.2013 .00185. PMID: 23882223; PMCID: PMC3713347.

20. G. Ribereau-Gayon, et al.: Effects of mistletoe (*Viscum album* L.) extracts on cultured tumor cells. *Experientia* 42, 594–599 (1986).

21. A. Büssing: Biological and pharmacological properties of *Viscum album* L. In Büssing A (Ed.). *Mistletoe: The Genus Vuscum*. Amsterdam: Harwood Academic, 2000, pp. 123–182.

22. J. E. Debreczeni, et al. "Structure of viscotoxin A3: Disulfide location from weak SAD data." *Acta. Cryst.* D59, 2125–2132 (2003).

23. H. Becker and J. M. Scher. "Short survey of the main components of European mistletoe (*Viscum album* L.)," in R. Scheer, et al. (ed.). *Fortschritte in Der Misteltherapie*. Essen: KVC Verlag, 2005, pp. 3–11.

24. U. Pfüller. "Chemical constituents of European mistletoe (Viscum album L.)," in A. Büssing A (ed.), *Mistletoe: The Genus Viscum*. Amsterdam: Harwood Academic, 2000, pp. 101–122.

25. M. Yang and W. J. Brackenbury. "Membrane potential and cancer progression," *Front. Physiol.* 2013 Jul 17;4:185. doi: 10.3389/fphys.2013 .00185. PMID: 23882223; PMCID: PMC3713347.

26. M. Giudici, et al. "Interaction of viscotoxins A3 and B with membrane model systems: Implications to their mechanism of action," *Biophys. J.* 2003 Aug;85(2):971-81. doi: 10.1016/S0006-3495(03)74536-6. PMID: 12885644; PMCID: PMC1303218. (AUTHOR NOTE: "[viscotoxins] bind with high affinity to membranes containing negatively charged phospholipids.")

27. S. Fischer. *In ivtro-Versuche zur T-Zellaktivität*. Stuttgart: Hippokrates Verlag, 1996, p. 168.

28. G. S. Kienle and H. Kiene. *Mistletoe in Oncology: Facts and Basic Concepts*. New York: Schatauer, 2003.

29. H. Becker and J. M. Scher. "Short survey of the main components of European mistletoe (*Viscum album* L.)," in R. Scheer, et al. (ed.). *Fortschritte in Der Misteltherapie*, Essen: KVC Verlag, 2005, pp. 3–11.

30. M. Hashemzaei, et al. "Anticancer and apoptosisinducing effects of quercetin in vitro and in vivo," *Oncol. Rep.* 2017 Aug;38(2):819-828. doi: 10.3892/or.2017.5766. Epub 2017 Jun 28. PMID: 28677813; PMCID: PMC5561933.

31. H. Becker and J. M. Scher. "Short survey of the main components of European mistletoe (*Viscum album* L.)." in R. Scheer, et al. (ed.). *Fortschritte in Der Misteltherapie*, Essen: KVC Verlag, 2005, pp. 3–11.

32. W. Dröge and R. Breitkreutz. "Glutathione and immune function," *Proc Nutr. Soc.* 2000 Nov;59(4):595–600. doi: 10.1017/s0029665100000847. PMID: 11115795.

33. K. Urech, et al. "Triterpenes of mistletoe (*Viscum album*) in the "birdlime" viscin and its antiproliferative activity," in R. Scheer, et al. (ed.). *Fortschritte in Der Misteltherapie*, Essen: KVC Verlag, 2005, pp. 3–11.

34. K. Hostanska, et al. "Recombinant mistletoe lectin induces p53-independent apoptosis in tumour cells and cooperates with ionising radiation," *Br J. Cancer.* 2003 Jun 2;88(11):1785-92. doi: 10.1038/sj.bjc .6600982. PMID: 12771996; PMCID: PMC2377150. (AUTHOR NOTE: This study used recombinant mistletoe lectin which means it was produced by bacteria as a specific, singular compound and not extracted from the plant at all.)

35. J. E. Felenda, et al. "Antiproliferative potential from aqueous Viscum album L. preparations and their main constituents in comparison with ricin and purothionin on human cancer cells," *Journal of Ethnopharmacology*, vol. 236, 2019, pp. 100–107; ISSN 0378-8741; https://doi .org/10.1016/j.jep.2019.02.047. (AUTHOR NOTE: This study found: "The complete mistletoe extract is more potent to inhibit tumor cell proliferation than isolated ML-1 at an equivalent concentration level.")

36. Table used with permission from Manufacturer Publication, in *Compendium of Mistletoe Therapy with Helixor® in Integrative Oncology* (n.d.), p. 8; https://docplayer.net/57758605-Helixor -compendium-of-mistletoe-therapy-with-helixor-in-integrative-oncology -mistletoe-therapy-for-tumor-patients-bringing-life-to-life.html.

37. G. Schrader-Fischer and K. Apel. "The anticyclic timing of leaf senescence in the parasitic plant viscum album is closely correlated with the selective degradation of sulfur-rich viscotoxins," *Plant Physiol.*, 1993; 101(3):745–749. doi:10.1104/pp.101.3.745.

38. K. Urech, et al. "Organ specific and seasonal accumulation of viscotoxinisoforms in Viscum album ssp. album," *Phytomedicine*, vol. 18, supp. 1. 2011, p. S7, ISSN 0944-7113; https://doi.org/10.1016/j.phymed.2011.09 .064. (http://www.sciencedirect.com/science/article/pii /S094471131100434X).

39. M Harmsma, et al. "Effects of mistletoe (Viscum album L.) extracts Iscador on cell cycle and survival of tumor cells," *Arzneimittelforschung*, Jun. 2006;56(6A):474–82. doi: 10.1055/s-0031-1296815. PMID: 16927529.

40.   J. Tabiasco, et al. "Mistletoe viscotoxins increase natural killer cell-medi-
      ated cytotoxicity," *Eur. J. Biochem.*, May 2002;269(10):2591–600. doi:
      10.1046/j.1432-1033.2002.02932.x. PMID: 12027898.

41.   Increase in CD8(+) cells: N. E. Gardin. "Immunological response to
      mistletoe (Viscum album L.) in cancer patients: A four-case series,"
      Phytother. Res., Mar. 2009;23(3):407–11. doi: 10.1002/ptr.2643. PMID:
      19003944.

42.   Increase in Cytotoxic T cells: J. Beuth, et al. "Behavior of lymphocyte
      subsets and expression of activation markers in response to immuno-
      therapy with galactoside-specific lectin from mistletoe in breast cancer
      patients," *Clin. Investig.*, Aug. 1992;70(8):658–61. doi: 10.1007
      /BF00180280. PMID: 1392440.

43.   W. B. Park, et al. "Inhibition of tumor growth and metastasis by
      Korean mistletoe lectin is associated with apoptosis and antiangio-
      genesis," *Cancer Biother. Radiopharm.*, Oct. 2001;16(5):439–47. doi:
      10.1089/108497801753354348. PMID: 11776761.

44.   J. M. Moon, et al. "Effect of mistletoe on endometrial stromal cell
      survival and vascular endothelial growth factor expression in patients
      with endometriosis," *Int. J. Med. Sci.*, Oct. 2018 20;15(13):1530–36. doi:
      10.7150/ijms.28470. PMID: 30443175; PMCID: PMC6216063.

45.   F. Stirpe, et al. "Inhibition of protein synthesis by a toxic lectin from
      Viscum album L. (mistletoe)," *Biochem. J.*, 1980;190(3):843–45.
      doi:10.1042/bj1900843.

46.   E. Kovacs, et al. "Improvement of DNA repair in lymphocytes of breast
      cancer patients treated with Viscum album extract (Iscador)." *Eur. J.
      Cancer*, 1991;27(12):1672-6. doi: 10.1016/0277–79(91)90443-h. PMID:
      1782081.

47.   J. M. Woynarowski and J. Konopa. "Interaction between DNA and
      viscotoxins: Cytotoxic basic polypeptides from Viscum album L," *Hoppe
      Seylers Z. Physiol. Chem.*, Oct. 1980;361(10):1535–45. doi: 10.1515/
      bchm2.1980.361.2.1535. PMID: 7192684.

48.   U. Elsässer-Beile, et al. "Biological effects of natural recombinant mistle-
      toe lectin and an aqueous mistletoe extract on human monocytes and
      lymphocytes *in vitro*," *J. Clin. Lab. Anal.*, 14, 255–59 (2000).

49.   G. M. Stein and P. A. Berg. "Evaluation of the stimulatory activity of
      a fermented mistletoe lectin-1 free mistletoe extract on T-helper cells
      and monocytes in healthy individuals in vitro." *Arzneimittelforschung*,
      Jun. 1996;46(6):635-9. PMID: 8767357.

50.   Lymphocytes and Neutrophils REF: N. E. Gardin. "Immunological
      response to mistletoe (Viscum album L.) in cancer patients: A four-case
      series," *Phytother. Res.*, Mar. 2009;23(3):407-11. doi: 10.1002/ptr.2643.
      PMID: 19003944.

51.   Neutrophil (granulocyte) REF: R. Huber, et al. "Mistletoe treatment
      induces GM-CSF- and IL-5 production by PBMC and increases blood
      granulocyte- and eosinophil counts: a placebo controlled randomized
      study in healthy subjects," *Eur. J. Med. Res.*, Oct. 2005 18;10(10):411–18.
      PMID: 16287602.

52.   G. S. Kienle and H. Kiene. *Mistletoe in Oncology: Facts and Basic
      Concepts*. New York: Schatauer, 2003.

53. G. M. Stein, et al. "Stimulation of the maturation of dendritic cells in vitro by a fermented mistletoe extract," *Anticancer Res.*, Nov.–Dec. 2002; 22(6C):4215–19. PMID: 12553059.

54. G. M. Stein, et al. "Activation of dendritic cells by an aqueous mistletoe extract and mistletoe lectin-3 in vitro," *Anticancer Res.* Jan.– Feb. 2002;22(1A):267–74. PMID: 12017301.

55. C. N. Baxevanis, et al. "Mistletoe lectin I-induced effects on human cytotoxic lymphocytes. I. Synergism with IL-2 in the induction of enhanced LAK cytotoxicity," *Immunopharmacol. Immunotoxicol.*, Aug. 1998; 20(3):355–72. doi: 10.3109/08923979809034819. PMID: 9736441.

56. J. E. Talmadge, et al. "Role of NK cells in tumour growth and metastasis in beige mice," *Nature*, Apr. 1980 17;284(5757):622–24. doi: 10.1038 /284622a0. PMID: 7366733.

57. E. Gorelik, et al. "Role of NK cells in the control of metastatic spread and growth of tumor cells in mice," *Int. J. Cancer*, Jul. 1982 15;30(1):107–12. doi: 10.1002/ijc.2910300118. PMID: 7118294.

58. C. Di Vito, et al. "NK cells to cure cancer," *Semin. Immunol.*, Feb. 2019;41:101272. doi: 10.1016/j.smim.2019.03.004. Epub 2019 May 10. PMID: 31085114.

59. S. Fischer, et al. "Oligoclonal in vitro response of CD4 T cells to vesicles of mistletoe extracts in mistletoe-treated cancer patients," *Cancer Immunol. Immunother.*, May 1997;44(3):150–56. doi: 10.1007/s002620050367. PMID: 9191874.

60. G. Nikolai, et al. "Effect of a mistletoe extract (Iscador QuFrF) on viability and migratory behavior of human peripheral CD4+ and CD8+ T lymphocytes in three-dimensional collagen lattices," *In Vitro Cell Dev. Biol. Anim.*, Oct. 1997;33(9):710–16. doi: 10.1007/s11626-997-0129-8. PMID: 9358287.

61. U. Hobohm. "Fever therapy revisited," *Br. J. Cancer*, 2005;92(3):421–25. doi:10.1038/sj.bjc.6602386.

62. P. Hegde, et al. "Viscum album exerts anti-inflammatory effect by selectively inhibiting cytokine-induced expression of cyclooxygenase-2," *PLoS One*, 2011;6(10):e26312. doi: 10.1371/journal.pone.0026312. Epub 2011 Oct 18. PMID: 22028854; PMCID: PMC3196571.

63. W. S. Chen, et al. "Tumor invasiveness and liver metastasis of colon cancer cells correlated with cyclooxygenase-2 (COX-2) expression and inhibited by a COX-2-selective inhibitor, etodolac," *Int. J. Cancer*, Mar. 2001 15;91(6):894-9. doi: 10.1002/1097-0215(200102)9999:9999<894 ::aid-ijc1146>3.0.co;2-#. PMID: 11275997.

64. F. Schad, et al. "Overall survival of stage IV non-small cell lung cancer patients treated with Viscum album L. in addition to chemotherapy: A real-world observational multicenter analysis," *PLoS One,* Aug. 2018 27;13(8):e0203058. doi: 10.1371/journal.pone.0203058. PMID: 30148853; PMCID: PMC6110500.

65. T. Ostermann, et al. "A systematic review and meta-analysis on the survival of cancer patients treated with a fermented viscum album L. extract (Iscador): An update of findings," *Complement Med. Res.*, 2020;27(4):260–71. English. doi: 10.1159/000505202. Epub 2020 Jan 10. PMID: 31927541.

66. B. K. Piao, et al. "Impact of complementary mistletoe extract treatment on quality of life in breast, ovarian, and non-small cell lung cancer patients: A prospective randomized controlled clinical trial," *Anticancer Research,* 24 no. 1 Jan.–Feb. 2004:303-9.

67. F. Pelzer, et al. "Complementary treatment with mistletoe extracts during chemotherapy: Safety, neutropenia, fever, and quality of life assessed in a randomized study," *J. Altern. Complement Med.,* 2018;24:954-961. DOI: 10.1089/acm.2018.0159.

68. V. F. Semiglazov, et al. "Quality of life is improved in breast cancer patients by standardised mistletoe extract PS76A2 during chemotherapy and follow-up: A randomised, placebo-controlled, double-blind, multicentre clinical trial," *Anticancer Research* 26 no. 2B (Mar.–Apr., 2006):1519-29.

CHAPTER 3

1. G. Bacci, et al., "Treatment and outcome of recurrent osteosarcoma: Experience at Rizzoli in 235 patients initially treated with neoadjuvant chemotherapy," *Acta. Oncologica,* vol. 44, no. 7, pp. 748–55, 2005.

2. S. S. Bielack, B. et al., "Second and subsequent recurrences of osteosarcoma: presentation, treatment, and outcomes of 249 consecutive cooperative osteosarcoma study group patients," *Journal of Clinical Oncology,* vol. 27, no. 4, pp. 557–65, 2009.

3. A. Briccoli, et al. "High-grade osteosarcoma of the extremities metastatic to the lung: long-term results in 323 patients treated combining surgery and chemotherapy, 1985- 2005," *Surgical Oncology,* vol. 19, no. 4, pp. 193–99, 2010.

4. E. Tirtei, et al., "Survival after second and subsequent recurrences in osteosarcoma: A retrospective multicenter analysis," *Tumori Journal,* vol. 104, no. 3, pp. 202–06, 2018.

5. A. A. Senerchia, et al., "Results of a randomized, prospective clinical trial evaluating metronomic chemotherapy in nonmetastatic patients with high-grade, operable osteosarcomas of the extremities: A report from the Latin American group of osteosarcoma treatment," *Cancer,* vol. 123, no. 6, pp. 1003–10, 2017.

6. R. Kebudi, et al. "Oral etoposide for recurrent/progressive sarcomas of childhood," *Pediatric Blood and Cancer,* vol. 42, no. 4, pp. 320–24, 2004.

7. S. S. Bielack, et al., "Second and subsequent recurrences of osteosarcoma: Presentation, treatment, and outcomes of 249 consecutive cooperative osteosarcoma study group patients," *Journal of Clinical Oncology,* vol. 27, no. 4, pp. 557–65, 2009.

8. G. Bacci, et al., "Treatment and outcome of recurrent osteosarcoma: experience at Rizzoli in 235 patients initially treated with neoadjuvant chemotherapy," *Acta Oncologica,* vol. 44, no. 7, pp. 748–55, 2005.

9. W. B. Coley, "Contribution to the knowledge of sarcoma," *Annals of Surgery,* vol. 14, pp. 199–222, 1891.

10. S. Kleinsimon, et al. "ViscumTT induces apoptosis and alters IAP expression in osteosarcoma in vitro and has synergistic action when combined with different chemotherapeutic drugs," *BMC Complementary and Alternative Medicine*, vol. 17, no. 1, p. 26, 2017.

11. M. op den Winkel, et al. "Prognosis of patients with hepatocellular carcinoma: Validation and ranking of established staging-systems in a large western HCC-cohort," *PLoS One*, 2012;7(10):e45066. doi:10.1371/journal.pone.: 0045066.

12. A. Tang, et al. "Epidemiology of hepatocellular carcinoma: Target population for surveillance and diagnosis," *Abdom. Radiol.* (NY), 2018 Jan;43(1):13–25. doi: 10.1007/s00261-017-1209-1. PMID: 28647765.

13. R. S. Finn, et al. "Atezolizumab plus Bevacizumab in unresectable hepatocellular carcinoma," *N. Engl. J. Med.*, 2020;382:1894-905. DOI: 10.1056/NEJMoa1915745.

14. L. Rimassa and A. Santoro. "Sorafenib therapy in advanced hepatocellular carcinoma: The SHARP trial," *Expert Review of Anticancer Therapy*, vol. 9,6 (2009): 739–45. doi:10.1586/era.09.41.

15. M. Kudo. "Targeted and immune therapies for hepatocellular carcinoma: Predictions for 2019 and beyond," *World J. Gastroenterology*, vol. 25,7 (2019): 789–807. doi:10.3748/wjg.v25.i7.789.

16. G. da Motta, et al. "Hepatocellular carcinoma: Review of targeted and immune rherapies," *J. Gastrointestinal Cancer*, vol. 49,3 (2018): 227–36. doi:10.1007/s12029-018-0121-4.

17. M. Pinter and M. Peck-Radosavljevic. "Review article: Systemic treatment of hepatocellular carcinoma," *Alimentary Pharmacology and Therapeutics*, vol. 48,6 (2018): 598–609. doi:10.1111/apt.14913.

18. R. S. Finn, et al. "Pembrolizumab as second-line therapy in patients with advanced hepatocellular carcinoma in keynote-240: A randomized, double-blind, phase III trial," *J. Clinical Oncology*, vol. 38,3 (2020): 193–202. doi:10.1200/JCO.19.01307.

19. T. Yau, et al, "LBA38_PR – CheckMate 459: A randomized, multi-center phase III study of nivolumab (NIVO) vs sorafenib (SOR) as first-line (1L) treatment in patients (pts) with advanced hepatocellular carcinoma (aHCC)," *Annals of Oncology*, vol. 30, supp. 5, Oct. 2019, 874–75.

20. A. Villanueva. "Hepatocellular carcinoma," *N. Engl. J. Med.*, Apr. 2019, 11;380(15):1450-1462. doi: 10.1056/NEJMra1713263. PMID: 30970190.

21. G. Falkson and W. Burger. "A phase II trial of vindesine in hepatocellular cancer," *Oncology*, Jan.–Feb. 1995;52(1):86-7. doi: 10.1159/000227434. PMID: 7800350.

22. S. Okada, et al. "A phase 2 study of cisplatin in patients with hepatocellular carcinoma," *Oncology*. 1993;50(1):22-6. doi: 10.1159/000227142. PMID: 7678453.

23. R. Wierzbicki, et al. "Phase II trial of chronic daily VP-16 administration in unresectable hepatocellular carcinoma (HCC)," *Ann. Oncol.*, 1994 May;5(5):466–7. doi: 10.1093/oxfordjournals.annonc.a058882. PMID: 8075054.

24. T. Yoshida, et al. "Phase II trial of mitoxantrone in patients with hepatocellular carcinoma," *Eur. J. Cancer Clin. Oncol.*, Dec.

1988;24(12):1897–98. doi: 10.1016/0277-5379(88)90104-6. PMID: 2851445.

25. R. Lee, et al. "Mistletoe extract viscum fraxini-2 for treatment of advanced hepatocellular carcinoma: A case series," *Case Rep. Oncol.,* 2021;14:224-231. doi: 10.1159/000511566.

26. P. Yang P, et al. "Clinical application of a combination therapy of lentinan, multi-electrode RFA and TACE in HCC ," *Advances in Therapy.* 25 (8): 787–94. (Aug. 2008). doi:10.1007/s12325-008-0079-x. PMID 18670743. S2CID 33140754.

27. H. Nimura, et al. "S-1 combined with lentinan in patients with unresectable or recurrent gastric cancer," *Gan. to Kagaku Ryoho* (in Japanese), (Jun. 2006). 33 (1): 106–9. PMID 16897983.

28. H. Nakano, et al. "A multi-institutional prospective study of lentinan in advanced gastric cancer patients with unresectable and recurrent diseases: Effect on prolongation of survival and improvement of quality of life Kanagawa Lentinan Research Group," *Hepatogastroenterology.* (1999). 46 (28): 2662–8. PMID 10522061.

29. K. Oba, et al. "Individual patient based meta-analysis of lentinan for unresectable/recurrent gastric cancer," *Anticancer Research* 29 (7): 2739–45. (July 2009). PMID 19596954.

30. S. Hazama, et al. "Efficacy of orally administered superfine dispersed lentinan (β-1,3-glucan) for the treatment of advanced colorectal cancer," *Anticancer Research* 29 (7): 2611–2617. (July 2009). PMID 19596936.

31. H. Kataoka, et al. "Lentinan with S-1 and paclitaxel for gastric cancer chemotherapy improve patient quality of life," *Hepatogastroenterology* 56 (90): 547–50. (2009). PMID 19579640.

32. N. Isoda, et al. "Clinical efficacy of superfine dispersed lentinan (β-1,3-glucan) in patients with hepatocellular carcinoma," *Hepatogastroenterology* 56 (90): (2009). 437–41. PMID 19579616.

33. K. Shimizu, et al. "Efficacy of oral administered superfine dispersed lentinan for advanced pancreatic cancer," *Hepatogastroenterology* 56 (89): 240–44. (2009). PMID 19453066.

34. Y. Zhang, et al. "Lentinan as an immunotherapeutic for treating lung cancer: A review of 12 years clinical studies in China," *J. Cancer Res. Clin. Oncol.,* 2018 Nov;144(11):2177–86. doi: 10.1007/s00432-018-2718-1; epub 2018 Jul 24. PMID: 30043277.

35. Portions of this study summary originally appeared at www.mistletoe -therapy.org (used with permission).

36. Some of these conclusions originally appeared at www.mistletoe-therapy .org (used with permission).

37. F. Pelzer, et al. "Complementary treatment with mistletoe extracts during chemotherapy: Safety, neutropenia, fever, and quality of life assessed in a randomized study," *J. Altern. Complement Med.,* 2018;24:954-961. DOI: 10.1089/acm.2018.0159.

38. V. Bocci. "Mistletoe (Viscum album) lectins as cytokine inducers and immunoadjuvant in tumor therapy: A review," *J. Biol. Reg. Homeos. Agents,* 7: 1-6, 1993.

39. U. Mengs, et al. "Mistletoe extracts standardized to mistletoe lectins in oncology: Review on current status of preclinical research," *Anticancer Res.*, 22: 1399-1408, 2002.

40. H. Stauder and E. D. Kreuser. "Mistletoe extracts standardised in terms of mistletoe lectins (MLI) in oncology: Current state of clinical research," *Onkologie* 25: 374–80, 2002.

41. D. F. Cella, et al. "The functional assessment of cancer therapy (FACT) scale: Development and validation of the general measure," *J. Clin. Oncol.*, 11: 570–79, 1993.

42. O. Krauss and R. Schwarz. "FACT—Functional assessment of cancer therapy," in J. Schumacher, et al. (eds.). *Diagnostische Verfahren zu Lebensqualität und Wohlbefinden*, Göttingen: Hogrefe-Verlag, 2003, pp. 97–101.

43. P. C. O'Brien. "Procedures for comparing samples with multiple endpoints," *Biometrics*, 40: 1079–87, 1984.

44. A. Coate, et al. "On the receiving end—III: Measurement of quality of life during cancer chemotherapy," *Ann. Oncol.*, 1: 213–17, 1990.

45. M. Pandey, et al. "Quality of life in patients with early and advanced carcinoma of the breast," *Eur. J. Surg. Oncol.*, 26: 20-24, 2000.

46. C. Hürny, et al. "Impact of adjuvant therapy on quality of life in women with node-positive operable breast cancer: International Breast Cancer Study Group," *Lancet*, 347: 1279–84, 1996.

47. Ibid.

48. C. Hürny, et al. "Quality of life assessment in the International Breast Cancer Study Group: Past, present, and future: Recent results," *Cancer Res.*, 152: 390–95, 1998.

49. M. Babjuk, et al. "EAU Guidelines on non-muscle-invasive urothelial carcinoma of the bladder: Update 2013," *Eur. Urol.*, 2013; 64: 639.

50. R. Sylvester, et al. "A single immediate postoperative instillation of chemotherapy decreases the risk of recurrence in patients with stage TaT1 bladder cancer: A meta-analysis of published results of randomized clinical trials," *J. Urol.*, 2004; 171: 2186.

51. R. Sylvester, et al. "High-grade Ta urothelial carcinoma and carcinoma in situ of the bladder," *Urology*, 2005; 66: 90.

52. R. L. Deresiewicz, et al. "Fatal disseminated mycobacterial infection following intravesical BCG," *J. Urol.*, 1990; 144: 1331.

53. D. L. Lamm, et al. "Incidence and treatment of complications of bacillus Calmette-Guerin intravesical therapy in superficial bladder cancer," *J. Urol.*, 1992; 147: 596.

54. M. Babjuk, et al. *Guidelines on non-muscle invasive bladder cancer (TaT1 and CIS)*, Arnhem, The Netherlands: European Association of Urology, 2013.

55. Per M. Debus, updates on EAU Guidelines may be found here: M. Babjuk, et al. "European Association of Urology guidelines on non-muscle-invasive bladder cancer (TaT1 and carcinoma in situ), 2019 update," *Eur. Urol.*, Nov. 2019;76(5):639-657. doi: 10.1016/j.eururo.2019.08.016. Epub Aug. 20, 2019. PMID: 31443960.

56. Assertions in this paragraph are based on authors' awareness of more recent studies (includes updates beyond the scope of what Tröger et. al. 2013).

57. A. Lambert, et al. "An update on treatment options for pancreatic adenocarcinoma," *Ther. Adv. Med. Oncol.*, 2019, vol. 2: 1–43. DOI: 10.1177/1758835919875568.

58. M. Rostock, et al. "Anticancer activity of a lectin-rich mistletoe extract injected intratumorally into human pancreatic cancer xenografts," *Anticancer Research*, 2005;25(3B): 1969-75.

59. H. Matthes, et al. "Intratumorale applikation von Viscum album L. (Mistelgesamtextrakt; Helixor M) in der therapie des inoperablen pankreaskarzinom" [Intratumoral application of Viscum album L. (whole mistletoe extract; Helixor M) as therapy for inoperable pancreatic cancer], *Z. Gastroenterology,* 2007;45, http://dx.doi.org/10.1055/s-2007-988162.

60. Much of this study summary originally appeared at www.mistletoe-therapy.org (used with permission).

61. K. Wode, et al. "Efficacy of mistletoe extract as a complement to standard treatment in advanced pancreatic cancer: Study protocol for a multicentre, parallel group, double-blind, randomised, placebo-controlled clinical trial (MISTRAL)," *Trials,* 21, 783 (2020). https://doi.org/10.1186/s13063-020-04581-y.

62. T. Nguyen, et al. "Cost and survival analysis before and after implementation of Dana-Farber clinical pathways for patients with stage IV non-small-cell. lung cancer," J. Oncol. Pract., 2017; 13:e346±e352. https://doi.org/10.1200/JOP.2017.021741 PMID: 28260402.

63. Administration USFD. Pembrolizumab (KEYTRUDA) Checkpoint Inhibitor. 2016. Available from: https://www.fda.gov/drugs/informationondrugs/approveddrugs/ucm526430.htm.

64. Administration USFD. FDA expands approved use of Opdivo in advanced lung cancer. 2015. Available from: https://www.fda.gov/newsevents/newsroom/pressannouncements/ucm466413.htm.

65. N. A. Rizvi, et al. "Nivolumab in combination with platinum-based doublet chemotherapy for first-line treatment of advanced non-small-cell lung cancer," *J. Clin. Oncol.*, 2016; 34:2969–79. https://doi.org/10.1200/JCO.2016.66.9861 PMID: 27354481.

66. T. Ostermann, et al. "A systematic review and meta-analysis on the survival of cancer patients treated with a fermented viscum album L. extract (Iscador): An update of findings," *Complement. Med. Res.*, 2020;27(4):260–71. English. doi: 10.1159/000505202. Epub 2020 Jan 10. PMID: 31927541.

67. Portions of this study summary originally appeared at www.mistletoe-therapy.org (used with permission).

68. R. Willemze, et al. "WHO-EORTC classification for cutaneous lymphomas," *Blood*, 2005 May 15;105(10):3768-85.

69. P. T. Bradford, et al. "Cutaneous lymphoma incidence patterns in the United States: A population-based study of 3,884 cases." *Blood*, 2009 May 21;113(21):5064-73.

70. D. N. Slater. "The new world health organization–European organiza-
     tion for research and treatment of cancer classification for cutaneous
     lymphomas: A practical marriage of two giants," *Br. J. Dermatol.*, Nov.
     2005;153(5):874–80.

71. X. F. Zhao, et al. "Pathogenesis of early leukemia and lymphoma," *Can-
     cer Biomark*, 2011; 9(1-6):341–74.

72. C. M. Magro, et al. "Cutaneous immunocytoma: A clinical, histologic,
     and phenotypic study of 11 cases," *App. Immunohistochem. Mol. Mor-
     phol.*, Sept. 2004;12(3):216–24.

73. J. H. Cho-Vega, et al. "Primary cutaneous marginal zone B-cell lym-
     phoma," *Am. J. Clin. Pathol.*, June 2006;125 Suppl:S38–49.

74. H. Takino, et al. "Primary cutaneous marginal zone B-cell lymphoma:
     A molecular and clinicopathological study of cases from Asia, Germany,
     and the United States," *Mod. Pathol.*, Dec. 2008;21(12):1517–26.

75. R. N. Hoover. "Lymphoma risks in populations with altered immunity: A
     search for mechanism," *Cancer Res.*, Oct. 1992 1;52(19 Suppl):5477s–8s.

76. A. Cozzio, et al. "Intra-lesional low-dose interferon alpha2a therapy for
     primary cutaneous marginal zone B-cell lymphoma," *Leuk. Lymphoma*,
     May 2006;47(5):865–69.

77. R. Dummer, et al. "Phase 2 clinical trial of intratumoral application of
     TG1042 (adenovirus-interferon-gamma) in patients with advanced cuta-
     neous T-cell lymphomas and multilesional cutaneous B-cell lymphomas,"
     Mol. Ther., June 2010;18(6):1244–47.

78. C. Yadav, et al. "Serum lactate dehydrogenase in non-Hodgkin's lym-
     phoma: A prognostic indicator," *Indian J. of Clinical Biochemistry*,
     vol. 31,2 (2016): 240–42. doi:10.1007/s12291-015-0511-3.

CHAPTER 4

1. A. Büssing, et al. "Differences in the apoptosis-inducing properties of Vis-
    cum album L. extracts," *Anti-Cancer Drugs*, Apr. 1997, vol. 8, p. S9-S14.

2. *Vademecum of Anthroposophic Medicines*. Association of Anthropo-
    sophic Medicine in Germany (GAAD), 2019, chap. 5.4.

3. According to data gathered by The Plant List Project: http://www
    .theplantlist.org/browse/A/Santalaceae/Viscum/. Accessed Apr. 24, 2021.

4. C. W. Barney, et al, "Hosts of Viscum album," *Forest Pathology*, June
    2007; 28(3):187–208.

5. *Vademecum of Anthroposophic Medicines*. Association of Anthropo-
    sophic Medicine in Germany (GAAD); 2019, chap. 5.7.1.

6. J. Wilkens and G. Böhm. *Mistletoe Therapy for Cancer* (Edinburgh:
    Floris Books, 2018), p. 53.

7. Per manufacturer data.

8. A. P. Simses-Wust, et al., "Sensitivity of primary cultures of breast cancer
    cells to different Iscador preparations," *Der Merkurstab*, 2011, 64(6);618.

9. T. Zuzak, et al. "Pediatric meduloblastoma cells are susceptible to viscum
    album (mistletoe) preparations," *Anticancer Research,* 2006, 26(5A).
    3485–92.

10. K. Mulsow, et al. "Quantifizierung des Mistellektins I aus Mistelextrakt-Fertigarzneimitteln [Quantification of mistletoe lectin I from mistletoe extract finished medicinal products]," *ZPT—Zeitschrift für Phytotherapie*, 2017; 38:148-151.

11. Original data set included a Helixor Pini batch with a higher reading of 2,100 ng/mL and 2,200 ng/mL of A-Chain and A-B Chain mistletoe lectins, respectively.

12. M. Girke, *Internal Medicine: Foundations and therapeutic concepts of Anthroposophic Medicine* (Berlin: Salumed-Verlag, 2016), chap. 14.3.5.6.

13. AUTHOR NOTE: This section is composed of general anthroposophic recommendations accumulated through decades of clinical practice, as well as from *Vademecum of Anthroposophic Medicines* (Association of Anthroposophic Medicine in Germany [GAAD], 2019), pp. 42–110. J. Wilkens and G. Böhm, *Mistletoe Therapy for Cancer*, Op. cit.

14. *Vademecum of Anthroposophic Medicines*. Association of Anthroposophic Medicine in Germany (GAAD), 2019, (chap. 5).

15. Ibid., chap. 9.

16. M. Girke, *Internal Medicine: Foundations and therapeutic concepts of Anthroposophic Medicine* (Berlin: Salumed-Verlag, 2016), chap. 14.3.5.6.

17. *Vademecum of Anthroposophic Medicines* (Association of Anthroposophic Medicine in Germany [GAAD], 2019), chap. 5.

18. R. Steiner, *Introducing Anthroposophical Medicine* (CW 312). Op. cit.

19. J. U. Umeafoekwe, et al. "Pulmonary effects of grain-dust observed in feedmill workers," Proceedings of the 6th National Conference of the Society for Occupational Safety and Environmental Health (SOSEH). Nov. 3–6, 2010. Princess Alexandra Auditorium, University of Nigeria, Nsukka, Enugu State, Nigeria.

20. J. Wilkens and G. Böhm, *Mistletoe Therapy for Cancer*, Op. cit., p. 53.

21. T. M. Dudenkov, et al. "SLCO1B1 polymorphisms and plasma estrone conjugates in postmenopausal women with ER+ breast cancer: Genome-wide association studies of the estrone pathway," *Breast Cancer Research and Treatment*, vol. 164,1 (2017): 189–99. doi:10.1007/s10549-017-4243-3.

22. C. A. Thomson, et al. "Chemopreventive properties of 3,3'-diindolylmethane in breast cancer: Evidence from experimental and human studies," *Nutrition Reviews*, vol. 74,7 (2016): 432–43. doi:10.1093/nutrit/nuw010.

23. J. Wilkens and G. Böhm. *Mistletoe Therapy for Cancer*, Op. cit., p. 75.

CHAPTER 5

1. N. Winters and J. H. Higgins Kelley. *The Metabolic Approach to Cancer Care: Integrating Deep Nutrition, the Ketogenic Diet, and Nontoxic Bioindividualized Therapies*, Hartford, VT: Chelsea Green, 2017.

2. H. A. Coller. "Is cancer a metabolic disease?" *The American Journal of Pathology*, vol. 184,1 (2014): 4-17. doi:10.1016/j.ajpath.2013.07.035.

3. G. P. Dunn, et al. "The immunobiology of cancer immunosurveillance and immunoediting," *Immunity*, vol. 21, no. 2, 2004, pp. 137–48.

4. F. M. Burnet. "The concept of immunological surveillance," *Prog. Exp. Tumor Res.*, 1970;13:1–27.

5. D. D. Chaplin. "Overview of the immune response," *Journal of Allergy and Clinical Immunology*, vol. 125,2 Suppl 2 (2010): S3–23. doi:10.1016/j .jaci.2009.12.980.

6. H. Gonzalez, et al. "Roles of the immune system in cancer: From tumor initiation to metastatic progression," *Genes and Development*, vol. 32,19–20 (2018): 1267-1284. doi:10.1101/gad.314617.118.

7. A. C. West, et al. "An intact immune system is required for the anticancer activities of histone deacetylase inhibitors," *Cancer Research*, Dec. 15, 2013; 73(24):7265-7276. doi:10.1158/0008-5472.CAN-13-0890.

8. A. A. Shafi and K. E. Knudsen, "Cancer and the circadian clock," *Cancer Res.*, Aug. 1 2019 79 (15) 3806–14. doi:10.1158/0008-5472.CAN-19-0566.

9. Salavaty, Abbas. "Carcinogenic effects of circadian disruption: an epigenetic viewpoint," *Chinese Journal of Cancer*, vol. 34,9 375–83. 8 Aug. 2015, doi:10.1186/s40880-015-0043-5.

10. G. Sulli, et al. "Interplay between circadian clock and cancer: New frontiers for cancer treatment." *Trends in Cancer*, vol. 5,8 (2019): 475–94. doi:10.1016/j.trecan.2019.07.002.

11. J. K. Kiecolt-Glaser and R. Glaser. "Psychoneuroimmunology and health consequences: Data and shared mechanisms," *Psychosomatic Medicine*, vol. 57,3 (1995): 269–74. doi:10.1097/00006842-199505000-00008.

12. R. H. Bonneau, et al. "Twenty years of psychoneuroimmunology and viral infections in brain, behavior, and immunity," *Brain, Behavior, and Immunity*, vol. 21,3 (2007): 273–80. doi:10.1016/j.bbi.2006.10.004.

13. E. Walter and M. Scott. "The life and work of Rudolf Virchow 1821– 1902: Cell theory, thrombosis and the sausage duel," *Journal of the Intensive Care Society*, vol. 18,3 (2017): 234–35. doi:10.1177 /1751143716663967.

14. M. J. Bissell. "Architecture is the message: The role of extracellular matrix and 3-d structure in tissue-specific gene expression and breast cancer," *The Pezcoller Foundation Journal: News from the Pezcoller Foundation World*, vol. 16,29 (2007): 2–17.

15. C. M. Nelson, et al. "Of extracellular matrix, scaffolds, and signaling: tissue architecture regulates development, homeostasis, and cancer," *Annual Review of Cell and Developmental Biology*, vol. 22 (2006): 287–309. doi:10.1146/annurev.cellbio.22.010305.104315.

16. M. Song, et al. "Neutrophil-to-lymphocyte ratio and mortality in the United States general population," *Scientific Reports*, vol. 11,1 464. 11 Jan. 2021, doi:10.1038/s41598-020-79431-7.

17. M. A. Cupp, et al. "Neutrophil to lymphocyte ratio and cancer prognosis: An umbrella review of systematic reviews and meta-analyses of observational studies," *BMC Medicine*, vol. 18,1 360. 20 Nov. 2020, doi:10.1186 /s12916-020-01817-1.

18. Y. Pascual-González, et al. "Defining the role of neutrophil-to-lymphocyte ratio in COPD: A systematic literature review." *International Journal of Chronic Obstructive Pulmonary Disease*, vol. 13 3651–62. Nov. 5, 2018, doi:10.2147/COPD.S178068.

19. M. A. Cupp, et al. "Neutrophil to lymphocyte ratio and cancer prognosis: An umbrella review of systematic reviews and meta-analyses of observational studies," *BMC Medicine*, 18, 360 (2020). https://doi.org/10.1186 /s12916-020-01817-1.

20. J. Fest, et al. "The neutrophil-to-lymphocyte ratio is associated with mortality in the general population: The Rotterdam study." *European Journal of Epidemiology*, vol. 34,5 (2019): 463–70. doi:10.1007/s10654 -018-0472-y.

21. M. U. Mushtaq, et al. "Prognostic significance of neutrophil-to-lymphocyte ratio and lymphocyte-to-monocyte ratio in myelodysplastic syndromes," *Journal of Clinical Oncology*, 2016 34:15; suppl, 7062.

22. S. Mallappa, et al. "Preoperative neutrophil to lymphocyte ratio >5 is a prognostic factor for recurrent colorectal cancer." *Colorectal Disease: The Official Journal of the Association of Coloproctology of Great Britain and Ireland*, vol. 15,3 (2013): 323–28. doi:10.1111/codi.12008.

23. G. Moon, et al. "Prediction of late recurrence in patients with breast cancer: Elevated neutrophil to lymphocyte ratio (NLR) at 5 years after diagnosis and late recurrence," *Breast Cancer* (Tokyo), vol. 27,1 (2020): 54–61. doi:10.1007/s12282-019-00994-z.

24. M. Gago-Dominguez, et al. "Neutrophil to lymphocyte ratio and breast cancer risk: Analysis by subtype and potential interactions," *Scientific Reports*, 10, 13203 (2020). https://doi.org/10.1038/s41598-020-70077-z.

25. M. U. Mushtaq, et al. "Prognostic significance of neutrophil-to-lymphocyte ratio and lymphocyte-to-monocyte ratio in myelodysplastic syndromes," *Journal of Clinical Oncology*, 2016 34:15; suppl, 7062.

26. G. Leone, et al. "The incidence of secondary leukemias," *Haematologica*, 1999 Oct;84(10):937–45. PMID: 10509043.

27. B. Zhang, et al. "How breast cancer chemotherapy increases the risk of leukemia: Thoughts about a case of diffuse large B-cell lymphoma and leukemia after breast cancer chemotherapy," *Cancer Biology and Therapy*, vol. 17,2 (2016): 125–28. doi:10.1080/15384047.2016.1139233.

28. AUTHOR NOTE: This effect on neutrophil and leukocyte numbers is primarily a clinically observed effect, but a fine discussion of this may also be seen here: C. Saha. "Unravelling the therapeutic intervention of inflammation and cancer by Viscum album: Understanding its anti-inflammatory and immunostimulatory properties," *Biotechnology*, Université de Technologie de Compiègne, 2015. English. NNT: 2015COMP2210. HAL ID tel-01214953.

29. AUTHOR NOTE: IL-6 is a marker of general inflammation that does not negate the use of VAE. In fact, VAE lowers that value. It is IL-8, however, that may negate our ability to use VAE, until we get IL-8 under control.

30. M. F. Sanmamed, et al. "Serum Interleukin-8 reflects tumor burden and treatment response across malignancies of multiple tissue origins," *Clin. Cancer Res.*, 20(22) Nov. 15, 2014, 5697–707.

31. R. Huber, et al. "Mistletoe treatment induces GM-CSF- and IL-5 production by PBMC and increases blood granulocyte- and eosinophil counts: A placebo-controlled randomized study in healthy subjects," *European Journal of Medical Research*, vol. 10,10 (2005): 411–18.

32. J. L. Sylman, et al. "A temporal examination of platelet counts as a predictor of prognosis in lung, prostate, and colon cancer patients." *Scientific Reports*, vol. 8,1 6564. Apr. 26, 2018, doi:10.1038/s41598-018 -25019-1.

33. B. Norbaini et al. "Cancer-associated thrombosis: An overview of mechanisms, risk factors, and treatment." *Cancers*, vol. 10,10 380. 11 Oct. 2018, doi:10.3390/cancers10100380.

34. S. Sen, et al. "Development of a prognostic scoring system for patients with advanced cancer enrolled in immune checkpoint inhibitor phase 1 clinical trials." *British Journal of Cancer*, vol. 118,6 (2018): 763-769. doi:10.1038/bjc.2017.480.

35. S. Shrotriya, et al. "C-reactive protein is an important biomarker for prognosis tumor recurrence and treatment response in adult solid tumors: A systematic review." *PloS One*, vol. 10,12 e0143080. Dec. 2015. doi:10.1371/journal.pone.0143080.

36. A. Katano, et al. "The impact of elevated C-reactive protein level on the prognosis for oro-hypopharynx cancer patients treated with radiotherapy," *Sci. Rep.*, 7, 17805 (2017). https://doi.org/10.1038/s41598-017 -18233-w.

37. J. J. Hu, et al. "Association between inflammatory biomarker c-reactive protein and radiotherapy-induced early adverse skin reactions in a multiracial/ethnic breast cancer population," *Journal of Clinical Oncology*, 36, no. 24 (Aug. 20, 2018) 2473-2482. DOI: 10.1200/JCO.2017.77.1790.

38. F. A. Mahmoud and N. I. Rivera. The role of C-reactive protein as a prognostic indicator in advanced cancer. *Current Oncology Report*, 4, 250–255 (2002). https://doi.org/10.1007/s11912-002-0023-1.

39. AUTHOR NOTE: CRP has also been examined as a diagnostic tool for cancer risk. For instance: J. Watson, et al. "Predictive value of inflammatory markers for cancer diagnosis in primary care: A prospective cohort study using electronic health records," *British Journal of Cancer*, 120 (2019), 1045–51. https://doi.org/10.1038/s41416-019-0458-x.

40. C. Yadav, et al. "Serum lactate dehydrogenase in non-Hodgkin's lymphoma: A prognostic indicator," *Indian Journal of Clinical Biochemistry*, vol. 31,2 (2016), 240-2. doi:10.1007/s12291-015-0511-3.

41. A. Farhana and S. L. Lappin. *Biochemistry, Lactate Dehydrogenase* (updated 2020 May 17); in StatPearls (online). Treasure Island, FL: StatPearls, 2021. https://www.ncbi.nlm.nih.gov/books/NBK557536/.

42. D. Mishra and D. Banerjee. "Lactate dehydrogenases as metabolic links between tumor and stroma in the tumor microenvironment," *Cancers*, vol. 11,6 750. 29 May. 2019, doi:10.3390/cancers11060750.

43. Ibid.

44. T. N. Seyfried, et al. "Cancer as a metabolic disease: Implications for novel therapeutics," *Carcinogenesis*, vol. 35,3 (2014): 515–27. doi:10.1093 /carcin/bgt480.

45. S. Shrotriya, et al. "C-reactive protein is an important biomarker for prognosis tumor recurrence and treatment response in adult solid tumors: A systematic review," *PloS One*, vol. 10,12 e0143080. 30 Dec. 2015, doi:10.1371/journal.pone.0143080.

46. AUTHOR NOTE: Regarding monitoring vitamin D levels, I routinely screen my patients' 1,25 and 25-OH levels prior to vitamin D supplementation and then watch their serum calcium levels monthly during supplementation to make sure there are no issues with hypercalcemia. I have yet to see D3 toxicity occur. If I see serum calcium rise, then we simply stop the D3 supplementation for a few days (but continue taking K2), then resume D3 at much lower doses. That's all that's needed.

47. A. J. van Ballegooijen, et al. "The Synergistic Interplay between vitamins D and K for bone and cardiovascular health: A narrative review," *International Journal of Endocrinology*, vol. 2017 (2017): 7454376. doi:10.1155/2017/7454376.

48. S. Goddek. "Vitamin D3 and K2 and their potential contribution to reducing the covid-19 mortality rate," *International Journal of Infectious Diseases: Official Publication of the International Society for Infectious Diseases*, vol. 99 (2020): 286-290. doi:10.1016/j.ijid.2020.07.080.

49. N. R. Parva, et al. "Prevalence of vitamin D deficiency and associated risk factors in the US population (2011–2012)," *Cureus*, vol. 10,6 e2741. 5 Jun. 2018, doi:10.7759/cureus.2741.

50. J. Chan, et al. "Serum 25-hydroxyvitamin D status of vegetarians, partial vegetarians, and nonvegetarians: The Adventist health study-2," *The American Journal of Clinical Nutrition*, vol. 89,5 (2009): 1686S-1692S. doi:10.3945/ajcn.2009.26736X.

51. L. Vranić, et al. "Vitamin D deficiency: Consequence or cause of obesity?" *Medicina* (Kaunas, Lithuania), vol. 55,9 541. 28 Aug. 2019, doi:10.3390/medicina55090541.

52. U. Gröber and K. Kisters. "Influence of drugs on vitamin D and calcium metabolism," *Dermato-endocrinology*, vol. 4,2 (2012): 158-66. doi:10.4161/derm.20731.

53. AUTHOR NOTE: 42 percent is the actual number noted in studies. But that is based on "average" findings, showing that 42 percent of the population has D3 levels *under 30*. The vitamin D deficiency percentage is closer to 70 percent when we look at those with levels under 50.

54. N. R. Parva, et al. "Prevalence of vitamin D deficiency and associated risk factors in the US population (2011–2012)," *Cureus*, vol. 10,6 e2741. 5 Jun. 2018, doi:10.7759/cureus.2741.

55. B. Loef, et al. "Immunological effects of shift work in healthcare workers," *Scientific Reports*, vol. 9,1 18220. 3 Dec. 2019, doi:10.1038/s41598-019-54816-5.

56. T. W. Kim et al. "The impact of sleep and circadian disturbance on hormones and metabolism," *Int. Journal of Endocrinology*, 2015;2015:591729. doi: 10.1155/2015/591729. Epub 2015 Mar 11. PMID: 25861266; PMCID: PMC4377487.

57. S. P. Megdal, et al. "Night work and breast cancer risk: A systematic review and meta-analysis," *European Journal of Cancer* (Oxford, UK: 1990), vol. 41,13 (2005): 2023-32. doi:10.1016/j.ejca.2005.05.010.

58. X. Yuan, et al. "Night shift work increases the risks of multiple primary cancers in women: A systematic review and meta-analysis of 61 articles," *Cancer Epidemiol Biomarkers Prev.*, 2018 Jan; 27(1):25-40.

59. E. Pukkala, et al. "Incidence of cancer among Finnish airline cabin attendants, 1967–92." *BMJ* (Clinical Research ed.), vol. 311,7006 (1995): 649–52. doi:10.1136/bmj.311.7006.649.

60. Oct. 2, 2017 Nobel Prize press release: https://www.nobelprize.org/prizes /medicine/2017/press-release/. Accessed Apr. 28, 2021.

61. J. C. Dunlap. "Molecular bases for circadian clocks," *Cell*, Jan. 22, 1999; 96(2):271-90. doi: 10.1016/s0092-8674(00)80566-8. PMID: 9988221.

62. D. Bell-Pedersen, et al. "Circadian rhythms from multiple oscillators: Lessons from diverse organisms," *Natural Reviews: Genetics*, Jul. 2005;6(7):544–56. doi: 10.1038/nrg1633. PMID: 15951747; PMCID: PMC2735866.

63. R. Pryor, et al. "The role of the microbiome in drug response," *Annual Review of Pharmacology and Toxicology*, vol. 60 (2020): 417–35. doi:10.1146/annurev-pharmtox-010919-023612.

64. W. Ma, et al. "Gut microbiota shapes the efficiency of cancer therapy," *Frontiers in Microbiology*, vol. 10 1050. Jun. 25, 2019, doi:10.3389/fmicb .2019.01050.

65. AUTHOR NOTE: Low D3 directly impacts hundreds of epigenetic switches, affecting metabolic function, hormonal regulation, and immune response, as shown in I. S. Fetahu, et al. "Vitamin D and the epigenome," *Front Physiol.*, Apr. 2014 29;5:164. doi: 10.3389/fphys.2014.00164. PMID: 24808866; PMCID: PMC4010791.

66. AUTHOR NOTE: Low D3 levels are also associated with depression and dopamine issues in particular, as shown in I. Anjum, et al. "The role of vitamin D in brain health: A mini-literature review," *Cureus*, Jul. 2018 10;10(7):e2960. doi: 10.7759/cureus.2960. PMID: 30214848. PMCID: PMC6132681.

67. B. S. McEwen. "Central effects of stress hormones in health and disease: Understanding the protective and damaging effects of stress and stress mediators," *European Journal of Pharmacology*, vol. 583,2-3 (2008): 174–85. doi:10.1016/j.ejphar.2007.11.071.

68. E. K. Adam, et al. "Diurnal cortisol slopes and mental and physical health outcomes: A systematic review and meta-analysis," *Psychoneuro-endocrinology*, vol. 83 (2017): 25-41. doi:10.1016/j.psyneuen.2017.05.018.

69. L. Fiorentino and S. Ancoli-Israel. "Sleep dysfunction in patients with cancer," *Current Treatment Options in Neurology*, vol. 9,5 (2007): 337–46.

70. A. S. Prasad. "Zinc in human health: Effect of zinc on immune cells," *Mol. Med.*, May–Jun. 2008; 14(5-6): 353–357.

71. E. Prado de Oliveira and R. C. Burini. "High plasma uric acid concentration: Causes and consequences," *Diabetol. Metab. Syndr.*, 4, 12 (2012). https://doi.org/10.1186/1758-5996-4-12.

72. M. Jung, et al. "Iron as a central player and promising target in cancer progression," *International Journal of Molecular Sciences*, vol. 20,2 273. Jan. 11, 2019, doi:10.3390/ijms20020273.

73. D. Galaris, et al. "Iron homeostasis and oxidative stress: An intimate relationship," *Biochimica et Biophysica Acta (BBA): Molecular Cell*

Research, vol. 1866, no. 12, 2019, 118535, ISSN 0167-4889, https://doi
.org/10.1016/j.bbamcr.2019.118535.

74. P. R. Bock, et al. "Targeting inflammation in cancer-related-fatigue:
A rationale for mistletoe therapy as supportive care in colorectal cancer patients," *Inflamm. Allergy Drug Targets,* 2014;13(2):105-11. doi:
10.2174/1871528113666140428103332. PMID: 24766319; PMCID:
PMC4133960.

75. M. Kröz, et al. "Mistletoe: From basic research to clinical outcomes
in cancer and other indications," *Evidence-based Complementary
and Alternative Medicine,* vol. 2014, Article ID 987527, 2 pages, 2014.
https://doi.org/10.1155/2014/987527.

76. S. C. Segerstrom, et al. "Psychological stress and the human immune
system: A meta-analytic study of 30 years of inquiry," *Psychological
Bulletin,* vol. 130,4 (2004): 601–30. doi:10.1037/0033-2909.130.4.601.

77. Ibid.

78. S. A. Font and K. Maguire-Jack, "Pathways from childhood abuse and
other adversities to adult health risks: The role of adult socioeconomic
conditions," *Child Abuse and Neglect,* 51, no. 2 (2016): 390–99.

79. L. LeShan, *Cancer as a Turning Point: A Handbook for People with
Cancer, Their Families, and Health Professionals,* New York: Plume,
1994.

80. K. Turner, *Radical Remission: Surviving Cancer Against All Odds,*
San Francisco: HarperOne, 2015.

81. Y. Balhara. "Diabetes and psychiatric disorders," *Indian Journal of
Endocrinology and Metabolism,* vol. 15,4 (2011): 274–83. doi:10.4103
/2230-8210.85579.

82. A. Felman. "How does diabetes affect mood and relationships?" *Medical
News Today* (medically reviewed by D. Weatherspoon, PhD, RN, CRNa)
May 24, 2019; published at https://www.medicalnewstoday.com/articles
/317458. Retrieved Apr. 30, 2021.

83. S. Penckofer, et al. "Vitamin D and depression: Where is all the
sunshine?" *Issues in Mental Health Nursing,* vol. 31,6 (2010): 385–93.
doi:10.3109/01612840903437657.

84. E. Golovina, et al. "GWAS SNPs impact shared regulatory pathways
amongst multimorbid psychiatric disorders and cognitive functioning,"
Frontiers in Psychiatry, Oct. 23 2020 https://doi.org/10.3389/fpsyt.2020
.560751.

85. Lin Chin-Chuen and Tiao-Lai Huang. "Brain-derived neurotrophic factor
and mental disorders," *Biomedical Journal,* vol. 43, no. 2, 2020,
pp. 134–42, ISSN 2319-4170, https://doi.org/10.1016/j.bj.2020.01.001.

86. A. M. Dlugos, et al. "Negative emotionality: Monoamine oxidase B
gene variants modulate personality traits in healthy humans," *Journal
of Neural Transmission* (Vienna, 1996), vol. 116,10 (2009): 1323–34.
doi:10.1007/s00702-009-0281-2.

87. "Genes may make some people more prone to anxiety," *American
Psychological Association,* Public Affairs Monograph (Washington DC,
2008), https://www.apa.org/news/press/releases/2008/08/genes-anxiety.
Retrieved Apr. 30, 2021.

88. B. M. Heiny, et al. (1998). "Correlation of immune cell activities and beta-endorphin release in breast carcinoma patients treated with galactose-specific lectin standardized mistletoe extract," *Anticancer Res.,* 18:583–86.

89. S. de Groot, et al. "Effects of short-term fasting on cancer treatment," *Journal of Experimental and Clinical Cancer Research: CR,* vol. 38,1 209. May. 22, 2019, doi:10.1186/s13046-019-1189-9.

90. S. K. Denduluri, et al. "Insulin-like growth factor (IGF) signaling in tumorigenesis and the development of cancer drug resistance," *Genes and Diseases,* vol. 2, no. 1, 2015, pp. 13–25, ISSN 2352-3042. https://doi.org/10.1016/j.gendis.2014.10.004.

91. Ibid.

92. C. C. Onunogbo, et al. 2013. "Effect of mistletoe (*Viscum album*) extract on the blood glucose, liver enzymes and electrolyte balance in alloxan induced diabetic rats," *American Journal of Biochemistry and Molecular Biology,* 3: 143–50. https://scialert.net/fulltext/?doi=ajbmb.2013.143.150.

93. A. E. Eno, et al. "Stimulation of insulin secretion by Viscum album (mistletoe) leaf extract in streptozotocin-induced diabetic rats," *Afr. Journal Med. Med. Sci,* Jun. 2008;37(2):141–47. PMID: 18939397.

CHAPTER 6

1. R. Steiner, lecture of Oct. 27, 1922 p.m. in *Physiology and Healing: Treatment, Therapy, and Hygiene* (CW 314), Op. cit.

2. M. Protsiv, et al. "Decreasing human body temperature in the United States since the Industrial Revolution," *eLife,* 2020; 9: e49555. Published online Jan 7, 2020.

3. Z. Obermeyer, et al. "Individual differences in normal body temperature: longitudinal big data analysis of patient records," *BMJ (Clinical research ed.),* vol. 359 j5468. Dec. 13, 2017, doi:10.1136/bmj.j5468.

4. D. B. Boivin, et al. "Circadian sex differences in sleep and alertness," *Proceedings of the National Academy of Sciences,* Sep 2016, 201524484. doi: 10.1073/pnas.1524484113.

5. D. B. Boivin, et al. "Diurnal and circadian variation of sleep and alertness in men vs. naturally cycling women," *Proceedings of the National Academy of Sciences of the United States of America,* vol. 113,39 (2016): 10980–5. doi:10.1073/pnas.1524484113.

6. J. E. Sullivan, et al. "Fever and antipyretic use in children," *Pediatrics,* vol. 127,3 (2011): 580–87. doi:10.1542/peds.2010-3852.

7. Ibid.

8. AUTHOR NOTE: Information about these kinds of lemon treatments for fever can be found at https://www.pflege-vademecum.de/anwendungen_bei_fieber.php.

9. H. J. Hamre, et al. "Antibiotic use in children with acute respiratory or ear infections: Prospective observational comparison of anthroposophic and conventional treatment under routine primary care conditions," *Evidence-based Complementary and Alternative Medicine: eCAM,* vol. 2014 (2014): 243801. doi:10.1155/2014/243801.

10. T. von Schoen-Angerer, et al. "Effect of topical rosemary essential oil on Raynaud phenomenon in systemic sclerosis," *Complementary Therapies in Medicine,* vol. 40, Oct. 2018, pp. 191–94.

11. T. Ostermann, et al. "Effects of rhythmic embrocation therapy with solum oil in chronic pain patients: A prospective observational study," *The Clinical Journal of Pain,* vol. 24,3 (2008): 237–43. doi:10.1097/AJP .0b013e3181602143.

12. P. Selg, *Helene von Grunelius und Rudolf Steiners Kurse für junge Mediziner: Eine biographische Studie* [Helene von Grunelius and Rudolf Steiner's course for young doctors: A biographical study], Dornach, Switzerland: Verlag am Goetheanum, 2003.

13. L. E. Williams and J. A Bargh. "Experiencing physical warmth promotes interpersonal warmth." *Science* (New York), vol. 322,5901 (2008): 606-7. OR Oct. 24, 2008: 322(5901):606–07 doi:10.1126/science.1162548.

14. L. K. Curran, et al. "Behaviors associated with fever in children with autism spectrum disorders," *Pediatrics,* vol. 120,6 (2007): e1386-92. doi:10.1542/peds.2007-0360.

CHAPTER 7

1. L. LeShan, *Cancer as a Turning Point: A Handbook for People with Cancer, Their Families, and Health Professionals,* New York: Plume, 1994.

2. M. Girke, *Internal Medicine: Foundations and therapeutic concepts of Anthroposophic Medicine* (Berlin: Salumed-Verlag, 2016), chap. 2; 1.0-1.5.

3. Ibid., chap. 14; 2.3.

4. Ibid., chap. 1.6 – 1.7.

5. Ibid., chap. 2.0-2.2.3.

6. Ibid., chap. 1.

7. M. Moreno-Smith, et al. "Impact of stress on cancer metastasis," *Future Oncology* (London), vol. 6,12 (2010): 1863–81. doi:10.2217/fon.10.142.

8. K. Esposito, et al. "Metabolic syndrome and risk of cancer: A systematic review and meta-analysis," *Diabetes Care,* vol. 35,11 (2012): 2402–11. doi:10.2337/dc12-0336. https://www.ncbi.nlm.nih.gov/pmc/articles /PMC3476894/#:~:text=Findings%20from%20this%20meta%2Danalysis ,by%20accompanying%20obesity%20of%20hyperglycemia.

9. S. P. Megdal, et al. "Night work and breast cancer risk: A systematic review and meta-analysis," *European Journal of Cancer* (Oxford, UK, 1990) vol. 41,13 (2005): 2023–32. doi:10.1016/j.ejca.2005.05.010.

10. E. McNeely, et al. "The self-reported health of U.S. flight attendants compared to the general population," *Environ. Health,* 13, 13 (2014). https: //doi.org/10.1186/1476-069X-13-13.

11. M. Girke, *Internal Medicine,* Op. cit., chap. 14.2 –14.4.

12. C. Tautz: *Kinderkrankheiten als Weg zur Immunkompetenz* [Childhood illnesses as a path toward immune competence] (Berlin: Der Merkurstab, 2002), pp. 24-29.

13. M. Girke. *Internal Medicine,* Op. cit., chap. 14.2.4.4.

14. S. C. Segerstrom and G. E Miller. "Psychological stress and the human immune system: A meta-analytic study of 30 years of inquiry," *Psychological Bulletin*, vol. 130,4 (2004): 601–30. doi:10.1037/0033-2909.130.4.601.

15. M. P. da Silveira, et al. "Physical exercise as a tool to help the immune system against covid-19: An integrative review of the current literature," *Clinical and Experimental Medicine*, vol. 21,1 (2021): 15–28. doi:10.1007/s10238-020-00650-3.

16. J. R. Infante, et al. "Levels of immune cells in transcendental meditation practitioners," *International Journal of Yoga*, vol. 7,2 (2014): 147–51. doi:10.4103/0973-6131.133899.

17. V. J. Felitti, et al. "Relationship of childhood abuse and household dysfunction to many of the leading causes of death in adults. The adverse childhood experiences (ACE) study," *American Journal of Preventive Medicine*, vol. 14,4 (1998): 245–58. doi:10.1016/s0749-3797(98)00017-8.

18. S. A. Font and K. Maguire-Jack, "Pathways from childhood abuse and other adversities to adult health risks: The role of adult socioeconomic conditions," *Child Abuse and Neglect,* 51, no. 2 (2016): 390–99.

19. H. Alcalá, et al. "Gender differences in the association between adverse childhood experiences and cancer," *Women's Health Issues*, 27, no. 6 (2017): 625–31.

20. B. von Laue. *Natur- und Geistesgeschichtliche Aspekte der Tumorentwicklung* [Natural and spiritual developmental aspects of tumor development] (Berlin: Der Merkurstab, 1999). p. 145.

21. R. Steiner, *Physiology and Healing: Treatment, Therapy, and Hygiene,* lect. 1, Dec. 7, 1920. Op. cit.

23. L. LeShan, *Cancer as a Turning Point,* Op cit.

24. X. Yuan, et al. "Night-shift work increases the risks of multiple primary cancers in women: A systematic review and meta-analysis of 61 articles," Op. cit.

25. E. Pukkala, et al. "Incidence of cancer among Finnish airline cabin attendants, 1967–92," Op cit.

26. S. P. Tsai, et al. (Apr. 2004). "Mortality patterns among residents in Louisiana's industrial corridor, USA, 1970–99," *Occup. Environ. Med.,* 61 (4): 295–304.

27. Centers for Disease Control. (2002). Cancer Prevention and Control "Cancer Burden Data Fact Sheets, Louisiana," Atlanta, GA.

28. A. D. Blodgett. "An analysis of pollution and community advocacy in 'Cancer Alley': Setting an example for the environmental justice movement in St James Parish, Louisiana," *Local Environment,* 11(6) (2007), 647–61, DOI: 10.1080/13549830600853700.

29. K. Turner, *Radical Remission: Surviving Cancer against All Odds*, San Francisco: HarperOne, 2015.

30. C. Tautz. *Kinderkrankheiten als Weg zur Immunkompetenz* [Childhood illnesses as a path toward immune competence] (Berlin: Der Merkurstab, 2002), pp. 24–29.

31. M. Orange, "Mistletoe fever with subcutaneously injected mistletoe," *Der Merkurstab*; 5/2017; pp 377–83.

32. D. Furman, et al. "Chronic inflammation in the etiology of disease across the life span," *Nature Medicine,* vol. 25,12 (2019): 1822-1832. doi:10.1038/s41591-019-0675-0.

33. M. Girke. *Internal Medicine,* Op. cit., chap. 5; 1.0-2.3.

34. K. H. Allin, et al. "Elevated C-reactive protein in the diagnosis, prognosis, and cause of cancer," *Critical Reviews in Clinical Laboratory Sciences,* vol. 48,4 (2011): 155-70. doi:10.3109/10408363.2011.599831.

35. AUTHOR NOTE: Such observations have been noticed by a group for rhythmic studies at the Carl Gustav Carus Institute in Niefern-Öschelbronn, Germany. I have also noticed some preliminary animal research here: A. Karakas, et al. "Effects of European mistletoe (*Viscum album* L. subsp. *album*): Extracts on activity rhythms of the Syrian hamsters (*Mesocricetus auratus*)," *Natural Product Research,* 22:11 (2008), 990–1000, DOI: 10.1080/14786410701654776.

36. M. Orange, et al. "Durable regression of primary cutaneous b-cell lymphoma following fever-inducing mistletoe treatment: Two case reports," *Phytomedicine,* 20, nos, 3–4 (Feb. 15, 2013): 324–27.

37. J. Blume, et al. "Immune suppression and immune activation in depression," *Brain, Behavior, and Immunity,* vol. 25,2 (2011): 221–29. doi:10.1016/j.bbi.2010.10.008.

38. E. Reiche et al. "Stress, depression, the immune system, and cancer," *The Lancet. Oncology,* vol. 5,10 (2004): 617–25. doi:10.1016/S1470-2045 (04)01597-9.

39. S. C. Segerstrom and G. E Miller. "Psychological stress and the human immune system: A meta-analytic study of 30 years of inquiry," Op cit.

40. V. J. Felitti, et al. "Relationship of childhood abuse and household dysfunction to many of the leading causes of death in adults: The adverse childhood experiences (ACE) study," Op. cit.

41. S. A. Font and K. Maguire-Jack, "Pathways from childhood abuse and other adversities to adult health risks: The role of adult socioeconomic conditions," Op. cit.

42. H. Alcalá, et al. "Gender differences in the association between adverse childhood experiences and cancer," Op. cit.

43. L. LeShan. *Cancer as a Turning Point,* Op. cit.

44. B. M. Heiny, et al (1998). "Correlation of immune cell activities and beta-endorphin release in breast carcinoma patients treated with galactose-specific lectin standardized mistletoe extract," *Anticancer Res.,* 18:583–86.

45. G. S. Kienle, et al. "Intravenous mistletoe treatment in integrative cancer care: A qualitative study exploring the procedures, concepts, and observations of expert doctors," *Evidence Based Complementary Alternative Medicine* (2016):4628287. ePub Apr. 24, 2016.

46. V. Bott. *Spiritual Science and the Art of Healing: Rudolf Steiner's Anthroposophical Medicine,* New York: Healing Arts Press,1996.

47. M. Gierke. *Internal Medicine,* Op. cit., chap. 1.2.

48. M. Debus. "Mistletoe induction therapy and advanced dosing protocols," *Mistletoe and Integrative Oncology: European Research and Best Practices 2020.* Presented by the Physicians' Association for Anthroposophic

Medicine (PAAM) and the Medical Section at the Goetheanum. Oct. 16, 2020. Denver, Colorado.

CHAPTER 8

1. H. F. Katharsis. *Reinigung als Heilverfahren: Studien zum Ritual der archaischen und klassischn Zeit sowie zum Corpus Hippocraticum* [Purification as a healing method: studies on the ritual in ancient times and the classical era as well as on the Hippocratic Corpus], 2001.

2. S. Hahnmann. *Dissertatio historico-medica de Helleborismo Vetrum* [Thesis on Helleborismo veterum, historical and medical aspects]. Leipzig, 1812.

3. P. Habermehl. Petronius, Satyrica 79-141: Sat.79-110: *Ein philologisch-literarischer Kommentar* (Texte und Kommentare) [A philological and literary commentary], 2006, p 135.

4. Fischer C. *Fleissiges Herren-Auge, oder, Wohl-Ab- und Angeführter Haus-Halter* [The industrious gentelman's gaze, or lessons in agriculture and economics], Frankfurt am Main: Zieger, 1696.

5. J. C. Sainty and R. O Buchholz. *Officials of the Royal Household, 1660–1837,* Part One: Department of the Lord Chamberlain, London, 1997.

6. E. Ben-Ayre, et. al. "Integrative oncology in the Middle East: From traditional herbal knowledge to contemporary cancer care," *Annals of Oncology,* 2012;23(1): 211–21, p. 214.

7. A. Skuse. *Constructions of Cancer in Early Modern England: Ravenous Natures,* Hampshire, UK: Palgrave Macmillan, 2015.

8. E. Ben-Ayre, et. al. "Integrative oncology in the Middle East: from traditional herbal knowledge to contemporary cancer care" (Op. cit.), p. 214.

9. B. Javadi, et al. "Anticancer plants in Islamic traditional medicine," in *Complementary Therapies for the Body, Mind and Soul,* 2015.

10. S. Hahnmann. *Dissertatio historico-medica de Helleborismo Vetrum,* Op. cit.

11. R. Steiner. *Introducing Anthroposophical Medicine* (CW 312), Op. cit.

12. W. Pelikan. *Healing Plants,* vols. 1 and 2, Spring Valley, NY: Mercury Press, 2012.

13. J. Wilkens, *The Healing Power of the Christmas Rose: The Medicinal Value of Black Hellebore,* Forest Row, UK: Temple Lodge 2017 (in association with Helixor Heilmittlel).

14. Zhi Pan, et al. "β-ecdysterone protects SH-SY5Y cells against 6-hydroxydopamine-induced apoptosis via mitochondria-dependent mechanism: Involvement of signaling pathway," *Neurotoxicity Research* vol. 30, pages 453–66 (2016).

15. A. Büssing, et al. "Immunomodulatory properties of Helleborus niger: 6th Inter-science World Conference on Inflammation, Antirheumatics, Analgetics, Immunomodulators," Mar. 28–30, 1995, Geneva, Switzerland: Palexpo, 1995.

16. F. A. Moharram, et al. "Antinociceptive and anti-inflammatory steroidal saponins from Dracaena ombet." *Planta medica,* vol. 73,10 (2007): 1101–06. doi:10.1055/s-2007-981565.

17. A. Büssing et al. "Immunomodulatory properties of Helleborus niger," Op. cit.

18. R. Rouf, et al. "Comparative study of hemagglutination and lectin activity in Australian medicinal mushrooms (higher Basidiomycetes)." *International Journal of Medicinal Mushrooms*, vol. 13,6 (2011): 493–504. doi:10.1615/intjmedmushr.v13.i6.10.

19. J. Wilkens, *Die Heilkraft der Christrose*, Op. cit., p. 40.

20. A. Bussing and K. Schweizer. "Effects of Phytopreparation from Helleborus niger on Immunocompetent cells in vitro," Op. cit., pp. 139–144.

21. Nhu Ngoc Quynh Vo, et al. "Structure and hemolytic activity relationships of triterpenoid saponins and sapogenins." *Journal of Natural Medicines*, vol. 71,1 (2017): 50-58. doi:10.1007/s11418-016-1026-9.

22. According to common principles in anthroposophic homeopathy. Primarily drawing from *Vademacum of Anthroposophic Medicines: Best Practices for Mistletoe Use in Cancer Care*, Association for Anthroposophic Physicians in Germany (GAAD), 2019 pp. 44–48: supp. to *Dr Merkurstab Journal of Anthroposophic Medicine*, vol. 72, 2019.

23. Jesse P, Mottke G, Eberle J, Seifert G, Henze G, Prokop A. "Apoptosis-inducing activity of *Helleborus niger* in ALL and AML." *Pediatric Blood and Cancer*, 2009;52(4): 464-469.

24. J. Wilkens, *Die Heilkraft der Christrose*, Op. cit., p. 49.

25. P. Jesse. "Praklinische Evaluationvon Helleborus Niger in Zellkuktturversuchen" Op. cit.

26. J. E. Felenda, et al. "Preclinical evaluation of safety and potential of black hellebore extracts for cancer treatment," *BMC Complementary and Alternative Medicine*, Op. cit., p. 11.

28. P. Jesse. "Praklinische Evaluation von Helleborus Niger in Zellkuktturversuchen," Op. cit.

29. A. Büssing, et al. "Effects of phytopreparation from Helleborus niger on Immunocompetent cells in vitro," Op. cit., pp 139–144.

30. A. Büssing, et al. "Immunomodulatory properties of Helleborus noiger," Op. cit.

31. P. Jesse, et al. "Apoptosis-inducing activity of Helleborus niger in ALL and AML," *Pediatric Blood and Cancer*, 2009;52(4): 464-469.

32. P. Jesse, et al. "Apoptosis induced by extracts of Helleborus niger in different lymphoma and leukemia cell lines and primary lymphoblasts of children with ALL is independent of smac-overexpression and executed via the mitochondrial pathway," *Blood* (2007) 110 (11): 4215. https://doi.org/10.1182/blood.V110.11.4215.4215.

33. AUTHOR NOTE: All information in this table draws from my clinical observations, the Homeopathic Pharmacopoeia (www.hpus.com), and observations by C. Schnürer, "Klinische Erfahrungen mit Helleborus niger bei Tumor- und AIDS-Kranken." [Clinical experience with Helleborus niger in cancer and AIDS patients.] *Der Merkurstab*. 1995;48(6):536-558. Article-ID: DMS-16797-DE DOI: https://doi.org/10.1427l/DMS-16797-DE.

34. J. Wilkens, *Die Heilkraft der Christrose*, Op. cit., p. 66.

35. J. E. Felenda, et al. "Preclinical evaluation of safety and potential of black Hellebore extracts for cancer treatment," *BMC Complementary and Alternative Medicine*, 21 May 2019;19(1). DOI: 10.1186/s12906 -019-2517-5.

36. P. Jesse, et al. "Apoptosis-inducing activity of Helleborus niger in AML and AML," Op. cit.

37. A. Büssing, et al. "Immunomodulatory properties of Helleborus niger," Op. cit.

38. J. Wilkens, *Die Heilkraft der Christrose* (*The Healing Power of the Christmas Rose*), Op. cit.

39. M. Debus. "Medikamentöse Begleitbehandlung bei onkologischen Erkrankungen" [Concomitant drug treatment for oncological diseases], *Der Merkurstab*, 2009;62(4):320–25. Article-ID: DMS-19466-DE. DOI: https://doi.org/10.14271/DMS-19466-DE.

40. C. Schnürer. "Klinische Erfahrungen mit Helleborus niger bei Tumor- und AIDS-Kranken," Op. cit.

41. P. Jesse, et al. "Apoptosis induced by extracts of Helleborus niger in different lymphoma and leukemia cell lines and primary lymphoblasts of children with ALL is independent of smac-overexpression and executed via the mitochondrial pathway," Op. cit.

43. Y. Arai, et al. "Enhancement of hyperthermia-induced apoptosis by local anesthetics on human histiocytic lymphoma U937 cells." *J. Biol. Chem.*, May 24, 2002;277(21):18986-93. doi: 10.1074/jbc.M108084200. Epub Feb 22, 2002.

44. T. Breitkreuz. "Helleborus niger in der Onkologie. Kasuistiken und Therapieerfahrungen aus dem Gemeinschaftskrankenhaus Herdecke" [Case reports and clinical experience from Herdecke Community Hospital 2001–2010], *Der Merkurstab*, 2010;63(6):526-534. Article-ID: DMS-19703-DE. DOI: https://doi.org/10.14271/DMS-19703-DE.

45. S. Kirste, et al. "Boswellia serrata acts on cerebral edema in patients irradiated for brain tumors: A prospective, randomized, placebo-controlled, double-blind pilot trial," *Cancer*, Aug 15, 2011;117(16):3788-95. doi: 10.1002/cncr.25945. Epub 2011 Feb 1.

46. P. G. Werthmann, et al. "Minor regression and long-time survival (56 months) in a patient with malignant pleural mesothelioma under Viscum album and Helleborus niger extracts: A case report," *Journal of Thoracic Disease*, vol. 9,12 (2017): E1064-E1070. doi:10.21037/jtd.2017.11.56.

47. T. Breitkreuz. "Helleborus niger in der Onkologie. Kasuistiken und Therapieerfahrungen aus dem Gemeinschaftskrankenhaus Herdecke 2001–2010," Op. cit. Article-ID: DMS-19703-DE. DOI: https://doi.org /10.14271/DMS-19703-DE.

48. M. Girke. *Internal Medicine*, Op. cit.

49. J. Wilkens, *The Healing Power of the Christmas Rose*, Op. cit.

50. Da-Cheng Hao. "Biodiversity, chemodiversity, and pharmacotherapy of ranunculus medicinal plants," *Ranunculales Medicinal Plants,* Academic Press. 23rd Apr. 2018. 357-386. Jan. 2019 DOI:10.1016/B978-0-12 -814232-5.00009-5 In book: (pp.357-386).

51. P. Jesse, et al, Apoptosis-inducing activity of Helleborus niger in AML and AML. Op. cit.

52. J. Wilkens, *The Healing Power of the Christmas Rose,* Op. cit.

53. Ibid.

54. M. Girke, *Internal Medicine,* Op. cit.

55. K. K. Auyeung, et al. "Astragalus membranaceus: A review of its protection against inflammation and gastrointestinal cancers," *The American Journal of Chinese Medicine,* vol. 44, No. 01, pp. 1–22 (2016) https://doi.org/10.1142/S0192415X16500014.

56. M. Girke. *Internal Medicine,* Op. cit., pp. 100, 218.

57. Ibid., pp. 110, 215, 279. 393.

58. Ibid., pp. 171, 1008, 1014.

59. Ibid., pp. 242, 319.

60. C. Scheffer, et al. "Potenzierte Organpräparate in der anthroposophischen Medizin. Teil 3: Goetheanistische Betrachtungen zu Schwein und Rind als Spendertiere" [Potentiated organ preparations in anthroposophic medicine. Part 3: Goetheanist considerations on pigs and cattle as donor animals], *Der Merkurstab,* 2019;72(1):12-20. Article-ID: DMS-21045-DE. DOI: https://doi.org/10.14271/DMS-21045-DE.

61. "Best Practices for Mistletoe Uses in Cancer Care," *Vademecum of Anthroposophic Medicines,* Association of Anthroposophic Medicine in Germany (GAAD), 2019, p. 139.

62. M. Girke, *Internal Medicine,* Op. cit., pp. 45, 506, 575.

63. R. Heine (ed.). *Anthroposophic Nursing Practice: Foundations and Indications for Everyday Caregiving.* Hudson, NY: Portal Books, 2020.

64. This case story was originally published by Fatima Zehra Raza, Smita Ranjan, Goetz H. Kloecker (University of Louisville), and James Graham (Brown Cancer Center, Louisville, KY), in *Journal of Clinical Oncology,* vol. 31, no. 15 supplement 2018.

CHAPTER 9

1. C. A. Buckner, et al. "Complementary and alternative medicine use in patients before and after a cancer diagnosis," *Curr. Oncol.,* 2018;25(4): e275-e281. doi:10.3747/co.25.3884.

2. J. Jou and P. J. Johnson. "Nondisclosure of complementary and alternative medicine use to primary care physicians: Findings from the 2012 National Health Interview Survey," *JAMA Internal Medicine,* vol. 176,4 (2016): 545-6. doi:10.1001/jamainternmed.2015.8593.

3. R. L. Smith, et al. "Metabolic flexibility as an adaptation to energy resources and requirements in health and disease," *Endocrine Reviews,* vol. 39,4 (2018): 489–517. doi:10.1210/er.2017-00211.

4. J. Araújo, et al. "Prevalence of optimal metabolic health in American adults: National Health and Nutrition Examination Survey 2009–2016," *Metabolic Syndrome and Related Disorders,* 2018. doi: 10.1089/met .2018.0105.

5. I. Spreadbury. "Comparison with ancestral diets suggests dense acellular carbohydrates promote an inflammatory microbiota, and may be the primary dietary cause of leptin resistance and obesity," *Diabetes, Metabolic Syndrome and Obesity: Targets and Therapy*, vol. 5 (2012): 175–89. doi:10.2147/DMSO.S33473.

6. C. Marbaniang and L. Kma. "Dysregulation of glucose metabolism by oncogenes and tumor suppressors in cancer cells," *Asian Pacific Journal of Cancer Prevention: APJCP*, vol. 19,9 2377–90. 26 Sep. 2018, doi:10.22034/APJCP.2018.19.9.2377.

7. K. A. Schwartz, et al. "Investigating the ketogenic diet as treatment for primary aggressive brain cancer: Challenges and lessons learned," *Front Nutr.*, 2018 Feb 23;5:11. doi: 10.3389/fnut.2018.00011. PMID: 29536011; PMCID: PMC5834833.

8. According to topical search at ClinicalTrials.gov, search conducted Apr. 24, 2021.

9. J. Tan-Shalaby. "Ketogenic diets and cancer: Emerging evidence," *Federal Practitioner: For the Health Care Professionals of the VA, DoD, and PHS*, vol. 34, Suppl 1 (2017): 37S–42S.

10. A. Poff et al. "Targeting the Warburg effect for cancer treatment: Ketogenic diets for the management of glioma," *Seminars in Cancer Biology*, 56 June 2019.

11. C. R. Marinac, et al. "Prolonged nightly fasting and breast cancer prognosis," *JAMA Oncology*, vol. 2,8 (2016): 1049–55. doi:10.1001/jamaoncol.2016.0164.

12. J. Fung, *The Cancer Code: A Revolutionary New Understanding of a Medical Mystery* (New York: Harper Wave, 2020), pp. 203–208, 229–238, 285–292.

13. "Hyperthermia in cancer treatment," National Institutes of Health (NIH), National Cancer Institute (NCI) monograph; reviewed Aug. 31, 2011 (https://www.cancer.gov/about-cancer/treatment/types/surgery/hyperthermia-fact-sheet). Accessed Apr. 29, 2021.

14. Z. Behrouzkia, et al. "Hyperthermia: How can it be used?" *Oman Medical Journal*, vol. 31,2 (2016): 89-97. doi:10.5001/omj.2016.19.

15. L. Wang, et al. "A systematic strategy of combinational blow for overcoming cascade drug resistance via NIR-light-triggered hyperthermia," *Advanced Materials* (Deerfield Beach, FL), e2100599. Apr. 8, 2021, doi:10.1002/adma.202100599.

16. B. E. Dayanc, et al. "Dissecting the role of hyperthermia in natural killer cell mediated anti-tumor responses," *International Journal of Hyperthermia: The Official Journal of European Society for Hyperthermic Oncology, North American Hyperthermia Group*, vol. 24,1 (2008): 41–56.

17. K. Jeziorski. "Hyperthermia in rheumatic diseases: A promising approach?" *Reumatologia*, vol. 56,5 (2018): 316-320. doi:10.5114/reum.2018.79503.

18. A. Thorne, et al. "Hyperthermia-induced changes in liver physiology and metabolism: a rationale for hyperthermic machine perfusion," *Gastrointestinal and Liver Physiology*, vol. 319, no. 1; July 2020:G43–50.

19. "Off target: Investigating the abscopal effect as a treatment for cancer," National Institutes of Health (NIH), National Cancer Institute (NCI) monograph. Reviewed Jan. 28, 2020. https://www.cancer.gov/news-events /cancer-currents-blog/2020/cancer-abscopal-effect-radiation -immunotherapy). Accessed Apr. 29, 2021.

20. Registered at https://clinicaltrials.gov/ct2/history/NCT02093871?V _4=View.

21. Described at "Clinical trial—ovarian cancer," Verthermia website: https://www.verthermia.net/clinical-science-ovarian.

22. J. Hussain and M. Cohen. "Clinical effects of regular dry sauna bathing: A systematic review," *Evidence-based Complementary and Alternative Medicine: eCAM*, vol. 2018 1857413. 24 Apr. 2018, doi:10.1155/2018/1857413.

23. S. J. Genuis, et al. "Clinical detoxification: elimination of persistent toxicants from the human body," *The Scientific World Journal*, vol. 2013 238347. Jun. 6, 2013, doi:10.1155/2013/238347.

24. A. Boretti and B. K. Banik. "Intravenous vitamin C for reduction of cytokines storm in acute respiratory distress syndrome," *Pharma. Nutrition*, vol. 12 (2020): 100190. doi:10.1016/j.phanu.2020.100190.

25. M. J. Gonzalez, et al. "High dose intravenous vitamin C and chikungunya fever: A case report," *Journal of Orthomolecular Medicine*, vol. 29,4 (2014): 154-156.

26. R. Chuen Fong, et al. "Effects of high doses of vitamin C on cancer patients in Singapore: Nine cases," *Integrative Cancer Therapies*, 2016, vol. 15(2) 197–204.

27. S. J. Padayatty, et al. "Vitamin C pharmacokinetics: Implications for oral and intravenous use," *Annals of Internal Medicine*, Apr. 6, 2004vol. 140, no. 7, Page: 533-537.

28. A. C. Carr, et al. "The effect of intravenous vitamin C on cancer- and chemotherapy-related fatigue and quality of life," *Front. Oncol.*, 2014 Oct 16;4:283. doi: 10.3389/fonc.2014.00283. PMID: 25360419; PMCID: PMC4199254.

29. Y. C. Raymond, et al. "Effects of high doses of vitamin C on cancer patients in Singapore: Nine cases," Op. cit.

30. E. Klimant, et al. "Intravenous vitamin C in the supportive care of cancer patients: a review and rational approach," *Curr. Oncol.*, Apr. 2018;25(2):139-148. doi: 10.3747/co.25.3790. Epub 2018 Apr 30. PMID: 29719430; PMCID: PMC5927785.

31. T. Hidenori, et al. "High-dose intravenous vitamin C improves quality of life in cancer patients," *Personalized Medicine Universe*, vol. 1, no. 1, 2012, pp. 49–53, https://doi.org/10.1016/j.pmu.2012.05.008.

32. S. Mousavi, et al. "Immunomodulatory and antimicrobial effects of vitamin C. *Eur. Journal of Microbiol. Immunology* (Bp). Aug. 2019 16;9(3):73-79. doi: 10.1556/1886.2019.00016. PMID: 31662885; PMCID: PMC6798581.

33. N. A. Mikirova, et al. "Anti-angiogenic effect of high doses of ascorbic acid," *Journal of Transl. Med.*, Sep. 2008, 12;6:50. doi: 10.1186/1479-5876-6-50. PMID: 18789157; PMCID: PMC2562367.

34. N. Mikirova, et al. "Effect of high-dose intravenous vitamin C on inflammation in cancer patients," *J. Transl. Med.,* 10, 189 (2012). https://doi.org /10.1186/1479-5876-10-189.

35. AUTHOR NOTE: I run the G6-PD test before initiating *any* IVC again for a patient if it has been more than six months since their last IVC and if a cytotoxic therapy has been used in the interim.

36. S. J. Padayatty, et al. "Vitamin C pharmacokinetics: implications for oral and intravenous use," Op. cit.

37. M. Di Rosa, et al. "Vitamin D3: A helpful immuno-modulator," *Immunology,* Oct. 2011;134(2):123-39. doi: 10.1111/j.1365-2567.2011.03482.x. PMID: 21896008; PMCID: PMC3194221.

38. C. F. Garland, et al. "The role of vitamin D in cancer prevention," *Am. J. Public Health,* Feb. 2006;96(2):252-61. doi: 10.2105/AJPH.2004.045260. Epub 2005 Dec 27. PMID: 16380576; PMCID: PMC1470481.

39. P. D. Chandler, et al. "Effect of vitamin D$_3$ supplements on development of advanced cancer: A secondary analysis of the VITAL randomized clinical trial," *JAMA Netw. Open,* 2020;3(11):e2025850. doi:10.1001 /jamanetworkopen.2020.25850.

40. S. Gutiérrez, et al. "Effects of omega-3 fatty acids on immune cells," *Int. J. Mol. Sci.,* Oct 11, 2019;20(20):5028. doi: 10.3390/ijms20205028. PMID: 31614433; PMCID: PMC6834330. AUTHOR NOTE: If omega-3 levels are low, the immune system is not responsive to modulation.

41. A. P. Simopoulos. "The importance of the ratio of omega-6/omega-3 essential fatty acids," *Biomedicine and Pharmacotherapy (Biomedecine and Pharmacotherapie),* vol. 56,8 (2002): 365–79. doi:10.1016/s0753 -3322(02)00253-6.

42. D. Friedmann-Morvinski and I. M. Verma. "Dedifferentiation and reprogramming: Origins of cancer stem cells," *EMBO Reports,* vol. 15,3 (2014): 244–53. doi:10.1002/embr.201338254.

43. E. Doldo, et al. "Vitamin A, cancer treatment and prevention: The new role of cellular retinol binding proteins," *BioMed research international* vol. 2015 (2015): 624627. doi:10.1155/2015/624627.

44. W. B. O'Shaughnessy (1838–40). "Case of tetanus, cured by a preparation of hemp (cannabis indica)," *Transactions of the Medical and Physical Society of Bengal.* 8: 462–469.

45. M. B. Bridgeman and D. T. Abazia. "Medicinal cannabis: History, pharmacology, and implications for the acute care setting," *P and T: A Peer-reviewed Journal for Formulary Management,* vol. 42,3 (2017): 180–188.

46. D. Downs. "The science behind the DEA's long war on marijuana," *Scientific American,* Apr. 19, 2016, online edition. https://www .scientificamerican.com/article/the-science-behind-the-dea-s-long-war-on -marijuana/ Retrieved Apr. 29, 2021.

47. M. A. Lee. *Smoke Signals: A Social History of Marijuana–Medical, Recreational and Scientific,* New York: Scribner, 2012.

48. K. Mackie. "Mechanisms of CB1 receptor signaling: Endocannabinoid modulation of synaptic strength," *Int. J. Obes.,* 30, S19–S23 (2006). https://doi.org/10.1038/sj.ijo.0803273.

49. A. Dhopeshwarkar and K. Mackie. "CB2 cannabinoid receptors as a therapeutic target—What does the future hold?" *Molecular Pharmacology*, vol. 86,4 (2014): 430-7. doi:10.1124/mol.114.094649.

50. S. Hryhorowicz, et al. "Pharmacogenetics of cannabinoids," *European Journal of Drug Metabolism and Pharmacokinetics*, vol. 43,1 (2018): 1-12. doi:10.1007/s13318-017-0416-z.

51. U. Reimann-Philipp, et al. "Cannabis chemovar nomenclature misrepresents chemical and genetic diversity: Survey of variations in chemical profiles and genetic markers in Nevada medical cannabis samples," *Cannabis and Cannabinoid Research*, vol. 5, No. 3, 2 Sep. 2020 https://doi.org/10.1089/can.2018.0063. https://www.liebertpub.com /doi/10.1089/can.2018.0063.

52. AUTHOR NOTE: Nutrition Genome is one of the epigenetic testing services that I rely on (see "Resources" in this volume). It is especially valuable for uncovering these SNPs.

53. S. Hryhorowicz, et al. "Pharmacogenetics of cannabinoids," *European Journal of Drug Metabolism and Pharmacokinetics*, vol. 43,1 (2018): 1-12. doi:10.1007/s13318-017-0416-z.

54. V. Di Marzo and C. Silvestri. 2019. "Lifestyle and metabolic syndrome: Contribution of the endocannabinoidome," *Nutrients*, 11, no. 8: 1956. https://doi.org/10.3390/nu11081956.

55. D. I. Abrams and M. Guzman. "Cannabis in cancer care," *Clinical pharmacology and therapeutics* vol. 97,6 (2015): 575-86. doi:10.1002/cpt.108.

56. Guillermo Velasco, Sonia Hernández-Tiedra, David Dávila, Mar Lorente, "The use of cannabinoids as anticancer agents," *Progress in Neuro-Psychopharmacology and Biological Psychiatry*, vol. 64, Jan. 2016, pp. 259–266, ISSN 0278-5846, https://doi.org/10.1016/j.pnpbp.2015.05.010.

57. A. Sainz-Cort, et al. "Anti-proliferative and cytotoxic effect of cannabidiol on human cancer cell lines in presence of serum," *BMC Res. Notes*, 13, 389 (2020). https://doi.org/10.1186/s13104-020-05229-5.

58. M. Scherma, et al. "The endogenous cannabinoid anandamide has effects on motivation and anxiety that are revealed by fatty acid amide hydrolase (FAAH) inhibition," *Neuropharmacology*, vol. 54,1 (2008): 129–40. doi:10.1016/j.neuropharm.2007.08.011.

59. Ibid.

60. R. N. Donahue, et al. "The opioid growth factor (OGF) and low dose naltrexone (LDN) suppress human ovarian cancer progression in mice," *Gynecologic Oncology*, vol. 122,2 (2011): 382-8. doi:10.1016/j.ygyno .2011.04.009.

61. D. Jackson, et al. "The effects of low dose naltrexone on opioid induced hyperalgesia and fibromyalgia," *Frontiers in Psychiatry*, vol. 12 593842. 16 Feb. 2021, doi:10.3389/fpsyt.2021.593842.

62. J. Younger, et al. "The use of low-dose naltrexone (LDN) as a novel anti-inflammatory treatment for chronic pain," *Clinical Rheumatology*, vol. 33,4 (2014): 451-9. doi:10.1007/s10067-014-2517-2.

63. T. Schwaiger. "The uses of low-dose naltrexone in clinical practice," *Natural Medicine Journal* (Apr. 2018), vol 10, no. 4 https://www

.naturalmedicinejournal.com/journal/2018-04/uses-low-dose-naltrexone
-clinical-practice. Retrieved Apr. 30, 2021.

64. L. A. Hammer, et al. "Opioid growth factor and low-dose naltrexone impair central nervous system infiltration by CD4 + T lymphocytes in established experimental autoimmune encephalomyelitis, a model of multiple sclerosis," *Experimental Biology and Medicine* (Maywood, NJ), vol. 241,1 (2016): 71–78. doi:10.1177/1535370215596384.

65. I. S. Zagon and P. J. McLaughlin. "Intermittent blockade of OGFr and treatment of autoimmune disorders," *Experimental Biology and Medicine*, vol. 243,17-18 (2018): 1323–30. doi:10.1177/1535370218817746.

66. AUTHOR NOTE: This is primarily a clinical observation (that LDN appears to calm over-zealous reactions in the immune system). Such reactions are often invoked in patients undergoing SOC immune therapy. Clinically, LDN has been a powerful tool to enhance outcomes and lower side effects to these drugs, which can otherwise wreak havoc in 80 percent or more of patients receiving them, as noted in "New drugs, new side effects: complications of cancer immunotherapy," National Institutes of Health (NIH), National Cancer Institute (NCI) monograph. May 10, 2019. At: https://www.cancer.gov/news-events/cancer-currents-blog/2019/cancer-immunotherapy-investigating-side-effects. Accessed Apr. 2021.

67. Z. Li, et al. "Low-dose naltrexone (LDN): A promising treatment in immune-related diseases and cancer therapy," *International immunopharmacology*, vol. 61, Op. cit.

68. N. Sharafaddinzadeh, et al. "The effect of low-dose naltrexone on quality of life of patients with multiple sclerosis: A randomized placebo-controlled trial," *Multiple Sclerosis* (Basingstoke, UK), vol. 16,8 (2010): 964-9. doi:10.1177/1352458510366857.

69. Washington State University. "Insights on how night shift work increases cancer risk," *ScienceDaily*, Mar. 8, 2021; www.sciencedaily.com/releases/2021/03/210308091744.htm>.

70. T. C. Erren, et al. IARC 2019: "Night shift work" is probably carcinogenic: What about disturbed chronobiology in all walks of life?" *J. Occup. Med. Toxicol.*, 14, 29 (2019). https://doi.org/10.1186/s12995-019-0249-6.

71. J. Hansen. "Night shift work and risk of breast cancer," *Current Environmental Health Reports*, vol. 4,3 (2017): 325-339. doi:10.1007/s40572-017-0155-y.

72. IARC Monographs, vol. 124 group. "Carcinogenicity of night shift work," *Lancet Oncol.*, 2019 Aug;20(8):1058–59. doi: 10.1016/S1470-2045(19)30455-3. Epub 2019 Jul 4. PMID: 31281097.

73. E. McNeely, et al. "The self-reported health of U.S. flight attendants compared to the general population," *Environ. Health*, 13, 13 (2014). https://doi.org/10.1186/1476-069X-13-13.

74. A. N. Viswanathan, et al. "Circulating melatonin and the risk of breast and endometrial cancer in women," *Cancer Letters*, vol. 281,1 (2009): 1–7. doi:10.1016/j.canlet.2008.11.002.

75. Y. Li, et al. "Melatonin for the prevention and treatment of cancer," *Oncotarget*, vol. 8,24 (2017): 39896-39921. doi:10.18632/oncotarget.16379.

76.   P. Lissoni, et al. "Five-year survival with high-dose melatonin and other antitumor pineal hormones in advanced cancer patients eligible for the only palliative therapy," *Research Journal of Oncology* (2018), vol. 2 no. 1: 2 (online) Mar. 26, 2018. Retrieved Apr. 29, 2021.

77.   R. J. Reiter, et al. "Melatonin, a full-service anti-cancer agent: Inhibition of initiation, progression and metastasis." *International Journal of Molecular Sciences*, vol. 18,4 843. 17 Apr. 2017, doi:10.3390 /ijms18040843.

78.   Ibid.

79.   B. Coiffard, et al. "A tangled threesome: Circadian rhythm, body temperature variations, and the immune system," *Biology,* vol. 10,1 65. 18 Jan. 2021, doi:10.3390/biology10010065.

CHAPTER 10

1.   M. Orange, et al. "Coley's lessons remembered: Augmenting mistletoe therapy," *Integrative Cancer Therapies,* vol. 15,4 (2016): 502–11. doi:10.1177/1534735416649916.

2.   L. K. Diamond and L. A. Luhby. "Pattern of 'spontaneous' remissions in leukemia of the childhood, observed in 26 of 300 cases," *Am. J. Med.,* 1951;10:238ff.

3.   R. Kleef, et al. "Fever, cancer incidence and spontaneous remissions," *Neuroimmunomodulation* (2001) 9:55–64. doi: 10.1159/000049008.

4.   M. Orange. "Mistletoe therapy for cancer patients. A thesis submitted to the University of Birmingham for the degree of Master of Science in Clinical Oncology," School of Cancer Sciences, University of Birmingham, 2010.

5.   R. Steiner. *Physiology and Healing: Treatment, Therapy, and Hygiene* (CW 314), Op. cit., lecture of Oct. 27, 1922,

6.   AUTHOR NOTE, DR. HANCOCK: For a little deeper examination of this matter, this webpage provides a calculator for calories burned while walking: https://caloriesburnedhq.com/calories-burned-walking/. This paper looks more closely at the toll fever takes on us: V. E. Baracos, et al. "The metabolic cost of fever," *Canadian Journal of Physiology and Pharmacology,* 65, no. 6 (June 1, 1987): 1248–54. https://doi.org/10.1139 /y87-199. Here is the math: 1 kcal will raise 1 kg of water 1 degree Celsius. We are, on average 80kg, and mostly H2O. So, it takes roughly 80 kcal to raise body temperature 1 degree. We burn about 70 calories per mile (1.6 kilometers). We can estimate a 10 percent increase in basal metabolic rate (BMR) for every 1-degree Celsius increase. An average woman has a BMR of 1,400; an average man has a BMR of 1,800. Average that out, and you see about 1,600 kcal per degree, of which 10 percent is 160 kcal. This seems to be 2 miles or 3.2 km!

7.   AUTHOR NOTE, DR. HANCOCK: The MFIT subcutaneous injection site will be large and palpable. Lymph nodes will still be activated. If necessary, one can do a PET in 2 weeks after MFIT and simply interpret the results in accordance with expected MFIT changes. As for IV, I usually allow a 2-week break between regular IV mistletoe and scans.

8. *Vademecum of Anthroposophic Medicines.* Association of Anthropo-sophic Medicine in Germany (GAAD); 2019.

9. AUTHOR NOTE, DR. HANCOCK: Although I've had a couple of patients who got significant fever with Helixor A, this was really an unintentional MFIT response.

10. R. Penter. "Der Injektionszeitpunkt und der Verlauf eines Zyklus der endogenen Hyperthermie bei der Mistelerstbehandlung" [The time of injection and the course of a cycle of endogenous hyperthermia in initial mistletoe treatment], *Der Merkurstab,* 2011(64):1.Jan.–Feb., 20–39.

11. M. Orange, et al. "Durable regression of primary cutaneous b-cell lym-phoma following fever-inducing mistletoe treatment: Two case reports," *Phytomedicine,* 20, nos. 3–4 (Feb. 15, 2013), 324–27.

12. *Vademecum of Anthroposophic Medicines,* Association of Anthropo-sophic Medicine in Germany, 2019, chap. 7.

13. M. Orange. "Mistletoe therapy for cancer patients: A thesis submitted to the University of Birmingham for the degree of master of science in clinical oncology," School of Cancer Sciences, University of Birming-ham, 2010.

14. M. T. Yilmaz, et al. "Abscopal effect, from myth to reality: From radia-tion oncologists' perspective," *Cureus,* vol. 11,1 e3860. Jan. 9, 2019, doi:10.7759/cureus.3860.

15. M. Zaric, et al. "Skin immunisation activates an innate lymphoid cell-monocyte axis regulating CD8+ effector recruitment to mucosal tissues," *Nat. Commun.,* 10, 2214 (2019). https://doi.org/10.1038/s41467-019 -09969-2.

16. F. Schad, et al. "Intratumoral mistletoe (Viscum album L) therapy in patients with unresectable pancreas carcinoma: A retrospective analysis," *Integr. Cancer Ther.,* Jul. 2014;13(4):332-40. doi: 10.1177 /1534735413513637. Epub 2013 Dec 19. PMID: 24363283.

17. *Vademecum of Anthroposophic Medicines.* Op. cit., chap. 7.

18. Jeong Su Cho, et al. "Chemical pleurodesis using mistletoe extraction (ABNOVAviscum® injection) for malignant pleural effusion," *Annals of Thoracic and Cardiovascular Surgery: Official Journal of the Associa-tion of Thoracic and Cardiovascular Surgeons of Asia,* 22, no. 1 (2016): 20–26, https://doi.org/10/f8swjk.

19. YongJin Chang, et al. "Viscum pleurodesis is as effective as talc pleurode-sis and tends to have less adverse effect," *Supportive Care in Cancer: Official Journal of the Multinational Association of Supportive Care in Cancer,* 28, no. 11 (Nov. 2020): 5463–67, https://doi.org/10.1007/s00520 -020-05405-0.

20. G. Bar-Sela, et al. "Reducing malignant ascites accumulation by repeated intraperitoneal administrations of a viscum album extract," *Anticancer Research,* 26, no. 1B (Feb. 2006): 709–13.

21. R. Stange et al. "Favourable course of persisting malignant ascites," *Forschende Komplementarmedizin* (2006) 16, no. 1 (Feb. 2009): 49–53, https://doi.org/10/d7kwcv.

22. *Vademecum of Anthroposophic Medicines.* Op. cit., chap. 9.3, p. 144.

23. M. Girke, et al. "Ascites bei Non-Hodgkin-Lymphom (V.a. splenales Lymphom): Remission nach viermaliger intraperitonealer Viscumalbum-Instillation" [Ascites in non-Hodgkin lymphoma (V.a. splenal lymphoma): Remission after four intraperitoneal instillation of the viscum album], *Der Merkurstab: Zeitschrift für Anthroposophische Medizin*, 2012;65(3):257-258. DOI: https://doi.org/10.14271/DMS-19967-de.

24. R. Achim, et al. "Mistletoe plant extract in patients with nonmuscle invasive bladder cancer: Results of a phase Ib/IIa single group dose escalation study," *The Journal of Urology*, 194, no. 4 (Oct. 2015): 939–43 (https://doi.org/10.1016/j.juro.2015.04.073).

25. H. Rexer and Geschäftsstelle der AUO, "Study on the treatment of non-muscle invasive bladder cancer: A phase-III efficacy study for intravesical instillation of mistletoe extract in superficial bladder cancer (TIM) AB 40/11 of the AUO," *Der Urologe. Ausg.*, A 54, no. 3 (Mar. 2015): 406–08, https://doi.org/10.1007/s00120-015-3781-8.

26. Vademecum of Anthroposophic Medicines. Published by Association of Anthroposophic Medicine in Germany (GAAD); 2019, chap. 7.9.

27. M. Debus. "Anwendungsmöglichkeiten von Helleborus niger in der Onkologie" [Possible uses of Helleborus in oncology.] *Der Merkurstab: Zeitschrift für Anthroposophische Medizin*, 2010;63(6):551–557.

28. K. M. Brintzenhofe-Szoc, et al. "Mixed anxiety/depression symptoms in a large cancer cohort: Prevalence by cancer type," *Psychosomatics*, 2009 Jul.–Aug. 50 (4):383–91.

29. S. Mayr, RM. "Depression in pancreatic cancer: Sense of impending doom," *Digestion*, 2010;82:1-3.

30. D. K. Andersen, et al. "Diabetes, pancreatogenic diabetes, and pancreatic cancer," *Diabetes*, May 2017, 66 (5) 1103–10. doi: 10.2337/db16-1477.

31. A. Marengo, et al. "Liver cancer: Connections with obesity, fatty liver, and cirrhosis," *Annual Review of Medicine*, vol. 67 (2016): 103–17. doi:10.1146/annurev-med-090514-013832.

32. G. J. Koelwyn, et al. "Exercise-dependent regulation of the tumour microenvironment," *Nat. Rev. Cancer*, 2017 Sep. 25;17(10):620-632. doi: 10.1038/nrc.2017.78. PMID: 28943640.

33. S. O. Dalton, et al. "Mind and cancer: Do psychological factors cause cancer?" *Eur. J. Cancer*, 2002JUI;38 (10):1313-23.

34. M. A. Nordstrom, et al. "Sick leave due to depressive disease: Not a risk factor for the development of malignant lymphoma," *Eur. J. Epidemiol.*, 2005;20 (9): 769–73.

35. J. R. Cerhan, et al. "Anthropometric characteristics, physical activity, and risk of non-Hodgkins lymphoma subtypes and B-cell chronic lymphocytic leukemia: A prospective study," *Am. J. Epidemiol.*, Sep. 15, 2002; 156 (6): 527–35.

36. L. Jachens. "Das maligne Melanom ausanthroposophisch-menschenkundlicher Sich" [The malignant melanoma from the anthroposophic point of view], *Der Merkurstab*, 2005(58):5 Sep.–Oct.; 375–89.

37. AUTHOR NOTE: Full ACS statement reads, "Breast cancer is the most common cancer in American women, except for skin cancers" (according to American Cancer Society statistics, at: https://www.cancer.org/cancer

/breast-cancer/about/how-common-is-breast-cancer.html. Accessed Apr. 22, 2021).

38.   American Cancer Society. *Cancer Facts and Figures 2020*, Atlanta, GA: American Cancer Society, 2020.

39.   "Blood Cancers," National Foundation for Cancer Research; monograph at: https://www.nfcr.org/cancer-types/blood-cancer. Accessed Apr. 22, 2021.

40.   N. Becker, et al. "Self-reported history of infections and the risk of non-Hodgkin lymphoma: An interlymph pooled analysis," Intl. *Journal of Cancer. Journal Intl. Du Cancer*, 131 no 10; Nov 15, 2012: 2342–48.

41.   S. Parodi, et al. "Childhood infectious diseases and risk of non-Hodgkin's lymphoma according to the WHO classification: A reanalysis of the Italian multicenter case-control study," *Int. J. Cancer*, 2020 Feb 15;146(4):977-986. doi: 10.1002/ijc.32393. Epub 2019 May 17. PMID: 31077355.

42.   H. F. Fischer, et al. "The effect of attending Steiner schools during childhood on health in adulthood: A multicentre cross-sectional study," *PLoS ONE*, 8, no. 9 (Sept. 12, 2013); https://doi.org/10.1371/journal .pone.0073135.

43.   M. Girke, *Internal Medicine*, Op. cit.

44.   A. C. Xavier, et al. "Down syndrome and malignancies: A unique clinical relationship," *Journal of Molecular Diagnostics: JMD*, 11, no. 5; 2009: 371–80.

45.   J. Grieco, et al. "Down syndrome: Cognitive and behavioral functioning across the lifespan," *American Journal of Med. Genetics, Part C: Sems. in Med. Genetics*, 169. No 2. 2015: 135-49.

46.   *Vademecum of Anthroposophic Medicines*, Association of Anthroposophic Medicine in Germany, 2019, chap. 9.

47.   C. Stumpf, et al. "Therapie mit Mistelextrakten bei malignen hämatologischen und lymphatischen Erkrankungen" [Mistletoe extract therapy for malignant haematological and lymphatic diseases], *Eine monozentrische retrospektive Analyse über 16 Jahre: Forschende Komplementärmedizin*, 2000; 7(3): 139–46.

48.   J. J. Kuehn. "Langfristig guter Verlauf unter Misteltherapie bei einem Patienten mit einem zentrozytisch-zentroblastischen non-Hodgkin-lymphom" [Long-term good progress with mistletoe therapy in a patient with centrocytic-centroblastic non-Hodgkins lymphoma], *Deutsche Medizinische Wochenschrift*, 1999; 124(47): 1414–18. http://doi.org/10 .1055/s-2007-1024555.

49.   G. Seifert, et al. "Response to subcutaneous therapy with mistletoe in recurrent multisystem Langerhans cell histiocytosis," *Pediatric Blood and Cancer*, 2005; 48(5): 591–92 (http://doi.org/10.1002/pbc.20649).

50.   This section, written by Debus, originally appeared in *Vademecum of Anthroposophic Medicines*, Op. cit., chap. 9.1.

51.   M. Girke. *Internal Medicine*, Op. cit., chap. 9.

53.   *Vademecum of Anthroposophic Medicines*, Op. cit., chap. 9, case description 142–143.

54. M. Orange, et al. "Durable regression of primary cutaneous b-cell lymphoma following fever-inducing mistletoe treatment: Two case reports," *Phytomedicine*, 20, nos. 3–4 (Feb. 15, 2013): 324–27.

55. T. Srdic-Rajic, et al. "Sensitization of K562 leukemia cells to Doxorubicin by the VAE: Viscum album enhances Doxorubicin antitumor effects," *Phytotherapy Research*, 30 no 3 2016: 483–95.

56. C. I. Delebinski, et al. "A natural comb. ext. of VA L. containing both triterpene acids and lectins is highly effective against AML in Vivo," *PloS One*, no. 8, 2015: e0133892.

57. M. P. Rausch and K. T. Hastings. "Immune checkpoint inhibitors in the treatment of melanoma: From basic science to clinical application," *Cutaneous Melanoma: Etiology and Therapy* (chap. 9), W. H. Ward, J. M. Farma (eds.); Brisbane (AU): Codon Publications, 2017 Dec 21.

58. G. Lahat, et al. "Sarcoma epidemiology and etiology: Potential enviro and genetic factors," *Surgical Clinics of North Am.*, 88, no 3; 2008: 451–81.

59. AUTHOR NOTE: Lymphoma and leukemia actually have two peaks: in youth and in older age. When such cancers appear in older age, we view the restraining/structuring forces as weakening.

60. R. Leroi. "Das Sarkom und seine Therapie, Teil I: Über die Bildung der Sarkome" [Sarcoma and its therapy, part I: On the formation of the sarcoma], *Beiträge zu einer Erweiterung der Heilkunst nach geisteswissenschaftlichen Erkenntnissen*, 1970;23(2):45–51. DOI: https://doi.org/10.14271/DMS-12805-DE.

61. Ibid., part 2: For Sarcoma Therapies.

62. R. D. Issels, et al. "Effect of neoadjuvant chemotherapy plus regional hyperthermia on long-term outcomes among patients with localized high-risk soft tissue sarcoma," *JAMA Oncology*, 4, no 4; 2018. 483-92.

63. A. Kirsch and T. Hajto. "Case reports of sarcoma patients with optimized lectin-oriented mistletoe extract therapy," *Journal of Alt. and Comp. Med.*, 17, 10; 2011: 973–79.

64. T. Waschakidze. "Intraläsionale Misteltherapie bei einer Patientin mit Liposarkom–eine Fallvignette aus Georgien" [Intralesional mistletoe therapy in a patient with liposarcoma–a case vignette from Georgia], *Der Merkurstab*, 69, no. 3 (2016): 205–7, https://doi.org/10.14271/DMS-20638-DE.

65. A. Longhi, et al. "Long-term follow-up of a randomized study of oral etoposide versus viscum album fermentatum pini as maintenance therapy in osteosarcoma patients in complete surgical remission after second relapse," *Sarcoma*, 2020;2020:8260730. Apr. 26, 2020. doi:10.1155/2020/8260730.

66. M. Reynel, et al. "Long-term survival of a patient with recurrent dedifferentiated high-grade liposarcoma of the retroperitoneum under adjuvant treatment with viscum album l. extract: A case report," *Integral Cancer Ther.*, 2021 Jan.–Dec.;20:1534735421995258. doi: 10.1177 /1534735421995258. PMID: 33618582; PMCID: PMC7905720.

67. A. Orton, et al. "A case of complete abscopal response in high-grade pleiomorphic sarcoma treated with radiotherapy alone," *Cureus*, vol. 8,10 e821. Oct. 7, 2016, doi:10.7759/cureus.821.

68. R. J. Brenneman, et al. "Abscopal effect following proton beam radio-therapy in a patient with inoperable metastatic retroperitoneal sarcoma," *Front Oncol.*, 2019 Sep 26;9:922. doi: 10.3389/fonc.2019.00922. PMID: 31616634; PMCID: PMC6775241. https://pubmed.ncbi.nlm.nih.gov /31616634.

69. E. Pennacchioli, et al. "Hyperthermia as an adjunctive treatment for soft-tissue sarcoma," *Expert Review of Anticancer Therapy*, vol. 9,2 (2009): 199-210. doi:10.1586/14737140.9.2.199.

70. R. D. Issels, et al. "Effect of neoadjuvant chemotherapy plus regional hyperthermia on long-term outcomes among patients with localized high-risk soft tissue sarcoma: The EORTC 62961-ESHO 95 randomized clinical trial," *JAMA Oncology*, vol. 4,4 (2018): 483-492.

71. *Cancer Facts and Figures 2020*, Atlanta: American Cancer Society, 2020.

72. Q. T. Ostrom, et al. "Adult glioma incidence and survival by race or ethnicity in the United States from 2000 to 2014," *JAMA Oncology*. 4, 9, 2018.

73. Q. T. Ostrom, et al. "The epidemiology of glioma in adults: A 'state of the science' review," *Neuro-oncology*, 16, 7; 2014: 896–913.

74. AUTHOR NOTE: By this definition nerve cells are undergoing tiny death-like states on a continuous basis (this also links to consciousness). Dr. Armin Husemann discusses this in some of his books. This principle has fascinating connections to the threefold human.

75. J. de Weille. "On the genesis of neuroblastoma and glioma," *International Journal of Brain Science*, vol. 2014, Article ID 217503, 14 pages.

76. "Glial cells–development and stem cells" *Embryonic Development and Stem Cell Compendium, LifeMap Discovery;* monograph at https: //discovery.lifemapsc.com/in-vivo-development/glial-cells. Accessed Apr. 23, 2021.

77. S. Jakel and L. Dimou. "Glial cells and their function in the adult brain: A journey through the history of their ablation," *Frontiers in Cellular Neuroscience*, 11: 2017.

78. I. S. Muskens, et al. "Germline genetic landscape of pediatric central nervous system tumors," *Neuro-oncology*, vol. 21,11 (2019): 1376–88. doi:10.1093/neuonc/noz108.

79. T. Bouzek. "Misteltherapie bei Patienten mit Hirntumoren: 3 Kasuis-tiken" [Mistletoe therapy in patients with brain tumors: 3 case reports], *Der Merkurstab* 2012;65(3):249-256. Article-ID: DMS-19966-DE. DOI: https://doi.org/10.14271/DMS-19966-DE.

80. N. Mckinney. *Naturopathic Oncology: An Encyclopedic Guide for Patients and Physicians* (4th ed.), Victoria, Canada: Liaison, 2020.

81. K. L. Pitter, et al. "Corticosteroids compromise survival in glioblastoma," *Brain*, 139, 5; 2016: 1458-71.

82. A. Poff, et al. "Targeting the Warburg effect for cancer treatment: Keto-genic diets for the management of glioma," *Seminars in Cancer Biology*, 56 June 2019.

83. T. N. Seyfried, et al. "Role of glucose and ketone bodies in the metabolic control of experimental brain cancer," *British Journal of Cancer*, 2003.

84. S. Khodadadi, et al. "Tumor cells growth and survival time with the ketogenic diet in animal models: A systematic review," *Int. J. Prev. Med.*, May 2017 25;8:35. doi: 10.4103/2008-7802.207035. PMID: 28584617; PMCID: PMC5450454.

85. K. Schwartz, et al. "Ketogenic diet therapy for aggressive primary brain tumors: stratification of survival by patients' age," *Current Developments in Nutrition*, vol. 4, issue supp. 2, June 2020, p. 350. https://doi.org/10.1093/cdn/nzaa044_049).

86. C. Tóth, et al. "38-month long progression-free and symptom-free survival of a patient with recurrent glioblastoma multiforme: A case report of the paleolithic ketogenic diet (PKD) used as a stand-alone treatment after failed standard oncotherapy," *Preprints*, 2019, 2019120264. doi: 10.20944/preprints201912.0264.v1.

87. A. Paoli, et al. "Beyond weight loss: A review of the therapeutic uses of very-low-carbohydrate (ketogenic) diets," *European Journal of Clinical Nutrition*, 67, 789–796 (2013). https://doi.org/10.1038/ejcn.2013.116.

CHAPTER 11

1. W. Tröger, et al. "Quality of life of patients with advanced pancreatic cancer during treatment with mistletoe: A randomized controlled trial," *Dtsch. Arztebl. Int.*, 2014;111:493–502. DOI: 10.3238/arztebl.2014.0493.

2. W. Tröger, et al. "Viscum album [L.] extract therapy in patients with locally advanced or metastatic pancreatic cancer: A randomised clinical trial on overall survival," *European Journal of Cancer*, 2013;49:3788–97. DOI: 10.1016/j.ejca.2013.06.043.

3. M. Loef and H. Walach. "Quality of life in cancer patients treated with mistletoe: A systematic review and meta-analysis" (pre-print published at medRxiv.org [Internet]. 2019). doi.org/10.1101/19013177.

4. M. Kröz, et al. "Reliability and validity of a new scale on internal coherence (ICS) of cancer patients," *Health Qual. Life Outcomes*, 2009;7:59. DOI:10.1186/1477-7525-7-59.

5. M. Kröz, et al. "Validation of a new scale in internal coherence (ICS) with mistletoe therapy-sensitive questions for cancer patients," in R. Scheer, et al. (eds.), *Die Mistel in der Tumortherapie*, 2, Aktueller Stand der Forschung und klinische Anwendung 2008.

6. W. Tröger, et al. "Quality of life and neutropenia in patients with early-stage breast cancer: A randomized pilot study comparing additional treatment with mistletoe extract to chemotherapy alone," *Breast Cancer*, 2009;16:35–45.

7. W. Tröger, et al. "Additional therapy with a mistletoe product during adjuvant chemotherapy of breast cancer patients improves quality of life: An open randomized clinical pilot trial," *Evidence-Based Complementary and Alternative Medicine*, 2014;2014:01. Sep. DOI: 10.1155/2014/430518.

8. W. Tröger, et al. "Quality of life of patients with advanced pancreatic cancer during treatment with mistletoe: A randomized controlled trial,"

Dtsch. Arztebl. Int., 2014;111:493–502, 433 p following 502.
DOI: 10.3238/arztebl.2014.0493.

9. H. Matthes, et al. "Supportive care in pancreatic carcinoma patients treated with a fermented mistletoe (Viscum album L.) extracts," in R. Scheer, et al (eds.), *Die Mistel in der Tumortherapie 2, Akuteller Stand der Forschung und klinische Anwendung.* Essen: KVC Verlag; 2008.

10. AUTHOR NOTE: Trial is registered at https://clinicaltrials.gov/ct2/show /NCT03051477. Updates on study publications will be available at http://mistletoebook.com.

11. T. Ostermann, et al. "A systematic review and meta-analysis on the survival of cancer patients treated with a fermented Viscum album L. extract (Iscador®): An update of findings," *Complementary Med. Res.*, 2020, DOI: 10.1159/000505202.

12. M. Loef and H. Walach. "Quality of life in cancer patients treated with mistletoe: A systematic review and meta-analysis," Op. cit.

CHAPTER 12

1. AUTHOR NOTE: According to data at Steiner Health, "By some estimates, 40 percent of French, and up to 60 percent of German cancer patients receive this botanical extract" (https://steinerhealth.org/articles/alternative -cancer-treatment/. Retrieved Apr. 29, 2021).

2. Trial details and registration at https://clinicaltrials.gov/ct2/show /NCT03051477.

3. M. E. Porter and T. H. Lee. "The strategy that will fix health care," *Harvard Business Review* (Oct. 2013); https://hbr.org/2013/10/the -strategy-that-will-fix-health-care Accessed Apr. 22, 2021.

4. M. E. Porter and E. Olmsted Teisberg. "Redefining health care: Creating value-based competition on results," *Harvard Business Review*, 2006.

5. A. Ladanie, et al. "Clinical trial evidence supporting US Food and Drug Administration approval of novel cancer therapies between 2000 and 2016," *JAMA Network Open*, 2020;3(11):e2024406. doi:10.1001 /jamanetworkopen.2020.24406.

6. Hyeongjun Yun, et al. "Growth of integrative medicine at leading cancer centers between 2009 and 2016: A systematic analysis of NCI-designated comprehensive cancer center websites," *JNCI Monographs*, vol. 2017, no. 52, Nov. 2017, lgx004, https://doi.org/10.1093/jncimonographs/lgx004.

7. S. J. Grant, et al. "Integrative oncology: International perspectives," *Integrative Cancer Therapies*, vol. 18 (2019): 1534735418823266. doi:10.1177/1534735418823266.

8. C. A. Buckner, et al. "Complementary and alternative medicine use in patients before and after a cancer diagnosis," *Current Oncology* (Toronto), vol. 25,4 (2018): e275-e281. doi:10.3747/co.25.3884.

9. Trial details and registration at https://clinicaltrials.gov/ct2/show /NCT03051477.

10. Per data published by Mistletoe-Therapy.org: "Currently 154 studies have been conducted on the anthroposophical mistletoe preparations

abnobaVISCUM, Helixor, Iscador and Iscucin (status May 2020)" (accessed Apr. 26, 2021).

11. A. Ladanie, et al. "Clinical trial evidence supporting US Food and Drug Administration approval of novel cancer therapies between 2000 and 2016," Op. cit.

12. P. Sharma, et al. "Primary, adaptive, and acquired resistance to cancer immunotherapy," *Cell*, 168, Feb. 9, 2017 a 2017 Elsevier Inc. 168(4): 707–23 (2017).

13. "Cancer: Key Statistics," World Health Organization. https://www.who .int/cancer/resources/keyfacts/en/. Retrieved Apr. 30, 2021.

14. A. S. Blevins Primeau, "Cancer recurrence statistics," *Cancer Therapy Adviser Factsheet,* Nov. 30, 2018, at: https://www.cancertherapyadvisor .com/home/tools/fact-sheets/cancer-recurrence-statistics/. Retrieved Apr. 30, 2021.

15. "Right to Try," *FDA Fact Sheet,* updated Jan. 14, 2020; https://www.fda .gov/patients/learn-about-expanded-access-and-other-treatment-options /right-try (retrieved Apr. 30, 2021).

Appendix B

1. S. C. Howard, et al. "The tumor lysis syndrome," *The New England Journal of Medicine,* vol. 364,19 (2011): 1844-54. doi:10.1056 /NEJMra0904569.

Appendix D

1. S. Sen, et al. "Development of a prognostic scoring system for patients with advanced cancer enrolled in immune checkpoint inhibitor phase-1 clinical trials," *British Journal of Cancer,* vol. 118,6 (2018): 763–69. doi:10.1038/bjc.2017.480.